Dawn Lambie, RN, MSN
Nancy Diehl, RN, MSN, CNS

CLINICAL HANDBOOK FOR

Medical–Surgical Nursing

Preparation for Practice

Kathleen S. Osborn, RN, MS, EdD

California State University
Sacramento, California

Cheryl E. Wraa, RN, MSN

University of California,
Davis Medical Center

California State University
Sacramento, California

Annita B. Watson, RN, MS, DNSc

California State University
Sacramento, California

Pearson

Boston Columbus Indianapolis New York San Francisco Upper Saddle River
Amsterdam Cape Town Dubai London Madrid Milan Munich Paris Montreal Toronto
Delhi Mexico City Sao Paulo Sydney Hong Kong Seoul Singapore Taipei Tokyo

Library of Congress Cataloging-in-Publication Data

Clinical handbook for medical–surgical nursing: preparation for practice/
   Kathleen S. Osborn . . . [et al.].
   p. ; cm.
Includes index.
Companion volume to: Medical–surgical nursing: preparation for practice/
   Kathleen S. Osborn, Cheryl E. Wraa, Annita Watson. c2010.
ISBN-13: 978-0-13-505203-7
ISBN-10: 0-13-505203-3
1. Nursing—Handbooks, manuals, etc. 2. Surgical nursing—Handbooks,
   manuals, etc. I. Osborn, Kathleen S.
[DNLM: 1. Perioperative Nursing—methods—Handbooks. 2. Nurse's
   Role—Handbooks. 3. Nursing Care—methods—Handbooks. WY 49
C64132 2010]
RT51.C644 2010
617'.0231—dc22
                                                                    2009031274

Notice: Care has been taken to confirm the accuracy of information
presented in this book. The authors, editors, and the publisher, however,
cannot accept any responsibility for errors or omissions or for
consequences from application of the information in this book and make
no warranty, express or implied, with respect to its contents. The authors
and publisher have exerted every effort to ensure that drug selections and
dosages set forth in this text are in accord with current recommendations
and practice at time of publication. However, in view of ongoing
research, changes in government regulations, and the constant flow of
information relating to drug therapy and drug reactions, the reader is
urged to check the package inserts of all drugs for any change in
indications of dosage and for added warnings and precautions. This is
particularly important when the recommended agent is a new and/or
infrequently employed drug.

                                            10 9 8 7 6 5 4 3 2 1
                                      ISBN 10: 0-13-505203-3

www.pearsonhighered.com   ISBN 13: 978-0-13-505203-7

Contents

Procedures and Therapies

Appendixes

PREFACE

This handbook has been developed as a reference tool for the bedside nurse. It complements the textbook *Medical–Surgical Nursing: Preparation for Practice*, by summarizing the key points related to diseases and disorders, allowing the nurse quick access to clinically relevant information.

The design of the book presents information in a logical sequence, offering the nurse a quick and clear picture of the patient's needs related to a specific disease or disorder. The first section of the handbook presents diseases and disorders organized according to the body system affected. For example, "Hepatitis" can be found in the "Gastrointestinal Disorders" section. This helps the reader access the information with ease and at the same time emphasizes the connection between a disease and the body system. The disorders are broken down into five categories: description of the disorder; signs and symptoms; diagnostics; patient care management; and nursing management.

The next section, "Procedures and Therapies," identifies those common interventions nursing needs to understand and/or be capable of performing. These interventions are seen in many different diseases and are referenced within each disorder section. Lastly are the appendixes, which contain charts and tables of pertinent patient care information such as care plans and pharmacology lists.

One of the most unique additions to this handbook is the "Critical Alert" feature. This feature is located within a disorder and identifies the crucial information a nurse needs to understand related to a specific disease.

The Critical Alert emphasizes the importance nursing places on assessing situations and the prioritization of information.

Nursing demands sharp assessment skills, recognition of patient changes, and an understanding of potential problems based on a patient's clinical diagnosis. Collaboration with the health care team provides nurses the opportunity to expand their knowledge base and thus provide quality patient care in a very rapidly changing environment. This handbook will assist the nurse in designing a plan of care that meets these expectations.

ACKNOWLEDGMENTS

I would like to recognize all of the individuals who contributed to my success in this project. Maureen Grealish, your editorial support and guidance has been invaluable. My colleagues, Sueann and Nancy, being a part of a team of professionals and excellent educators has motivated me throughout this entire experience. Finally, my dear family, Paul and Erin, my life would be lost and incomplete without you. I love you dearly.

Dawn Lambie, RN, MSN

I would like to thank the entire team for its leadership and support during this project. Special thanks to Dawn Lambie, who made this opportunity possible. My experience working with Dawn on the handbook has strengthened our professional and personal relationship and I will be forever grateful. Last, but not least, I thank my husband, Gregory, for his love and support that makes every new day a gift. I love you!

Nancy Diehl, RN, MSN, CNS

ARTHRITIS AND CONNECTIVE TISSUE DISORDERS

Arthritis

Arthritis is a common descriptive term that applies to the collection of rheumatic diseases that can be localized, self-limiting conditions or systemic, autoimmune processes.

Ankylosing Spondylitis

Ankylosing spondylitis (AS) is a type of arthritis that affects the spine and the sacroiliac joints and is progressive in nature.

Signs and Symptoms

- Pain (sacroiliac area)
  - Low back pain and stiffness in the morning that improves with activity
- Loss of flexibility in the lumbar spine
- Impaired lung capacity
  - Due to $\uparrow$ inflammation and healing occurs that causes new bone growth to fuse together
- Impaired activities of daily living
- Fatigue, weight loss
- Fever
- Diarrhea
- Eye pain and photophobia

Gouty Arthritis

Gouty arthritis is a condition in which there is an imbalance in purine metabolism, which increases uric acid in the joints with the formation of uric acid crystals. It can affect any joint but most commonly affects those of the feet, especially the great toe.

Risk Factors

- Heredity
- Enzyme defect
- Exposure to lead

Signs and Symptoms

- Asymptomatic
    - ↑ serum uric acid
- Acute gout
    - ↑ uric acid crystals accumulating in the space of the joints
    - Tophi (uric acid crystals in the earlobes)
    - Sudden onset of severe pain, usually in the night
        - Knifelike pain in the earlobe, elbow, or feet
    - ↑ swelling and inflammation
    - Affected part is hot to the touch
    - Triggered by stress, illness, or the consumption of alcohol or drugs
- Interval gout
    - Condition is in remission
- Chronic tophaceous gout
    - Occurs when the illness is not treated
    - Disabling effects such as permanent damage to the joints and kidneys

Osteoarthritis (OA)

Osteoarthritis, the most common form of arthritis, is a chronic condition that accompanies aging, most commonly affecting weight-bearing joints. The disease can occur as a primary idiopathic disorder that is localized or generalized (involves more than three joints). Secondary OA is due to an underlying cause such as congenital defects of joint structure, single severe trauma or multiple traumas, inflammatory diseases, or metabolic disorders. Joint degeneration with OA occurs on the articular surfaces of the cartilage with bony formations at the edges of weight-bearing joints.

Contributing Factors

- Joint integrity
- Genetic predisposition
- Local inflammation
- Mechanical forces
- Cellular and biochemical processes

Signs and Symptoms

- Brief interval of morning stiffness
- Pain on motion with overuse of affected joint
- Joint bone deformity (occurs over time)

Psoriatic Arthritis

Psoriatic arthritis is an inflammatory process associated with psoriasis, although it has been known to develop even in the absence of detectable psoriasis. It affects the ligaments, tendons, fascia, and joints. Factors that contribute to the disease are genetic, immunologic, and environmental (bacterial and viral infections, and trauma).

Signs and Symptoms

- Pain and stiffness in the affected joints
  - Worsens with prolonged immobility
  - Improves with physical activity
  - Local effusions
- Dactylitis ("sausage digit")
  - Occurs 50% of time
  - Uniform swelling of the soft tissues between the metacarpophalangeal and interphalangeal joints
  - Diffuse swelling of the entire digit
- Pits in the nail plate and onycholysis (separation of the lateral edges of the nail plate from the nail bed)

Reactive Arthritis (Reiter's syndrome or undifferentiated spondylarthropathy)

Reactive arthritis is caused by a reaction to an infection somewhere else in the body. Causes include *Chlamydia trachomatis* (spread through sexual contact) and gastrointestinal infections, such as *Salmonella, Shigella, Yersinia,* and *Campylobacter.* Reactive arthritis characteristically causes inflammatory response in the genitourinary tract, the joints, and the eyes.

Signs and Symptoms

- Asymmetrical joint swelling (knees and ankles)
- Enthesopathy
  - Inflammation around the insertion of ligaments, tendons, joint capsule, or fascia near the bone
- Dactylitis
- Inflammation of the neck and low back
- Circinate balanitis (painless skin lesions)
- Unilateral uveitis
- Crohn's-like bowel inflammation
- Aortic regurgitation
- Amyloidosis
- Rheumatic infections

Rheumatoid Arthritis (RA)

Rheumatoid arthritis is a chronic inflammatory process that affects the peripheral joints and surrounding muscles, ligaments, tendons, and blood vessels. It is thought to be an autoimmune disorder that not only involves tissue hypersensitivity but also has a genetic component. Antiglobulin antibodies combine with immunoglobulin in the synovial fluid and form complexes. Neutrophils are then attracted to the joint space and perpetuate the inflammatory response.

Signs and Symptoms

The remissions and exacerbations of RA allow for a varying degree of signs and symptoms.

- Redness, heat
- Swelling, deformity
- Pain
- Fatigue, low-grade fever, anorexia
- Pannus
  - Development of an extensive network of new blood vessels in the synovial membrane that causes destruction
  - Differentiates RA from other arthritis conditions
- Lymph node swelling
- Dry mouth
- Pleuritis (due to RA nodules in lungs)
- Anemia
- Spleen enlargement causing ↓ WBC
- Vasculitis (potentially causes necrosis of tissues of the nail beds and dermal ulcers)

Septic Arthritis

Septic arthritis (non-gonococcal bacterial arthritis) is the most destructive form of acute arthritis and can result from trauma, from direct inoculation of bacteria during joint surgery, from spread of infection from another part of the body (hematogenous), or when an infection from an adjacent bone extends through the cortex into the joint space

Signs and Symptoms

- Single swollen and painful joint (effusion)
  - Knee
  - Wrist
  - Ankles
  - Hips
- Fever and chills
- ↑ WBC
- Evidence of an associated skin, urinary, or respiratory infection. The definitive diagnostic test is the

identification of bacteria via a culture of the synovial fluid obtained from joint aspiration.

Diagnostics (for all arthritis disorders)

- Health history and physical examination
- Laboratory
  - Rheumatoid factor (for rheumatoid arthritis)
  - Sedimentation rate (SED rate)
  - CBC (evaluates for anemia and leukocytosis)
  - Serum uric acid (for gouty arthritis)
  - Joint aspiration to evaluate for infection or presence of uric acid crystals (for gouty arthritis)
  - HLA-B27 (for reactive arthritis and ankylosing spondylitis)
  - Immunoglobin A (IgA) antibodies (for reactive arthritis)
  - Urine protein (for reactive arthritis)
  - Stool cultures (for reactive arthritis)
  - Culture of the synovial fluid (for septic arthritis)
- Imaging
  - X-rays, CT scan, MRI, bone scans
  - Slit lamp examination (for reactive arthritis)

Patient Care Management

The goals of care for all arthritis disorders are very similar: control pain and progression of disease so patient can have a functional normal life. The following identifies management strategies for all disorders.

- Medical
  - Rest and exercise
  - Dietary modifications (for gouty arthritis)
  - Nonsteroidal anti-inflammatory agents (NSAIDs)
  - Cyclooxygenase-2 (COX-2) inhibitors (Celebrex)
  - Anti-malarial agents (Plaquenil)

- Antineoplastics (Methotrexate) (for rheumatoid arthritis)
- Immunosuppressants (Imuran) (for rheumatoid arthritis)
- Cyclophosphamide (Cytoxan) (for rheumatoid arthritis)
- Tumor necrosis factor (TNF) inhibitors (Enbrel, Remicade) (for rheumatoid arthritis, psoriatic arthritis, ankylosing spondylitis)
- Glucocorticoids (Prednisone) (for rheumatoid arthritis)
- Antigout agents (Colchicine, Allopurinol)
- Antibiotics (for reactive and septic arthritis)
- Surgical
  - Considered only when the patient exhausts previous options and the patient's quality of life is further compromised
  - Synovectomy (removal of the swollen synovial casing prior to damage to the bone and cartilage taking place)
  - Arthrodesis (fusion of the joint when there is severe destruction at the surface)
  - Reconstructive surgery (total knee or total hips are done when these weight-bearing joints have been completely damaged)
- Multidisciplinary
  - Clinical nutritionist (to help with weight reduction)
  - Physical therapist (to develop an exercise program to include range-of-motion exercises)

Nursing Management

Regardless of the type of arthritis the nursing plan of care has similar components.

- Pain, Acute and Chronic
  - Assess pain thoroughly using numeric scale and patient self-report

- Monitor uric acid levels (gout)
- Alternative pain interventions: rest, gentle exercise (swimming) position, elevation, ice, heat, distraction, ROM, PROM
- Provide pain medications
- Mobility: Physical, Impaired
  - Prevention of contractures: exercise, sleep on a firm mattress, and use splints to maintain alignment
  - ROM and PROM (walking and swimming)
- Falls, Risk
  - Implement fall protocol
- Body Image, Disturbed
  - Establish rapport with the patient so they feel comfortable to verbalize feelings or concerns
  - Listen actively
  - Assist the patient in making realistic short- and long-term goals
  - Refer to local chapters of the American Arthritis Association and other organizations
- Nutrition: Imbalanced, More than Body Requirements
  - Encourage consumption of foods that decrease uric acid, such as grains, fruits, vegetables, and beans (Gout)
  - Teach the patient to avoid the following foods high in purines: cheese, wine, organ meats, and shellfish (Gout)
  - Encourage the patient to drink plenty of liquids, about 2,000–3,000 milliliters daily, to reduce potential creation of kidney stones (Gout)
  - Consult nutritionist to assist with developing a low-calorie, balanced, appealing diet plan to reduce weight
- Knowledge Deficit
  - Instruct patient/family regarding maintaining safe environment in the home (e.g., removing

scatter rugs, removing clutter, and providing assistance when the patient is ambulatory)

- Explain the purpose of surgical treatment options so patient can make an informed decision (health care provider will need to perform the informed consent)

- Explain adverse effects of medications and when to notify health care provider

- Encourage patient to keep appointments with specialists (e.g., ophthalmologist, orthopedist, rheumatologist, physical/occupational therapist)

- Instruct patient to notify health care provider if experiencing signs of infection (e.g., ↑ temperature and WBC, worsening pain and swelling)

Lyme Disease

Lyme disease is caused by bacteria, called *Borrelia burgdorferi,* which are found in infected black-legged ticks. This bacterium affects the organs and joints.

Signs and Symptoms

There are three stages (and associated symptoms) of the disease, which are:

- Early localized disease:
  - Occurs a few days to 1 month after the tick bite
  - Erythema chronicum migrans (reddened area where the tick bite occurred)
  - Headache, confusion, forgetfulness, stiff neck, irregular heartbeat, painful and swollen joints, and swollen lymph glands
- Early disseminated disease:
  - Occurs days to 10 months after the tick bite
  - Carditis (generalized inflammation of heart), conduction defects, mild cardiomyopathy, or myopericarditis
  - Neurological symptoms include lymphocytic meningitis; encephalitis; cranial neuropathy (most often facial, can be bilateral), peripheral neuropathy, radiculoneuropathy; or myelitis.

- Late or chronic disease:
  - Occurs months to years after the tick bite
  - Intermittent monoarticular or oligoarticular arthritis, persistent monoarthritis, usually affecting the knee
  - Neurological symptoms are subtle but can include encephalopathy, encephalomyelitis, and/or peripheral neuropathy.

Diagnostics
- Health history and physical examination
- Laboratory
  - Serum antibody

Patient Care Management
- Medical

  Antibiotics (oral or intravenous)
  - Antipyretics
  - NSAIDs for joint pain

Nursing Management
Nursing management focuses on treatment of the infection and education of the patient and family on ways to avoid exposure to ticks and possible re-infection.

- Infection, Risk
  - Monitor for ↑ temperature
  - Assess for localized signs of infection (worsened inflammation, exudate, pain)
  - Monitor for ↑ WBC
- Pain, Acute
  - Assess pain using numeric scale (0–10) and patient self-report
  - Administer pain medications (NSAIDs, analgesics) and re-assess accordingly
- Knowledge, Deficient
  - Instruct patient and family regarding strategies to avoid exposure to ticks (e.g., wearing

protective clothing, application of repellent, avoiding known infested areas)

- Instruct patient and family regarding course of disease, including chronic stage and associated symptoms

Scleroderma

Scleroderma is a progressive autoimmune disease where the immune system stimulates the production of an excess of fibroblasts, the cells that produce collagen. Fibrotic changes occur in connective tissue throughout the body, involving any of the following systems: integumentary, circulatory, joints, alimentary canal, cardiac, respiratory, renal, and/or gastrointestinal tract.

Signs and Symptoms

The disease is characterized by inflammatory and then degenerative and fibrotic changes in the skin, blood vessels, synovial membranes, skeletal muscles, and internal organs.

- Joint pain
- Muscle weakness
- Hard skin that fixes to underlying structures
- General body movements are rigid
- Telangiectases are noted on the lips, fingers, face, and tongue
- Dysphagia
- Raynaud's-type symptoms (see Peripheral Vascular Disorders)

CREST syndrome (signs of disease progression)

- C: calcium deposits in organs
- R: Raynaud's type symptoms
- E: esophageal dysfunction
- S: sclerodactyly (scleroderma of the fingers and toes)
- T: telangiectasia (vascular lesion formed by dilation)

Diagnostics

- Health history and physical examination
- Laboratory

- Positive LE prep
- ↑ gamma globulin levels
- Antinuclear antibodies (ANA)
- Imaging
  - Chest x-rays
  - Lung function testing
  - CT scan (to examine the lungs)
- Other
  - ECG
  - Echocardiogram
  - Cardiac catheterization

Patient Care Management

- Medical
  - Corticosteroids for inflammation
  - Salicylates or narcotics for joint pain
  - Vasodilators for Raynaud's-type symptoms
    - nifedipine (Procardia, Adalat), nicardipine (Cardene), or topical nitroglycerin
  - Immunosuppressants and D-penicillamine
  - Prilosec, Prevacid, and antacids (for heartburn and esophageal irritation)
  - Irritated, itchy dry skin can be helped by emollients such as Lubriderm, Eucerin, or Bag Balm
  - Hand warming and protection from cold temperatures (mild Raynaud's disease)

Nursing Management

Scleroderma requires that the nurse assess each body system affected by the disease for decrease in function, including cardiac, pulmonary, integumentary, and gastrointestinal. The following are additional nursing interventions required when caring for a patient with scleroderma.

- Pain, Chronic
  - Assess pain using numeric scale (0–10) and patient self-report
  - Administer pain medications and reassess accordingly
  - ROM and PROM to maintain mobility
- Skin Integrity, Impaired
  - Inspect skin and oropharyngeal areas for lesions
  - Use mild soap, lotion, emollients, and sunscreen
- Body Image, Disturbed
  - Explain the expected physical changes to prepare paitent and begin coping process
- Knowledge Deficit
  - Explain the purpose of each medication and advise the patient about the adverse effects of all of the medications
  - Encourage patient to avoid exposure to the cold due to vasoconstriction of vessels, thereby decreasing peripheral circulation
  - Instruct patient to avoid smoking
  - Encourage patient to keep scheduled appointments and notify health care provider when changes are noted

Sjögren's Syndrome

Sjögren's syndrome (SS) is an autoimmune disease where immune cells attack and destroy the glands that produce tears and saliva. The result is dry eyes and dry mouth.

Signs and Symptoms
- Dry eyes and dry mouth
- Inflammation in other systems (kidneys, gastrointestinal tract, lung, and blood vessels)

Diagnostics
- Health history and physical examination
- Laboratory

- ANA
- Rheumatoid factor
- Sjögren's syndrome antigens (SSA and SSB)
- SED rate
- Imaging
  - Sialography (x-ray of the salivary duct system)
- Other
  - Schirmer's test (measures tear production)
  - Rose Bengal and Lissamine green (uses dyes to observe abnormal cells on the surface of the eye)
  - Slit lamp exam
  - Parotid gland flow (measures the amount of saliva produced over a certain period of time)

Patient Care Management
- Medical
  - Most replacement therapies for symptoms of dryness
  - NSAIDs
  - Corticosteroids and immunosuppressive therapies for severe complications

Nursing Management
- Nutrition: Imbalanced, Less than Body Requirements
  - Provide foods that are moist and easy to swallow during episodes of stomatitis
- Pain, Chronic
  - Increasing fluid intake, using oral sprays, and chewing sugarless gum may help oral dryness.
  - Wearing sunglasses to protect the eyes and using artificial tears
  - Assess pain using numeric scale (0–10) and patient self-report
  - NSAIDs or analgesics

- Knowledge, Deficit
  - Instruct patient and family to notify health care provider if experiencing signs of infection ($\uparrow$ temperature, fatigue, chills)
  - Encourage patient and family to use strategies to reduce effect of dryness

Systemic Lupus Erythematosus (SLE)

Systemic lupus erythematosus is a chronic inflammatory autoimmune disease where autoantibodies attack connective tissue or organs. Certain immune complexes deposit in blood vessels, among collagen fibers, and on organs that cause necrosis and inflammation in the major organs, such as the kidneys, brain, eyes, lymphatic system, gastrointestinal (GI) tract, lungs, and skin. SLE is characterized by remissions and exacerbations, which are common during the spring and summer months.

For a patient who is genetically susceptible, there are multiple predisposing factors including physical or mental stress, exposure to sunlight or ultraviolet light, viral or streptococcal infections, pregnancy, and abnormal estrogen metabolism.

Signs and Symptoms

- Weakness
- Sensitivity to light
- Pain in the joints
- $\uparrow$ temperature
- Butterfly rash on the face and the palms of the hands
- Weight loss
- Organ dysfunction (renal, GI, cardiac, respiratory, or neurological)

Diagnostics

- Health history and physical exam
- Laboratory
  - Lupus erythematosus preparation (LE prep)

- Antinuclear antibodies (ANAs)
- Urinalysis (evaluates for evidence of kidney involvement)

Patient Care Management

- Medical
  - Rest and exercise
  - Nonsteroidal anti-inflammatory agents (NSAIDs)
  - Anti-malarial agents (Plaquenil)
  - Antineoplastics (Methotrexate)
  - Immunosuppressants (Imuran)
  - Cyclophosphamide (Cytoxan)
  - Rituximab (Rituxan)
  - Glucocorticoids (Prednisone)
- Other
  - Plasmapheresis (for serious brain or kidney disease)
  - Dialysis
  - Kidney transplantation

Nursing Management

- Mobility, Impaired
  - PROM or ROM
  - Encourage rest alternating with exercise
- Pain, Chronic
  - Assess pain using numeric scale (0–10) and patient self-report
  - Administer pain medications and reassess accordingly
- Activity Intolerance
  - Patients should try to sleep between 8 and 10 hours a night.
  - Encourage the patient to pace activities and plan rest

- Tissue Perfusion, Ineffective
  - Daily weights
  - $\downarrow$ specific gravity, $\downarrow$ urine output
  - Limit sodium intake to reduce edema
  - Monitor for $\uparrow$ HR, $\downarrow$ BP
  - Assess skin for temperature, color, and moisture (e.g., cool, pale, moist)
- Knowledge Deficit
  - Teach the patient and family the importance of rest and decreased stress
  - Instruct patient regarding proper skin care, which includes hygiene, use of mild soap, use of sunscreen when outdoors, and avoidance of exposure to the sunlight
  - Instruct patient and family regarding action of medications, adverse effects, and any interactions with food or other medications
  - Encourage patient to seek pregnancy counseling

BURNS

Burns

Burn injuries are a traumatic, dehumanizing injury that can be fatal, disfiguring, and incapacitating. They occur when there is direct or indirect contact with a heat source causing a loss of skin integrity that ranges from a minor superficial injury to a deep full-thickness injury that extends into the underlying structures and organs.

Classification

- Minor
  - Partial-thickness injuries < 15% of total body surface area (TBSA) (adults)
  - Full-thickness injuries < 2% of TBSA not involving ears, eyes, face, hands, feet, and perineum

- Moderate
  - Partial-thickness injuries 15–25% of TBSA (adults)
  - Full-thickness injuries 10% of TBSA not involving ears, eyes, face, hands, feet, and perineum

- Major
  - Electrical injuries
  - Inhalation injuries
  - Complicated injuries (multiple trauma)
  - High-risk patients such as older adults and those with chronic illnesses

- All burns involving ears, eyes, face, hands, feet, and perineum
- Partial-thickness injuries > 25% of TBSA (adults)
- Full-thickness injuries 10% or greater of TBSA

Types

Thermal Burns

- Most common
- Occur when heat is transferred to the body from an external source; for example, flames from a fire
- The depth of the injury is related to the length of exposure and the temperature of the heat source.
- Scalds
  - Type of thermal injury that occurs from contact with hot foods or liquids, including steam
  - The severity of the burn is related to the temperature of the hot liquid and the length of time it is in contact with the body.
  - 120°F (48°C): requires 5 minutes for a full-thickness burn to occur
  - 140°F (60°C): requires 5 seconds or less for a serious burn to occur

Electrical Burns

- Tend to be deeper than most burn injuries
- The depth and severity of the injury depends on the amount of voltage, the length of exposure, the type of current, the pathway of flow, and the local tissue resistance.
- Example: Entry wound is the hand and the exit is the bottom of the foot, the current traveled through most of the major organs
- Acute tubular necrosis occurs when myoglobin is released into the blood stream after deep muscle injury.

- Tetanic muscle contractions cause fractures of long bones and vertebrae and suffocation (due to effect on respiratory muscles) and cardiac conduction system disturbances.

Radiation Burns

- Result of overexposure to the sun or are associated with radiation treatment for cancer
- May also occur from industrial accidents such as at nuclear power plants
- The cells most susceptible to injury are those that divide rapidly such as bone marrow, skin, and the gastrointestinal tract.

Chemical Burns

- Occur when the skin is in contact with caustic chemical compounds such as strong acids, alkalis, or organic compounds
- Common agents are bleach, boric acid, creosote, paint thinner, and plumbing pipe decloggers such as Drano or Liquid-Plumr.

Inhalation Burns

- Result from inhalation of heated air and smoke
- Diagnosing injury includes knowing if the injury occurred in an enclosed area; there are burns of the face and neck; and there are singed nasal hairs, a hoarse, dry cough, bloody/sooty sputum, and labored respirations.
- Edema, blisters, and ulcerations along the mucosal lining of the oropharynx and larynx may be present.
- Signs of respiratory distress may be present (e.g., stridor, use of accessory muscles, hypoxia).

Signs and Symptoms

The clinical presentation for each type of burn depends on the body area involved and the extent of burn. Refer to the causes of burns section.

Diagnostics

- Health history and physical examination
  - Size of injury
  - Depth of injury
  - Age of patient
  - Part of body burned
- Laboratory (See Appendix #34 Diagnostic Tests for Burns)
- Imaging (to diagnose other injuries)

Patient Care Management

Management of the patient with a burn injury is specific according to the phase of the injury.

Emergency Phase (time of injury to 2–3 days):

- Maintain an airway and oxygen levels
- Treat concurrent injuries
- Correct fluid imbalance
- Prevent wound infection
- Conserve body heat
- Pain management
- Provide emotional support

Acute Phase

The acute period of burn management begins when the patient is hemodynamically stable and ends with closure of the burn wounds.

- Wound care
  - Cleansing and debridement
  - Escharotomies
  - Dressings (topical antibiotic dressing, temporary dressings)
  - Skin grafting
- Pain management
- Temperature control (preserving body heat)

- Prevention of infection
- Nutritional support
- Mobility
  - Splinting and positioning
  - Exercising affected joints

Rehabilitative Phase

The rehabilitative phase typically begins when there is less than 20% open wound and the patient is functioning at the highest possible level since admission. Collaboration with the entire multidisciplinary team (PT, OT, Clinical Nutrionalist, and Discharge Planner) optimizes the patient's chance of achieving his or her highest functional level.

- Physical therapy to increase strength, endurance, function, and ROM
- Ongoing functional and cosmetic reconstruction
- Pain management
- Nutritional support
- Psychological recovery

Nursing Management

Effective nursing management requires understanding the key interventions for each phase of treatment. The following interventions encompass all phases of burn care.

- Deficient Fluid Volume
  - Large-bore intravenous (IV) catheter through nonburned tissue
  - Administer and titrate IV fluids per ordered formulas and parameters
    - Provide oral fluids if tolerated
  - Accurate I&O and daily weight
  - Assess vital signs and urine output at least hourly (to determine adequacy of fluid replacement)
  - Monitor central venous pressure (CVP) and pulmonary artery wedge pressure (PAWP)

(to determine adequacy of fluid replacement and cardiac output)

- Monitor arterial blood gases (to assess acid–base balance and presence of shock)
- Test all stools and emesis for blood (to monitor for blood loss from stress ulcers)
- Maintain a heated environment (to prevent loss of body heat due to loss of skin integrity)
- Monitor serum electrolytes, hemoglobin, and hematocrit, and report critical abnormalities to the health care provider (to monitor hematologic changes associated with fluid loss and tissue destruction)

Critical Alert

A hemoglobin (Hgb) of > 20 g/dL and/or a hematocrit (HCT) of > 60% is an indication that fluid resuscitation is inadequate and needs to be increased. The Hgb and HCT are not the best indicators of fluid balance because many blood cells are destroyed with the initial tissue injury. Use other indicators of fluid balance, such as heart rate, central venous pressure (CVP), and blood pressure (BP), because they are more reflective of the adequacy of hydration.

- Monitor for blood loss from burns or other injuries (to assess need for blood replacement therapy)
- Assess orientation frequently and regularly
- Risk for Imbalanced Fluid Volume
    - Monitor lung sounds (to assess for fluid build-up)
- Ineffective Peripheral Tissue Perfusion
    - Elevate affected extremities above the heart to reduce edema formation
    - Monitor arterial pulses by palpation and/or ultrasound every hour during the first 24–48 hours
    - Assess pain and capillary permeability on both burned and unburned areas
    - Assess for numbness or tingling

- Remove constricting clothing, jewelry, and dressings to promote tissue perfusion
- If pulses diminish or become absent, if pain increases, or if capillary refill slows, notify the health care provider immediately.

Critical Alert
Assessment of pulses, capillary refill, and color of the area distal to the escharotomy is critical. Any changes in the circulatory status need to be reported to the health care provider immediately. If an escharotomy is done in the chest area, close monitoring of lung sounds is essential to assess gas exchange. Until the swelling subsides, the need for repeated escharotomies continues.

- Impaired Gas Exchange and Ineffective Airway Clearance
  - Assess for adventitious or diminished breath sounds
  - Note presence of cough and sputum (amount, color, consistency)
  - Monitor ABG's, O_2 sat, respiratory rate and depth, presence of cyanosis

Critical Alert
Continuous monitoring of arterial blood gases (ABGs) is necessary to assess the need for intubation and ventilatory support. Have necessary supplies ready for emergent intubation with inhalation injuries.

- Monitor restlessness and confusion
- Turn, cough, deep breathe, elevate head of bed, and instruct on use of incentive spirometry
- Administer humidified oxygen as prescribed
- Report respiratory distress to the health care provider
- Assess need for suctioning and/or endotracheal intubation
- Impaired Skin Integrity
  - Assess extent of (TBSA) of burn

- Assess wound for depth, location, and dimensions
- Wound care per orders
- Elevate affected areas to decrease edema
- Position therapeutically to prevent contracture formation
- Assess for infection
- Establish a skin breakdown prevention plan
- Monitor blood glucose
- Monitor white blood count (WBC) daily to assess for infection
- Monitor donor sites for infection

Critical Alert

Nurses are primarily responsible for prevention of infection in a donor site. Early detection and reporting will help prevent conversion of a donor site from a partial-thickness to a full-thickness injury.

- Nutritional support, including vitamins and minerals
- Risk for Infection
  - Assess for infection (drainage: exudate, color, odor) and document with each dressing change
  - Cleanse and shave wound per protocol
  - Culture wounds and body secretions per protocol
  - Use strict aseptic technique
  - Notify health care provider of presence of infection or wound enlargement
  - Monitor serum WBC
  - Maintain nutritional therapies
  - Monitor and record temperature hourly
- Imbalanced Nutrition: Less than Body Requirements
  - Consult nutritionist to establish calorie, protein, carbohydrate, and nutrient needs
  - Record accurate intake and output, and calorie count every shift

- Maintain oral hygiene
- Monitor elimination patterns and bowel sounds
- Administer enteral feedings per protocol (See Procedures and Therapies)
- Allow patient to select desired foods
- Provide high-calorie, high-protein, high-carbohydrate diet, including snacks
- Avoid painful procedures near mealtime and make the environment pleasant for eating
- Monitor laboratory values; e.g., total protein levels, complete blood count, glucose, iron, and pre-albumin
- Administer antacids, stool softeners, laxatives, and antiulcer agents per health care provider orders
- Assess dietary patterns in culturally diverse populations
- Acute Pain
  - Use pain scale (0–10) to quantify pain level
  - Use pain control measures before pain becomes severe and reassess accordingly
  - Assess cultural and religious impact on patient's responses
  - Explain, prepare, and medicate patient for painful procedures (dressing change) and anticipated discomforts

---

Critical Alert

Assess adequacy of pain management for dressing changes daily. Secure health care provider's orders for more medication, and have these orders available as backup if needed. Be sensitive to cultural diversity in response to pain and medicate accordingly.

- Teach nonpharmacologic method of control; e.g., guided imagery and massage, diversional activities, and breathing exercises

- Cover wounds and elevate affected areas
- Provide rest periods between procedures to assist with coping with ongoing pain
- Impaired Physical Mobility
  - Consult with physical therapist and occupational therapist to formulate a plan for maintaining and increasing mobility
  - Perform active and passive range-of-motion (ROM) exercises every 2 hours
  - Apply splints as prescribed
  - Maintain anti-deformity positions and reposition hourly
  - Elevate affected extremities
  - Maintain limbs in functional alignment
  - Anticipate need for analgesia
  - Ambulate when stable
  - Assess for loss of ROM and muscle atrophy related to immobility
  - Educate patient/family regarding rationale for imposed activity restrictions; e.g., recent skin grafting
  - Provide diversional activities to increase compliance with immobility
- Ineffective Thermoregulation
  - Minimize heat loss by covering patient with dressing and blankets
  - Apply heat lamps and radiant heat shields
  - Keep room temperature elevated, especially during dressing changes
  - Monitor rectal and core temperatures as per orders and report changes
- Fear and Anxiety
  - Assess and document level of anxiety
  - Explore with the patient/family techniques to reduce anxiety

- Provide factual information concerning diagnosis, treatment, disfigurement, disabilities, and prognosis
- Instruct patient on use of relaxation techniques
- Assess need for and administer anti-anxiety and pain medication
- Assist patient/family in setting realistic goals for progress
- Consider psychiatric counseling for patients/families who exhibit inability to accept situation
- Powerlessness
  - Determine knowledge of health and injury
  - Discuss realistic options for self-care
  - Reinforce personal strengths
  - Encourage verbalization of feeling of powerlessness
  - Assist patient to increase independence when realistic
  - Allow control over surroundings and schedule when possible
- Disturbed Body Image and Risk for Complicated Grieving
  - Assess patient's level of anxiety and knowledge related to body image changes
  - Encourage discussion of meaning of loss
  - Observe interaction with significant people
  - Assess for signs of grieving
  - Establish therapeutic environment with an atmosphere of acceptance
  - Explain expected appearance
  - Offer mirror for viewing of facial burns
  - Be realistic and positive during explanations
  - Set realistic goals for future

- Deficient Knowledge
    - Assess patient/family's readiness and ability to learn, and individual learning needs
    - Determine level of existing knowledge
    - Provide factual information about diagnosis, treatments, and prognosis
    - Explain all procedures in simple, concise language—allowing for questions
    - Encourage questions
    - Ongoing education of treatment plan and rationale
    - Document response to teaching

CARDIAC INFLAMMATORY DISORDERS

Cardiac disorders caused by either inflammation or structural changes and abnormalities impact tissue perfusion due to either altered myocardial pumping ability or abnormal blood flow through the heart. All three layers of the heart, the pericardium, myocardium, and endocardium, can be subject to inflammation and structural abnormalities. The inflammatory conditions affecting the heart are rheumatic heart disease, pericarditis, myocarditis, and endocarditis. A collaborative care approach is optimal for management of patients with inflammatory heart disease as these are chronic requiring lifelong management.

Cardiomyopathies (CMPs)

Diseases of the myocardial muscle fibers resulting in progressive structural and functional abnormalities of the myocardium. There are four types of CMPs: dilated, hypertrophic, restrictive, and arrhythmogenic. All types of cardiomyopathy can lead to cardiomegaly and heart failure.

- Primary CMPs: etiology unknown and affects only the heart muscle itself
- Secondary CMPs: caused by other disease processes such as ischemia, viral infections, alcohol intake and drug abuse, inherited disorders, and pregnancy.

Arrhythmogenic Right Ventricular Cardiomyopathy (ARVC)

ARVC is also referred to as arrhythmogenic right ventricular dysplasia/cardiomyopathy (ARVD/C) and arrhythmogenic right ventricular dysplasia (ARVD).

Defined as an electrical disturbance that develops when the muscle tissue in the right ventricle is replaced with fibrous scar and fatty tissues. Cause unknown, there is a possible familial link in some patients.

- The onset of the disease typically between the late teens to early 20s
- Affects men and women of any ethnic origin
- Although condition is reported more frequently among athletes, generally believed that sporting activities do not cause ARVC

Signs and Symptoms

- Many patients report little to no difficulties or manifestations.
- Others have life-threatening symptoms—sudden death.
- Palpitations, light-headedness, syncope, and fatigue
- ECG abnormalities
    - Complete or incomplete right bundle branch block
    - Ventricular tachycardia with left bundle branch block contour, and inverted T waves inverted over the right precordial leads
    - The ventricular tachycardia may be due to reentry
    - Supraventricular arrhythmias
    - Exercise can induce the ventricular tachycardia in some patients.
    - Sudden cardiac death the most serious complication of ARVC and at times the very first sign of the disease
- Heart failure is a less common symptom and appears to occur later in the disease. Right heart failure is more common than left heart failure.

Diagnostics

- MRI is a useful noninvasive test for diagnosis detection of right ventricular myocardial fibro-fatty changes in ARVD/C.
- Chest x-ray—Cardiomyopathy

- Echocardiogram—Dilated right and left ventricles with diminished contractility
- ECG—Repolarization and depolarization abnormalities; intraventricular conduction delay; complete or incomplete right bundle branch block
- Serial ECGs are indicated to detect rhythm changes and serious life-threatening ventricular dysrhythmias. 24-hour Holter monitoring or stress testing to determine the effect of life activities and stress on arrhythmic events
- Cardiac catheterization—r/o CAD; Right ventricular dilation and dysfunction
- Electrophysiology Study (EPS)—Induce dysrhythmias for therapy
- Endomyocardial biopsy—Fibrous scars and fatty infiltration changes to right ventricular myocardium
- Exercise radionuclide study—Detect exercise-induced ventricular dysrhythmias and assess functional capacity

Patient Care Management

- Controlling clinical manifestations and progression of the disease
- In-depth medical and family history; assess any personal or family history of palpitations, light-headed sensation, or collapse
- No precise guidelines to determine which patients need to be treated and which is the best management approach

---

Critical Alert
Due to the chronic and progressive nature of cardiomyopathy and the increased risk of sudden cardiac death as the disease progresses, a collaborative care approach is optimal for management.

- Nurse: Plays pivotal role in coordinating the efforts of the health care team and facilitate communication between members of the team and the patient/family

- Health care provider: Monitors the progression of the cardiomyopathy; determines the treatment plan
- Pharmacist: Crucial in educating patient about managing medications and their side effects
- Dietitian: Advises dietary changes needed to control congestion exacerbated by excess salt and fluid intake
- Physical therapist: Assists in maintenance of optimum conditioning given the activity restrictions
- Occupational therapist: Helps facilitate realistic occupational goals
- Social Services: Assists patient with end-of-life wishes and an advance directive
- Psychiatric counseling: Assists in lifestyle adjustments necessitated by a chronic disease process

- Medication Therapy
  - Beta-adrenergic blockers and class I and III antiarrhythmic drugs (sotalol or amiodarone) alone or in combination with beta-adrenergic blockers
  - Heart failure therapy if indicated
- Procedural Therapy

Reserved for those patients with life-threatening ventricular dysrhythmias in whom drug treatment is either ineffective or is associated with serious side effects.

  - Electrophysiology (EPS) guided drug testing
  - Radio-frequency catheter ablation
  - Implantable cardioverter defibrillator ICD
- Curative Therapy
  - Heart transplantation

Nursing Management
Alterations in Cardiac Output and Tissue Perfusion

- Continuous monitoring for changes in systemic perfusion, noting trends in order to pick up ominous changes and worsening signs of heart failure

- Monitored carefully for cardiac dysrhythmias
- Maintain proper hydration—Dehydration decreases preload and cardiac output which may lead to syncope, serious cardiac arrhythmias (ventricular tachycardia), and sudden death
- Limit workload of the heart by pacing and restricting activity

(See Appendix #18, Nursing Process: Patient Care Plan for Cardiomyopathy.)

Knowledge Deficit
- Prevention of disease progression
- Compliance with therapy
- Prevent exacerbation of heart failure
- Reportable conditions
  - Clinical manifestations of heart failure
  - Clinical manifestations of infective endocarditis
  - New onset chest pain
- Teach importance of avoiding strenuous exercise in preventing symptoms, dehydration, and possibly lethal complications
- Teach compliance with the medication regimen and dietary sodium restrictions to prevent the progression of the disease process and potentially improve the quality of life for the chronic disease

(See Appendix #19, Patient Teaching for Cardiomyopathies.)

Dilated Cardiomyopathy (DCM)

Chronic noncurable disease is the most common form of cardiomyopathy. Characterized by dilation and impaired contraction of one or more ventricles and an increase in myocardial wall thickness (hypertrophy). Results in hypocontractility, reduced stroke volume, ejection fraction, and ultimately decreased cardiac output. Blood flows more slowly through the enlarged heart, causing mural thrombi (blood clots on the heart wall) to form, increasing the risk of atrial and ventricular emboli formation.

Risk Factors

- Long-term uncontrolled hypertension
- Hypocalcemia; hypophosphatemia; uremia
- Hyperlipidemia; stress and sedentary lifestyle
- Alcohol abuse; obesity; smoking; cocaine, sleep apnea
- Cardiac valve disease; coronary artery disease; cardiac surgery
- Congenital heart disease; familial cardiomyopathies
- Viral myocarditis; bacterial/parasitic infections; amyloidosis and sarcoidosis
- Antiviral medications; chemotherapeutic agents; radiation therapy
- Toxins (lead, mercury, carbon monoxide, arsenic)
- Pregnancy and postpartum period
- Connective tissue disorders (SLE, scleroderma, giant cell arthritis)
- Neuromuscular disorders (Duchenne's muscular dystrophy)
- Nutritional deficiency (decreased thiamine, selenium, carnitine)
- Endocrine disorders (diabetes, Cushing's disease)

Signs and Symptoms

DCM has an insidious onset; some may be asymptomatic for months or even years after diagnosis and others have pronounced symptoms from the onset.

- Increasing fatigue, dyspnea, and activity intolerance, classic symptoms of both right- and left-sided heart failure
- Mitral and/or tricuspid insufficiency due to ventricular dilation
- Sudden death can occur at any stage of the disease

Diagnostics

- Chest x-ray—Cardiomegaly, heart enlargement, pulmonary congestion
- ECG—Dysrhythmias, axis deviation, LBBB, ST segment changes
- Echocardiogram—Enlarged chambers, ventricular wall thickness, sluggish wall motion, decreased systolic and diastolic function
- Cardiac catheterization to r/o CAD and evaluate cardiac output
- Endomyocardia biopsy—To r/o other causes
- Radionuclide study—Deficits in myocardial muscle perfusion

Patient Care Management

- Determine cause, improve contractile efficiency, and manage the symptoms and complications
- Control progression of structural dysfunction that leads to heart failure
- Medication Therapy
  - Anticoagulants for the blood stasis problems
  - Diuretics and fluid/sodium-restricted diets to decrease fluid overload and pulmonary congestion activity
  - Heart failure therapy with ACE inhibitors (or angiotensin receptor blockers), beta-blockers, and aldosterone blockers. May slow, stop, or even reverse tissue remodeling that occurs
  - Antiarrhythmic medications to decrease dysrhythmias
- Procedural Therapy
  - Implantable cardioverter defibrillator (ICD) to prevent sudden cardiac death
  - Cardiac resynchronization therapy (CRT)—Biventricular pacemaker to help increase cardiac output if ejection fraction less than 35%

Nursing Management
Alterations in Cardiac Output

- Continuous monitoring for changes in systemic perfusion, noting trends to detect ominous changes and worsening signs of heart failure
- Monitored carefully for cardiac dysrhythmias

Activity Intolerance

- Limit workload of the heart by pacing and restricting activity
- Activity restriction is essential during the acute illness, but resuming activities that increase strength and endurance should be promoted.

(See Appendix #18.)

Knowledge Deficit

- Prevention of disease progression
- Compliance with therapy
- Prevent exacerbation of heart failure
- Reportable conditions
  - Clinical manifestations of heart failure
  - Clinical manifestations of infective endocarditis
  - New onset chest pain

(See Appendix #19.)

Hypertrophic Cardiomyopathy (HCM)

A disorder of the contractile element of the cardiac muscle that is characterized by left ventricular and occasionally right ventricular hypertrophy, with greater hypertrophy occurring in the septum. HCM can be caused by hypertension or hypoparathyroidism, and it frequently is idiopathic. Men and the black population are affected more by HCM; it is usually diagnosed in young athletic individuals and is a genetic disorder in more than 50% of cases. Changes result in a decreased ventricular chamber size and cause the ventricles to take a longer period of time to relax. This has a direct negative effect on cardiac output and, thus, tissue perfusion.

Hypertrophic Obstructive Cardiomyopathy (HOCM)

Hypertrophic Obstructive Cardiomyopathy (HOCM), also referred to as idiopathic hypertrophic subaortic stenosis (IHSS), has the same etiology as HCM, although these patients also have obstruction to the outflow tract of the left ventricle (LV) leading into the aorta. The hypertrophy distorts the septum, and in some patients the anterior leaflet of the mitral valve, causing it to meet the septum, narrowing the left ventricular outflow tract during systole. Significant LV outflow obstruction is present in some patients at rest, while in others it is evident only during increased activity such as exercise.

Signs and Symptoms

Clinical manifestations of HCM and HOCM are similar to dilated cardiomyopathy.

- Typically begins in late adolescence or early adulthood, but may appear at any age
- Hypertrophic cardiomyopathy may occur without symptoms.
- Symptoms appear gradually, will progress over time, and are associated with deterioration of LV function resulting in right- and left-sided heart failure.
- Exercise tends to precipitate the symptoms and increases the risk of sudden death, which appears most often in young adults.
- Sudden death or severe heart failure may be the first clinical manifestations.
- Dyspnea, most common symptom
- Other symptoms include chest pain, dizziness, presyncope or syncope, fatigue, orthopnea and paroxysmal nocturnal dyspnea, and palpitations.

- Dysrhythmias—Supraventricular (primarily atrial fibrillation) and ventricular (tachycardia and fibrillation), along with sudden death
- Abnormally forceful LV apical pulse, S_4
- Systolic murmur—Harsh crescendo–decrescendo heard best at the left lower sternal border and the apex
- Systolic thrill palpable at the apex or lower left sternal border
- Severe cases of hypertrophic obstructive cardiomyopathy (HOCM)
  - Elevated pulmonary artery pressures due to an inability of the left ventricle to empty, increasing right ventricular pressure, causing the interventricular septum to shift to the left. The leftward shift causes further obstruction to the ventricular outflow tract.
  - Reduced preload decreases chamber size and increased heart rate will increase LV outflow obstruction. Dehydration and suddenly sitting upright (orthostatic hypotension) are two examples of factors that will decrease preload, and fever and exercise are two factors that increase heart rate. The end result is a reduction in cardiac output that may range from minimal to severe and may lead to syncope, serious cardiac arrhythmias (ventricular tachycardia), and sudden death.

Diagnostics

- Echocardiogram is the most useful tool when diagnosing both HCM and HOCM for visualization of the LV hypertrophy, wall motion abnormalities, and diastolic dysfunction.
- Chest x-ray—Cardiomegaly, specifically left atrial enlargement, pulmonary congestion
- ECG—(Resting and Ambulatory)
  - Resting—Increased voltage and duration of QRS, atrial, and ventricular dysrhythmias

- Ambulatory—ST segment changes that occur with increased activity. Increased hypercontractility that increases with activity.
- Echocardiogram enlarged chambers, ventricular wall thickness, sluggish wall motion, decreased systolic and diastolic function
- Cardiac catheterization to r/o CAD and to assess hemodynamic status, and chamber size/function and valve function
- Radionuclide study—Increased left ventricular and septal wall size; asymmetrical hypertrophy and hypercontractility
- Cardiac Biopsy—Test for infiltrations and fibrosis

Patient Care Management

- Finding and treating the underlying cause, if possible
- Control clinical manifestations, prevent progression of the disease, and improve the quality of life
- Improving cardiac output by reducing ventricular contractility and relieving LV outflow obstruction
- Fluid stabilization, prevent dehydration
- Medication Therapy
  - Negative inotropic medications, such as beta-adrenergic blocking agents and calcium antagonists to decrease the hypercontractility and outflow obstruction; decrease heart rate, which decreases cardiac workload and oxygen consumption
  - Anticoagulants to prevention of clot formation in the presence of atrial fibrillation
  - Antiarrhythmic medications
    - Prevent life-threatening dysrhythmias
  - Prophylactic antibiotics before dental work or invasive procedures to prevent endocarditis
- Procedural Therapy
  - Implantable cardioverter defibrillator (ICD) to prevent sudden cardiac death

- Cardiac resynchronization therapy (CRT)— Biventricular Pacemaker to help increase cardiac output if ejection fraction less than 35%
- Surgical Therapy

  Surgical procedures are performed when the patient has not responded to medical therapy and marked obstruction to the aortic outflow tract occurs due to the mitral valve meeting the enlarged septum.
  - Ventriculomyotomy involves excising some of the hypertrophied septal muscle, widening the LV outflow tract, and improving cardiac output, and relieving symptoms.
  - Replacement of the mitral valve with an artificial valve. Reduces the space taken up by the mitral valve and supporting structures, allowing blood to move more easily around the enlarged septum.
- Nonsurgical Therapy
  - Alcohol ablation involves injection of alcohol down a small branch of the coronary artery feeding the area of muscle hypertrophy (septum). The alcohol destroys the extra cardiac muscle.
- Curative Therapy
  - Heart transplantation is the only long-term cure for HCM.

Nursing Management
Alterations in Cardiac Output

- Continuous monitoring for changes in systemic perfusion, noting trends to detect ominous changes and worsening signs of heart failure
- Monitored carefully for cardiac dysrhythmias
- Maintain proper hydration—Dehydration decreases preload and cardiac output, which may lead to syncope, serious cardiac arrhythmias (ventricular tachycardia), and sudden death.

Activity Intolerance
- Limit workload of the heart by pacing and restricting activity
- Activity restriction is essential during the acute illness, but resuming activities that increase strength and endurance should be promoted.

(See Appendix #18.)

Knowledge Deficit
- Prevention of disease progression
- Compliance with therapy
- Prevent exacerbation of heart failure
- Reportable conditions
  - Clinical manifestations of heart failure
  - Clinical manifestations of infective endocarditis
  - New onset chest pain
- Inform patient that close blood relatives (parents, children, or siblings) may also have enlarged ventricular septum, testing is recommended.

(See Appendix #19.)

Restrictive Cardiomyopathy

Restrictive cardiomyopathy (RCM) is the least common type of cardiomyopathy found in the United States. Ventricles have normal wall thickness, but are rigid, producing elevated filling pressures and dilated atria. Involvement of the valve is common, but the outflow tract is spared. Contractility is unaffected by restrictive cardiomyopathy, however intraventricular pressures increase and cardiac output decreases, resulting in heart failure.Typically progresses rapidly, resulting in high mortality.

- Primary restrictive cardiomyopathy is idiopathic.

- Secondary restrictive cardiomyopathy is thought to be caused by:
  - Cocaine-use, amyloidosis, endomyocardial fibrosis, disorders in glycogen storage, hemochromatosis, and sarcoidosis

Signs and Symptoms
- Dyspnea
- Pulmonary and systemic congestion
- Palpitations, fatigue, syncope, angina, generalized weakness, and exercise intolerance
- In the advanced stages, both right- or left-sided heart failure
- S_3 frequently present
- Systolic murmur from mitral and tricuspid regurgitation

Diagnostics
- Chest x-ray—Cardiomegaly, specifically atrial enlargement; pulmonary venous congestion; pleural effusions may be present with heart failure.
- Echocardiogram—Thickened cardiac wall, small ventricular chamber size, dilated atria
- ECG—(Resting and Ambulatory)—Atrial fibrillation, tachycardia; complex ventricular dysrhythmias
- Radionuclide study—Increased ventricular volume mass, decreasing chamber size; areas of decreased perfusion
- Endomyocardial biopsy—Presence of amyloidosis and/or sarcoidosis

Patient Care Management
There is no specific treatment or cure for RCM. Therapy is aimed at controlling symptoms to improve the quality of life.

- Reduce the workload of the heart to diminish heart failure
- Medication Therapy
  - Calcium channel blockers and beta-adrenergic blockers to decrease heart rate and increase ventricular filling time
  - Diuretics reduce pulmonary and systemic congestion, although the patient has to be monitored closely to prevent dehydration
  - Antiarrhythmic medications
  - Anticoagulants are indicated for patients in atrial fibrillation to prevent thromboembolism
- A low-sodium diet will decrease fluid retention and pulmonary congestion
- Procedural Therapy
  - Implantable cardioverter defibrillator (ICD) to prevent sudden cardiac death
  - Cardiac resynchronization therapy (CRT)—Biventricular pacemaker to help increase cardiac output if ejection fraction less than 35%

Nursing Management

Alterations in Cardiac Output

- Continuous monitoring for changes in systemic perfusion, noting trends to detect ominous changes and worsening signs of heart failure
- Monitored carefully for cardiac dysrhythmias
- Maintain proper hydration—Dehydration decreases preload and cardiac output, which may lead to syncope, serious cardiac arrhythmias (ventricular tachycardia), and sudden death.

Activity Intolerance

- Limit workload of the heart by pacing and restricting activity
- Activity restriction is essential during the acute illness, but resuming activities that increase strength and endurance should be promoted.

(See Appendix #18.)

Knowledge Deficit
- Prevention of disease progression
- Compliance with therapy
- Prevent exacerbation of heart failure
- Reportable conditions
  - Clinical manifestations of heart failure
  - Clinical manifestations of infective endocarditis
  - New onset chest pain
- Teach importance of avoiding strenuous exercise in preventing symptoms, dehydration, and possibly lethal complications.

(See Appendix #19.)

Infective Endocarditis (IE)

Infective endocarditis is an infection of the cardiac endocardial layer of the heart, which may include one or more heart valves, the mural endocardium, and/or a septal defect. It is a life-threatening disease that occurs most often in persons with structural abnormalities of the heart or great vessels, but it also can occur with normal hearts.

Two Types: Acute IE and Subacute IE
- Acute IE—Rapid onset, caused by a virulent organism following infections of the respiratory, gastrointestinal, and genitourinary tracts, and open heart surgery. If untreated can lead to death within days to weeks.
- Subacute IE—Most common form; organism present in an inactive state for long periods of time; common in people with preexisting valve disease.

Risk Factors
- Recent dental surgery; bleeding gums

- Nosocomial infections; rheumatic fever; history of endocarditis
- Congenital heart disease; Marfan's syndrome
- Hypertrophic cardiomyopathy
- Weakened cardiac valves; mitral valve prolapse with murmur; aortic valve leaflet abnormalities; degenerative valvular lesions; prosthetic heart valve; narrowed valve orifice
- Long-term central line placement; urinary tract infection
- Invasive procedures—Oral surgery; gynecologic procedures; implantation of a cardioverter-defibrillator; hemodynamic catheters; insertion of an indwelling urinary catheter, or renal shunt
- Pneumonia; HIV; chest trauma; cellulitis
- Illegal intravenous drug use

Signs and Symptoms
- Fever, tachycardia, fatigue, malaise, anorexia, weight loss, headache, and chills; back pain; abdominal discomfort; anorexia and weight loss
- Heart murmur, usually on the aortic or mitral valves
- Dyspnea, cough, and chest pain, especially if heart failure and decreased cardiac output have occurred
- ECG changes include conduction delays (first-, second-, and third-degree heart blocks), diffuse ST segment changes, and PR interval depression
- Pericardial effusion and tamponade due to accumulation of serous, purulent, and/or hemorrhagic fluid in the pericardial sac
- Vascular changes
  - Splinter hemorrhages are black longitudinal streaks on the nail beds
  - Petechiae on the lips, buccal mucosa, palate, ankles, feet, antecubital space, and popliteal areas
  - Painful, red or purple, pea-size lesions, referred to as Osler's nodes, present on the fingertips or toes

- Janeway's lesions, flat, painless, small, red spots, found on the palms of the hand and soles of the feet
- Roth's spots, round white spots surrounded by hemorrhage, on the retina
- Focal neurological complaints and stroke syndromes from tiny emboli

Diagnostics

Based on a constellation of clinical findings

- Blood cultures that are repeated two to three times over a 24-hour period
- Transesophageal echocardiography (TEE)
- If right-sided IE is suspected, a ventilation/perfusion (V/Q) scan
- CT scan

Patient Care Management

The goals are making a rapid diagnosis and initiating treatment to eradicate the infecting organism to minimize valve damage, and prevent heart failure. Underdiagnosis can lead to clinical catastrophe and death.

- Medication Therapy
    - Intravenous antibiotics for 2 to 8 weeks depending on the organism
    - Supportive treatments for the clinical manifestations
- Surgical Therapy
    - Repair valvular regurgitation
    - Replacement of a severely damaged valve or valve that is a continuing source of infection

Prophylactic treatment for all persons who have the medical indications:

(See Appendix #21, Indications for Prophylactic Antibiotic Therapy with Infective Endocarditis.)

Nursing Management

Nursing care for patients with endocarditis focuses on prevention of life-threatening complications.

Infection

- Monitor vital signs
- Administer antibiotics
- Reduce fever, headache, and chills with medications

Alterations in Cardiac Output and Tissue Perfusion

- Assess
  - Vital signs
  - Dysrhythmias
  - Fluid status
  - Anxiety
  - Lung sounds
  - Monitor for presence or changes in murmur

Activity Intolerance

- Monitor patient activity tolerance
- Space activities and visitors to allow for periods of rest

Risk of Life-threatening and Long-term Complications

- Monitor and report
  - New or changing murmurs, indicating valve malfunction
  - Clinical manifestations of heart failure
  - Embolic events
    - Spleen—Localized abdominal tenderness and rigidity, sharp upper left quadrant pain, and splenomegaly
    - Kidneys—Flank pain, hematuria, and azotemia
    - Neurological deficits
    - Pulmonary emboli

- Splinter hemorrhages on the nail beds; petechiae on the lips, buccal mucosa, palate, ankles, feet, antecubital space, and popliteal areas; Osler's nodes and Janeway's lesions (late finding)
- Knowledge Deficit
  - Discharge medications with patient's understanding of the regimen
  - Prevention of recurrent infection
    - Avoid infection sources
    - Good dental hygiene
    - Prophylactic treatment as prescribed

(See Appendix #17, Patient Teaching & Discharge Priorities for Inflammatory Heart Disease.)

> **Critical Alert**
> This is a life-threatening illness, with the potential for permanent cardiac damage that has a significant impact on the quality of life. Patients and their families must inform health care providers of a valve disorder, history of infective endocarditis, or a prosthetic valve each time dental or invasive diagnostic procedures are performed. A medic alert bracelet is also advisable.

Myocarditis

Myocarditis, a focal or diffuse inflammation of the myocardium or heart muscle, is an uncommon disorder that is frequently associated with pericarditis. Most originate from a viral infection, and often remain undiagnosed, due to the general lack of initial symptoms. Immunosuppressed patients are at a higher risk. In some cases the disease presents as an acute catastrophic illness requiring immediate attention.

- Affects the heart's ability to pump blood normally, thereby affecting cardiac output.

- Scarring and permanent myocardial damage from myocarditis vary from none to severe heart failure leading to death or cardiomyopathy, requiring a heart transplant.

- Myocarditis may be mistaken for ischemic, valvular, or hypertensive heart disease and can be both acute and chronic.

Risk Factors

- Autoimmune and connective tissue diseases
- Drug hypersensitivity or toxicity
- Sarcoidosis
- Hypersensitive immune reactions such as rheumatic fever
- Postcardiotomy syndrome
- Toxins
- Chemicals
- Alcohol use
- Nosocomial infections
- Large doses of radiation to the chest for treatment of malignancy

Signs and Symptoms

- Early cardiac symptoms typically appear 7 to 10 days after the initial infection.
- Range from no overt symptoms to severe heart involvement
  - Flu-like symptoms—Fatigue, malaise, shortness of breath, fever, gastrointestinal upset, and aching joints
  - Suddenly with manifestations of heart failure or sudden cardiac death without prior symptoms

Diagnostics

(See Appendix #14, Diagnostic Tests for Cardiac Inflammatory Disorders.)

Patient Care Management

- Health history and physical examination
- Assessment of the risk factors

- Early diagnosis and treatment to mitigate the damage to the myocardial cells
- Bed rest to decrease metabolic demand and reduce myocardial workload
- Activity restrictions of varying levels may continue for up to 6 months
- Oxygen when heart failure symptoms are present in the setting of hypoxemia
- Medication Therapy
  - Antibiotics
  - Nonsteroidal antinflammatory agents
  - Steroids
  - Cardiac medications
  - Diuretics
  - Anticoagulants
  - Antianxiety

(See Appendix #15, Pharmacology Summary of Medications to Treat Inflammatory Heart Disease.)

Critical Alert

Digoxin: Patients with myocarditis are sensitive to the effects of digoxin. Digoxin increases the force of cardiac contractions, thus increasing the workload and oxygen demand of the heart muscle. These patients must be monitored closely for heart failure. Vital signs, lungs sounds, increasing shortness of breath, and peripheral edema need to be monitored on a frequent and ongoing basis.

Nursing Management
Alterations in Cardiac Output

- Assess for clinical manifestations of heart failure
  - Vital signs
  - Dysrhythmias
  - Fluid status
  - Anxiety
  - Lung sounds

- Activities for energy conservation
  - Monitor patient activity tolerance
  - Space activities and visitors to allow for periods of rest

(See Appendix #16, Nursing Process: Patient Care Plan for Inflammatory Heart Disease.)

Knowledge Deficit

(See Appendix #17.)

Pericarditis

Pericarditis, an inflammation of the pericardial sac, is the most common pathologic process affecting the pericardium. Due to an inflammatory process, the two layers of the pericardium become inflamed and roughened, and the amount of fluid in the pericardial sac increases. Pericarditis can be acute and/or chronic constrictive (recurrent). Causes can be infectious, noninfectious, or hypersensitive or autoimmune.

- Infectious
  - TB: Bacterial: tuberculosis, streptococcus, staphylococcus, meningococcus, syphilis, pneumococcus, Lyme disease
  - Viral: coxsackie virus B, echoviruses, endoviruses, adenoviruses, HIV, hepatitis
  - Fungal
  - Parasitic
- Noninfectious
  - Chest trauma or injury
  - Cardiac surgery
  - Uremia
  - Radiation therapy
  - Cancer that has metastasized to the pericardium

- MI (48–72 hr)
- Dissecting aortic aneurysm
- Hypersensitive or autoimmune
  - Systemic lupus erythematosus
  - Rheumatoid arthritis
  - Scleroderma
  - Polyarteritis nodosa
  - Ankylosing spondylitis
  - Myxedema
  - MI (1–4 weeks, Dressler's syndrome)
  - Drug reactions: procainamide, hydralazine, minoxidil

Acute Pericarditis

Acute pericarditis can be either dry or exudative. If exudative, the pericardial sac fills with the serofibrinous exudate. Anywhere from 100 to 3,000 mL of fluid or exudate has been known to accumulate in the pericardial sac. This excess fluid accumulation restricts cardiac filling and emptying, decreasing cardiac output and tissue perfusion.

Critical Alert
Without prompt treatment, shock and death will occur.

Chronic Constrictive Pericarditis

Chronic constrictive pericarditis occurs when the pericardial layers adhere to each other as a result of fibrosis of the pericardial sac. The scarring and thickening of the pericardium, which decreases cardiac filling and contracting, leads to decreased cardiac output and heart failure. Occurs as a result of tuberculosis, typically found in the immigrant and prison populations, and people with acquired immunodeficiency syndrome

(AIDS). Constrictive pericarditis also may develop secondary to surgery, uremia, or radiation.

Signs and Symptoms

- Chest Pain
  - Sudden, often on the left side of the chest and radiates to the left shoulder, neck, and back
  - Mild to severe anginal-type or sharp pleuritic type. Worse with inspiration, coughing, movement of the trunk, deep breathing, and when lying flat. Decreasing pain when sitting up and leaning forward. (*Note*: Key factor in the diagnostic assessment)
- Dyspnea
- Fever, chills
- Malaise, anorexia, weight loss, and nausea in acute stages
- Joint pain
- ECG Changes
  - Transient PR interval depression
  - Tachycardia, bradycardia, and atrial fibrillation
  - ST elevation (I, II, AVF, V4, V6 followed by T wave inversion without Q waves)
  - Decreased amplitude of QRS complexes
- Pericardial friction rub (*Note*: Key factor in the diagnostic assessment)
  - Best heard over the left sternal border in the 2nd, 3rd, or 4th intercostal space with the stethoscope diaphragm
  - Louder when the patient is sitting up and leaning forward
  - Described as a grating, scraping, squeaking, or crunching sound resulting from friction between the roughened, inflamed layers of the pericardium
  - Heard even while patient is holding breath—confirming that it is cardiac in nature

- Transient and may vary in intensity from hour to hour
- Pericardial Effusion
  - An excess of pericardial fluid as a result of an accumulation of infectious exudates or toxins, and/or blood; a threat to normal cardiac function
  - Gradual buildup and stretch can accommodate 1 to 2 liters without causing cardiac compression
  - Rapid buildup of fluid with only 80 to 200 mL of fluid causes cardiac compression
  - Heart sounds typically muffled and may be difficult to auscultate
  - Large pleura effusions with pulmonary compression causes coughing, dyspnea, and tachypnea. Compression of the laryngeal nerve causes hoarseness, and compression of the phrenic nerve may induce hiccups.
  - Treatment focuses on decreasing inflammation and treating the pain. NSAIDs such as aspirin treat the inflammation, and opioids are used to treat the pain.
- Cardiac Tamponade
  - Occurs when there is a rapid and large accumulation of fluid in the pericardial space. Drop in cardiac output and subsequent loss of tissue perfusion make this a life-threatening situation.
  - The hallmark signs are:
    - Narrowing of the pulse pressure (systolic minus diastolic blood pressure to less than 30 mmHg)
    - Tachycardia
  - Classic assessment findings are referred to as Beck's triad
    - ↓ blood pressure
    - Muffled heart sounds
    - Jugular venous distention

- Other findings:
  - Weak peripheral pulses
  - Pulsus paradoxus (greater than 10 mmHg drop in systolic BP during inspiration) (*Note*: Key factor in the diagnostic assessment)
  - Restless
  - Decreased level of consciousness
  - Decrease amplitude of the QRS complex

> **Critical Alert**
> The sudden onset of pulsus paradoxus indicates that cardiac tamponade is occurring. Assess the patient for other signs of tamponade: tachycardia, diminished heart sounds, narrowed pulse pressure, and distended neck veins. The health care provider must be notified to institute diagnosis and treatment immediately. Cardiac tamponade is a life-threatening complication of pericardial effusion.

Diagnostics

- CT scans and MRI used to identify pericardial effusions or pericardial thickening
- Hemodynamic monitoring to evaluate pulmonary artery pressure and cardiac output
- Pericardiocentesis—Removal of pericardial fluid
  - Relieves pressure causing tamponade
  - Culture of fluid, sensitivity and cytology

(See Appendix #14.)

Patient Care Management

- Determine cause and prevent complications
- Differentiate from MI (pain may be similar)
- Medication Therapy
  - NSAIDS and aspirin for inflammation and pain
  - Antibiotics if bacterial; no curative for viral
  - Steroids if secondary to systemic lupus erythematosus
  - TB drugs if caused by tuberculosis

(See Appendix #15.)

- If renal cause, more frequent and intense dialysis is indicated.
- Pericardiocentesis to relieve constriction and prevent cardiac tamponade
- Pericardiectomy (pericardial window) for recurrent effusions, tamponade or adhesions from chronic constrictive pericarditis

Nursing Management

Alterations in Cardiac Output and Tissue Perfusion

- Assess
  - Vital signs
  - Dysrhythmias
  - Fluid status
  - Anxiety
  - Lung sounds
  - Monitor for presence or changes in murmur

Activity Intolerance

- Monitor patient activity tolerance
- Space activities and visitors to allow for periods of rest

Monitor for Complications

- Pericardial Effusion
  - Muffled heart sounds
  - Coughing, dyspnea, tachypnea, hoarseness and hiccups
- Cardiac Tamponade
  - Classic assessment findings are referred to as Beck's triad
    - ↓ Blood pressure—Pulsus paradoxus (greater than 10 mmHg drop in systolic BP during inspiration)

- Muffled heart sounds
- Jugular venous distention
- Other findings:
  - Restless
  - Decreased level of consciousness
  - Weakened pulses

Critical Alert

Pulsus paradoxus is a greater than 10 mmHg drop in systolic BP during inspiration. The BP normally decreases during inspiration but does so by less than 10 mmHg. A paradox of greater than 10 mmHg is present when there is increased thoracic pressure as a result of pericardial swelling. This is an important diagnostic clue most frequently picked up by the nurse. The patient typically becomes restless and may have a decreased level of consciousness as the fluid accumulates and the cardiac output drops. Finally, the amplitude of the QRS complex of the ECG is low.

Pain Management

- Assess pain using numeric scale (0–10) to quantify pain
- Use pain control measures before the pain becomes severe to intervene early and with less medication
- Careful pain assessment and differentiation from angina-type chest pain

---

Critical Alert

Anginal pain is typically described as a burning, pressure-type pain that is not associated with position change or deep breathing. It is relieved by nitroglycerin and rest. The chest pain associated with pericarditis is often described as sharp and gets worse with deep breathing. It is relieved by sitting up and taking anti-inflammatory drugs.

(See Appendix #16.)

Knowledge Deficit
(See Appendix #17.)

Rheumatic Heart Disease

Rheumatic heart disease is a complication of rheumatic fever, thought to be caused by an abnormal autoimmune response to the original infection. The infection results in long-term scarring and malfunction of the heart valves.

- Rheumatic fever, thought to be eradicated in developed countries, in recent years has made a comeback. Risk factors include: poor inner-city neighborhoods; crowded living conditions; damp weather; malnutrition; immunocompromised state; poor access to health care.

- Once rheumatic fever has occurred, a person is more susceptible to recurrent infections and more valve damage.

- Rheumatic fever follows untreated pharyngitis from Lancefield group A beta-hemolytic streptococcus. The infecting organism produces enzymes that cause thickening and fusion of the valve leaflets resulting in stenosis or regurgitation.

- Valve dysfunction symptoms begin about one to six weeks after the infection.

Rheumatic Heart Disease, Signs and Symptoms

Acute Rheumatic Fever	Rheumatic Heart Disease
• Fever • Headache • Malaise • Weakness • Polyarthritis—Swollen, painful joints—Most common symptom and in 70–75% cases occurs as the earliest manifestation	• New murmur or change in existing murmur—Major sign of cardiac involvement. Apical pansystolic—mitral regurgitation; apical diastolic—severe mitral insufficiency; basal diastolic—aortic regurgitation

(continued)

Rheumatic Heart Disease, Signs and Symptoms
(*continued*)

Acute Rheumatic Fever	Rheumatic Heart Disease
• Erythema marginatum—red, raised, lattice-like rash • Shortness of breath • Syndenham chorea—sudden, irregular, aimless involuntary movements • Elevated WBC count	• Chest pain • Tachycardia • Cardiac dysrhythmias • ECG changes—Prolonged PR interval • Pericardial friction rub • Pericarditis • Cardiomegaly • Mitral and aortic stenosis • Heart failure secondary to myocarditis and/or valve insufficiency

Diagnostics

(See Appendix #14.)

Patient Care Management

Prevention is the primary goal in the management of rheumatic heart disease.

- Early treatment of the streptococcal infection with antibiotics. Aggressive early treatment is essential in this population in patients with previous streptococcal infections due to increased susceptibility.
- Bed rest to reduce cardiac workload
- Medication Therapy
  - Antibiotics
  - Nonsteroidal anti-inflammatory agents
  - Cardiac medications
  - Antianxiety

(See Appendix #15.)

Nursing Management

Alterations in Cardiac Output

- Continuous monitoring for changes in systemic perfusion, noting trends to detect ominous changes and signs of heart failure
- Report any change in the loudness of the murmur as this may indicate a progression of cardiac valve disorders

Activity Intolerance

- Strict bedrest to decrease myocardial oxygen demand and cardiac workload
- Activity restriction is essential during the acute illness, but resuming activities that increase strength and endurance should be promoted.

Infection

- Administration of antibiotics to eradicate the infecting organism

Knowledge Deficit

(See Appendix #17.)

Cardiac Valvular Disorders

Cardiac valvular disorders are classified according to the valve involved and the functional alterations, which include stenosis and regurgitation.

Valvular Regurgitation

- Regurgitant valve is one that is unable to close normally, causing a backward flow of blood, referred to as insufficiency or incompetence.

- Inability of a valve to completely close during systole, resulting in a back flow of blood through the incompetent valve orifice into the previous chamber

- Malfunction in any one of the structures, leaflets, chordae tendineae, papillary muscles, and the valve annulus will cause valvular regurgitation.

- Affects the aortic, mitral, and on rare occasions the tricuspid valve

- Both of the chambers dilate and hypertrophy due to extra workload and hypoxemia, leading to progressive chamber failure and a decreased cardiac output.

Valvular Stenosis

- Stenotic valve is unable to open normally, causing an impedance of blood flow.

- Obstructs blood flow through the valve orifice and decreases cardiac output

- Occurs in the mitral, aortic, and tricuspid valves

- Degree of stenosis determines the reduction in cardiac output, the presence and severity of clinical manifestations.

- Mild to moderate stenosis maintains cardiac output at rest, but causes symptoms with exercise because of the increased need for oxygen.

Aortic Valve Disease
Aortic Valve Stenosis (AVS)

AVS is a progressive chronic disease that results in an obstruction to blood flow from the left ventricle to the aorta during systole. Eventually ventricular hypertrophy, pulmonary hypertension, and ventricular failure occur. Causes include congenital leaflet malformation, rheumatic endocarditis, and degenerative changes associated with the aging process.

Signs and Symptoms
- Dyspnea
- Angina
- Fatigue
- Syncope
- Palpitations
- Harsh crescendo–decrescendo systolic murmur
- Prominent S_4
- Increased pulmonary artery pressure and decreased cardiac output
- Lung congestion
- Left- and right-sided heart failure

Aortic Valve Regurgitation (AVR)

AVR can be acute or chronic. Blood regurgitates back into the left ventricle through aortic valve that is unable to completely close. The increased blood in the left ventricle causes dilation, hypertrophy, and eventually left ventricular dysfunction.

Chronic AVR

May remain asymptomatic for as long as 20 years. Common causes are rheumatic heart disease (67%), congenital valve malformation, and cardiomyopathy. Other causes include connective tissue disorders (Marfan's syndrome), rheumatoid arthritis, ankylosing spondylitis, chronic hypertension, and syphilitic aortitis.

With chronic AVR, the left ventricle increases stroke volume in an attempt to increase cardiac output. Untreated, AVR will lead to increased left atrial pressures and dilation, pulmonary hypertension and congestion, and finally right-sided heart failure.

Acute AVR

Most common cause is abrupt dilation of the aortic root caused by a descending dissecting aortic aneurysm. Other causes are blunt chest trauma and endocarditis. In acute AVR the left ventricle has not had time to develop the compensatory mechanisms. The extra blood volume dramatically increases the cardiac workload resulting in rapid decline in hemodynamic status, and development of fulminant pulmonary edema.

Signs and Symptoms

- Palpitations and exaggerated carotid artery pulsations; bounding heartbeat is due to the large ventricular stroke volume and rapid diastolic runoff.
- High-pitched blowing, crescendo–decrescendo diastolic murmur
- Exertional dyspnea, orthopnea, and paroxysmal nocturnal dyspnea
- Dizziness and exercise intolerance
- Nocturnal angina with diaphoresis
- Widened pulse pressure with an increased systolic pressure and a decreased diastolic pressure
- Left- and right-sided heart failure

Mitral Valve Disease

Three diseases affect the mitral valve: stenosis, regurgitation, and prolapse.

Mitral Valve Stenosis (MVS)

- The stenosis narrows the opening of the valve, which obstructs blood flow to the left ventricle eventually backing up into the pulmonary system leading to pulmonary hypertension and pulmonary edema.

- Obstruction may be mild or severe; stenosis is progressive and chronic.
- Causes include rheumatic heart disease, infectious endocarditis, congenital mitral stenosis, rheumatoid arthritis, thrombus formation, calcification of the annulus, atrial myxoma (tumor), and SLE.

Signs and Symptoms

Symptoms typically appear gradually, early symptoms appear with exercise. Later-stage symptoms occur with rest.

- Atrial fibrillation (occurs 50% of the time)
- Dyspnea, dyspnea on exertion, orthopnea, all due to pulmonary hypertension
- Diastolic murmur
- Loud first heart sound heard (S_1) reflecting high atrial pressures
- Dry cough, dysphasia, and bronchitis due to bronchial irritation
- Fatigue and weakness due to decreased cardiac output
- Clinical manifestations of right-sided heart failure
- Palpitations and angina
- Crackles in the lung bases
- Hemoptysis

Mitral Valve Regurgitation (MVR)

Fibrotic changes and calcification of the mitral valve result in an inability to close completely during systole; often present with mitral valve stenosis.

- Chronic MVR, the left atrium, left ventricle, and pulmonary vasculature dilate to accommodate the chronic volume overload.

- Acute MVR occurs with myocardial infarction causing rupture of the papillary muscle and a sudden increase in left atrial distention and pressure backing up into the pulmonary system, causing pulmonary edema.
- Causes: Rheumatic heart disease (most common); connective tissue disorders (Marfan's syndrome), congenital valve malformation, coronary artery disease, endocarditis, dilated cardiomyopathy, mitral valve prolapse, amyloidosis, ankylosing spondylitis, and myocardial infarction

Signs and Symptoms
Chronic MVR
- Symptoms take years to appear; remaining asymptomatic until left ventricular failure occurs
- Gradual onset of dyspnea, weakness, and fatigue gradually progressing to orthopnea, paroxysmal nocturnal dyspnea, and peripheral edema
- S_3 and pansystolic (both systole and diastole) murmur
- Cough, pulmonary crackles

Acute MVR
- Symptoms of pulmonary edema and shock appear quickly
- Sudden onset of dyspnea, thready peripheral pulses, and cool clammy skin
- Pulmonary crackles
- Decreased cardiac output
- Atrial fibrillation with thrombus formation (occurs 75% of the time)
- Blowing high-pitched, systolic murmur
- Left- and right-sided heart failure

Mitral Valve Prolapse (MVP)
MVP is the most common form of heart valve disease, more common in women, and often benign. MVR results from abnormalities of the valve leaflets, chordae

tendineae, papillary muscles, and left ventricular dysfunction. MVP occurs when one or more of the valve leaflets bulge or prolapse into the left atrium during systole resulting in valvular regurgitation.

May be genetically inherited, related to Marfan's syndrome, Graves' disease; idiopathic or caused by endocarditis, coronary artery disease, myocarditis, connective tissue disorders, cardiomyopathy, hyperthyroidism, and cardiac trauma.

Signs and Symptoms

- Onset of symptoms is often due to a major physiological stressor.

- Palpitations and irregular heartbeat; paroxysmal atrial tachycardia, premature ventricular contractions, and ventricular tachycardia, precipitated by stress, caffeine, alcohol, and over-the-counter stimulants

- Light-headedness, dizziness, especially with position change; low blood pressure

- Fatigue, weakness, dyspnea

- Sharp stabbing chest pain, especially during periods of stress, usually at rest but may occur with exercise. Chest pain may last for hours or days.

- Pansystolic murmur; midsystolic to late-systolic click heard between S_1 and S_2

Pulmonic Valve Disease

Disorders of the pulmonic valve are rare, and usually caused by a congenital valvular malformation, although endocarditis, tumors, and rheumatic heart disease have been implicated as causes.

Pulmonic Valve Stenosis (PVS)

In PVS, the blood from the right ventricle is obstructed from flowing into the pulmonary vasculature during systole and backs up into the right ventricle.

Pulmonic Valve Regurgitation (PVR)

PVR causes blood to regurgitate back into the right ventricle. Pulmonic regurgitation is typically caused by infective endocarditis, pulmonary artery aneurysm, syphilis, and pulmonary hypertension, which dilates the pulmonary orifice.

Signs and Symptoms

- Decreasing cardiac output due to decrease blood flow
- Hypertrophy from ventricular volume and pressure
- Right-sided heart failure
- Dyspnea and fatigue
- PVS: ECG has tall peaked T waves from atrial hypertrophy
- Atrial fibrillation
- PVR: high-pitched diastolic blowing murmur along the left sternal border
- PVS: systolic crescendo–decrescendo murmur heard in the second left intercostal space (pulmonic area)

Tricuspid Valve Disease
Tricuspid Valve Stenosis (TVS)

Tricuspid valve stenosis is an extremely rare and uncommon disorder caused by rheumatic heart disease, IV drug use, and concurrently with mitral stenosis.

Tricuspid Valve Regurgitation (TVR)

Tricuspid valve regurgitation increases right atrial pressure causing venous congestion and right-sided heart failure. It is usually the result of pulmonary hypertension, but may occur with rheumatic heart disease, inferior myocardial infarction, blunt chest trauma, and infective endocarditis.

Signs and Symptoms

- Right-sided heart failure
- Low cardiac output
- Fatigue and weakness
- Prominent waves in the neck veins due to vigorous atrial contraction

- Atrial fibrillation—Decreases cardiac output 20–25% and increases risk of thrombus formation
- High-pitched blowing systolic murmur

Cardiac Valvular Disorders (all)

Diagnostics

- A heart murmur is usually the first indication of valve disease.
- Transesophageal echocardiography best diagnostic tool

  (See Appendix #11, Diagnostics Cardiac Valvular Disorders.)

Patient Care Management

The focus of medical and surgical intervention is to prevent heart failure and serious cardiac muscle damage. Despite differences in pathophysiology the clinical management of patients with valve disease is similar.

- Find and treat the cause of the disorder and prevent complications and death
- Maintaining cardiac output and activity level
- Treatment of heart failure
- Medication Therapy
  - Cardiac medications
  - Diuretics
  - Antibiotics
  - Anticoagulants
  - Nitrates

  (See Appendix #12, Summary of Medications for Cardiac Valvular Disorders.)

- Invasive Therapy

  When hemodynamic status becomes unstable and a negative impact on the quality of life occurs, invasive management may be necessary to cure the problem or relieve symptoms. Valve repair options include (annuloplasty, valvuloplasty, or commissurotomy) or valve replacement with a prosthesis.

- Annuloplasty repairs the enlarged annulus. Open heart surgery and cardiopulmonary bypass are required for an annuloplasty.

- Valvuloplasty repairs the valve leaflet rather than replaces it. Can be done with or without cardiopulmonary bypass.

- Percutaneous transluminal balloon valvuloplasty is used to dilate stenosed mitral and aortic valves. Performed in the heart catheterization laboratory under local anesthesia using a balloon-dilating catheter.

- Prosthetic heart valve replacement—The goal is to replace the valve before permanent left ventricular damage occurs. Valve replacement surgery is done under general anesthesia using cardiopulmonary bypass.

  - Mechanical Valves—The most frequently cited complications of mechanical valves are thromboembolism and anticoagulation-related problems. Most mechanical valves are expected to last 20 to 30 years.

  - Biological valves, most commonly come from pigs (porcine valves); although cow valves (bovine), and human valves also are used. Decreased incidence of clot formation compared to mechanical valves; therefore, long-term anticoagulation is not necessary. Biological valves are expected to last 7 to 10 years.

Due to the chronic and progressive nature of cardiac valve disease, a collaborative care approach is optimal for management. Utilizing a multidisciplinary team approach, will facilitate the best possible quality of life for the patient and family.

Nursing Management
Alterations in Cardiac Output

- Assess for clinical manifestations of right- and left-sided heart failure

- Vital signs
- Dysrhythmias
- Fluid status
- Anxiety
- Lung sounds
- Monitor for atrial fibrillation
- Monitor for changes in murmur
- Activities for energy conservation
  - Monitor patient activity tolerance
  - Space activities and visitors to allow for periods of rest

  (See Appendix #20, Postoperative Nursing Care of the Valve Surgery Patient.)

Knowledge Deficit
- Teach patient and family purpose and importance of treatment regime.
- Teach medication regime—Dosages, frequency, side effects, and special considerations.
- If applicable, teach patient and family about anticoagulation medication.
  - Report bruising, bleeding, epistaxis, hemoptysis, dark stool; follow dietary restrictions, continue regular laboratory follow-up.
- Teach patient and family about the disease and progression of clinical manifestations. Instruct patient to seek medical help when unable to perform ADLs.
- To prevent complications, teach patient the importance of informing health care providers of a valve disorder, history of infective endocarditis, or a prosthetic valve each time dental or invasive diagnostic procedures are performed. A medic alert bracelet would be useful.
- Assess the patient's support systems as these are chronic debilitating disorders.

- Provide patient and family with resources to assist with coping with progression of chronic illness.
- Nursing plays a pivotal role in coordinating the efforts of the health care team and facilitates communication between the members of the team and the patient/family.

Critical Alert

After valve replacement surgery, if the patient experiences fever, increased heart rate, fatigue, malaise, anorexia, weight loss, headache, chills, or night sweats, he/she must notify the health care provider. The clinical manifestations are a sign of postoperative infective endocarditis, which needs immediate medical attention.

COMPLEX RESPIRATORY DISORDERS

Acute Respiratory Distress Syndrome (ARDS)

Acute Lung Injury (ALI)

Acute respiratory distress syndrome (ARDS) is a progressive form of respiratory failure that leads to alveolar capillary, inflammation, pulmonary edema, and lung injury that results in hypoxemia. The term *acute lung injury* (ALI) is sometimes used when referring to ARDS, but ALI is less severe. ARDS has a mortality rate of 40%; patients usually die from multiple-organ failure complications rather than from the respiratory failure. There is no cure for ALI/ARDS or treatment that prevents the patient from developing this disease.

ARDS is caused by injury to the alveolar-capillary membrane that allows fluids, proteins, and cell products to flow into the alveoli. Inflammation in the lungs adds to the damage. As alveoli collapse, the lungs become heavy and stiff and difficult to ventilate. Hypoxemia, low lung compliance, and increased minute ventilation (V_E) (volume of gas ventilated in 1 minute) are the classic features of respiratory failure caused by ARDS. ARDS is similar to the pathophysiology of pulmonary edema with injury to the A-C membrane. The injury is multifactorial, related to other diseases or caused by mechanical ventilation. The complexity, interrelatedness, and mechanism of action of these host defense mediators are reasons why no cure for ARDS has been found since the disease was first recognized as a syndrome.

Injury can be the result of direct and indirect causes:

- Direct causes injury to the airways and parenchyma of the lung.
- Indirect requires the action of intermediary substances to cause injury.
  - Intermediary substances are host defenses that are released when tissue is injured and when inflammation occurs. In the case of ALI and ARDS these substances become "overactivated" and become part of the problem instead of the solution. A-C membrane occurs when pro-inflammatory mediators, oxygen free radicals, and other cytokines are activated in response to injury.
  - Systemic inflammatory response syndrome (SIRS) describes the syndrome when these substances of inflammation are activated. When SIRS is caused by infection, it is called sepsis, and with significant hypotension, and septic shock. If other organ systems are involved such as the renal or cardiovascular system, then multiple-organ dysfunction syndrome (MODS) might develop. There is a proposed link between sepsis and lung injury. ALI develops in 10% to 45% of patients who develop severe sepsis syndrome.

Critical Alert
Almost any disease process that generates a large-scale inflammation and injury pattern can cause ALI and ARDS.

Risk Factors Predictive of Increased Mortality in Patients with ALI/ARDS:

- Liver dysfunction
- Sepsis
- Nonpulmonary organ dysfunction
- Age
- Organ transplantation
- HIV infection
- Active malignancy

- Length of mechanical ventilation prior to ARDS
- Oxygenation index
- Mean airway pressure $\times$ FiO$_2$ $\times$ 100/PaO$_2$
- Mechanism of lung injury
- Right ventricular dysfunction
- PaO$_2$/FiO$_2$ ratio $<$ 100
- Chronic alcoholism

Clinical Causes/Diagnoses for ARDS/ALI

Types of Disorders	Diagnoses/Clinical Causes
Infectious causes	Gram-negative sepsis or gram-positive sepsis:
	Bacterial pneumonia
	Viral pneumonia
	Mycoplasmal pneumonia
	Fungal pneumonia
	Parasitic infections
	Mycobacterial disease
Aspiration	Gastric acid:
	Food and other particulate matter
	Fresh or sea water (near drowning)
	Hydrocarbon fluids
Trauma	Lung contusion:
	Fat emboli
	Nonthoracic trauma
	Overdistention (mechanical ventilation)
	Blast injury (explosion, lightning)
	Thermal injury (burns)
	Inhaled gases (phosgene, ammonia)
Hemodynamic disturbances	Shock of any etiology:
	Anaphylaxis
	High-altitude pulmonary edema
	Reperfusion
	Air embolism
	Amniotic fluid embolism

(*continued*)

Clinical Causes/Diagnoses for ARDS/ALI (*continued*)

Types of Disorders	Diagnoses/Clinical Causes
Drugs	Suicide gesture (aspiration):
	Heroin
	Methadone
	Propoxyphene
	Naloxone
	Cocaine
	Barbiturates
	Colchicine
	Salicylates
	Ethchlorvynol
	Interleukin-2
	Protamine
	Hydrochlorothiazide
	Obstruction or its release
	Disseminated intravascular coagulation:
	Incompatible blood transfusion
	Rh incompatibility
	Antileukocyte antibodies
	Leukoagglutinin reactions
	Postcardiopulmonary bypass pump oxygenator
	Pancreatitis
	Uremia
	Diabetic ketoacidosis
Metabolic disorders	Head trauma
	Grand mal seizures
	Increased intracranial pressure (any cause)
	Subarachnoid or intracerebral hemorrhage
Neurological disorders	Lung reexpansion
	Upper airway obstruction
Miscellaneous disorders	

Source: From Murray, J., & Nadel, J. (Eds.). (2005). *Textbook of respiratory medicine* (4th ed., p. 1511, Table 51-4). Philadelphia: W. B. Saunders. Used with permission.

ARDS Phases

Early Phase—Acute Exudative Phase occurs within the first 7 to 10 days after injury.

- Extensive edema is produced in response to the lung injury

- This fluid is high in protein content and floods the interstitial space, collapses alveoli, causes hemorrhage and diffuse alveolar damage.

- Decreased functional residual capacity (FRC) (the amount of gas in the lungs after a normal expiration) due to fluid filled alveoli

- Lung stiffness because many alveoli have collapsed or are flooded with fluid; on expiration, the lung recoils to a smaller volume. Some alveoli remain normal in function and structure. If high pressures are used in an attempt to ventilate the patient, these pressures are transmitted to the "normal" alveoli injuring them.

- Decreased ability of the lungs to exchange oxygen and carbon dioxide

- Increased polymorphonuclear neutrophils (PMNs) in the capillaries, in the interstitial spaces and in the alveoli, adding to the disruption of gas exchange at the A-C membrane

- Once activated by lung injury, neutrophils cause damage by blocking the air spaces, and in their mission to destroy bacteria and limit inflammation, they destroy alveolar endothelial cells in the process

- Pulmonary hypertension occurs caused by refractory hypoxemia and excretion of endothelin-1, a powerful vasoconstrictor.

Proliferative Phase of ARDS begins approximately 7 to 10 days postinjury.

- The air spaces have been filled with fluid are narrowed and filled with fibroblasts, the A-C membrane is thick and not efficient in gas exchange.

- Fibroblasts are present in the interstitial spaces and even in the air spaces that continue to collapse at an alarming rate.

- The compliance of the lung is decreased now, and high pressures are needed to ventilate through narrowed air spaces and collapsed alveoli.

Fibrotic Phase, the final phase of ARDS, can begin as early as 10 days after initial insult.

- Marked by fibrotic stiffness of the alveolar ducts, alveoli, and interstitial space as the result of the body's attempt at repair
- Requires long-term ventilator support until the lung damaged is repaired
- Increased CO_2 retention due to fibrotic changes in the lungs, not present until this final stage of the disease
- Stiff fibrotic structures seen on chest x-ray and their "honeycombed" appearance

Signs and Symptoms
- Hyperventilation with a corresponding respiratory alkalosis
- Chest x-ray may appear normal and this rapid respiratory rate is the only clinical sign that is present.
- Hypoxemia quickly becomes refractory to standard oxygen therapies, and the patient requires intubation and mechanical ventilation to maintain oxygenation and ventilation.
- Respirations are rapid and shallow with use of accessory muscles.
- Skin appears cyanotic or mottled, and does not improve with oxygen administration.
- Bilateral crackles are heard in the bases or throughout the lung fields.
- Coarse rhonchi and wheezes, depending on the severity of the fluid in the alveoli
- Pink frothy sputum of classic pulmonary edema is seen in some cases.
- Respiratory alkalosis in the early stage
- Respiratory acidosis in the advanced stage

- Chest x-ray exhibits the bilateral patchy infiltrates—"whiteout" can cover the entire lung field.
- Late findings include hypotension and decreased cardiac output.

Diagnostics

- ABG values to detect and document hypoxemia and pH imbalances
  - Hypocapnia is a typical finding early in ARDS.
  - Hypercapnia can be seen as ventilatory failure progresses.
  - PaO_2 of less than 50 mmHg is a typical finding.
- Sputum should be collected for Gram stain and cultures (e.g., bacterial, fungal, viral).
- Chest CT may be helpful in advanced cases but is not necessary for diagnosis.
- Echocardiography may be helpful to exclude a cardiogenic etiology for pulmonary edema.

Patient Care Management

- Treat the underlying cause of the precipitating event
- Supportive treatment
  - Oxygen
  - Early mechanical ventilation–modes employ very high respiratory rates and small tidal volumes to prevent further lung injury.
- Fluid management
  - Restrict fluids in order to limit the lung edema and at the same time prevent hypotension and renal failure
- Vasopressor drugs (dopamine and norepinephrine and other agents that increase blood pressure)
  - Prevent hypotension and tissue hypoxia and increase cardiac output in shock unresponsive to fluid resuscitated
- Promote healing and prevent complications
  - Nutrition either enterally or parenterally (enteral preferred)

> **Critical Alert**
> Research continues to identify therapies to limit the inflammation and the activation of neutrophils and monocytes in ARDS.

Nursing Management

Ineffective Gas Exchange, Risk of Life-threatening Hypoxia

- Frequent and ongoing assessment
- Airway and oxygenation status
- Respiratory rate
- Work of breathing
- ABGs
- Oxygen saturation
- Vital signs
- Anxiety assessment related to respiratory distress
- Assess skin and nail beds for cyanosis and pallor
- Lung sounds
- Notify health care provider for changes in oxygenation and assessment

Risk for Complications

- Deep breathing and coughing, use of incentive spirometer
- Frequent turning and repositioning
- Note oxygen desaturation with turning from one side to the other
- Careful attention to preoxygenation prior to suctioning or to the grouping of nursing activities can prevent decreased SpO_2 and allow turning and other care activities.

> **Critical Alert**
> Patients with ARDS frequently have little respiratory reserve and develop hypoxemia when turned, suctioned, or bathed. If desaturation is related to turning on a certain side or after an activity, the effect is documented, so it is not repeated.

- Management of the ventilated patient to optimize oxygenation and prevention complications

(See Procedures and Therapies: Endotracheal Intubation; Mechanical Ventilation; Noninvasive Positive Pressure Ventilation; and Suctioning.)

Acute Respiratory Failure (ARF)

Acute respiratory failure (ARF) is a condition defined as a failure of gas exchange (oxygenation or ventilation or both) due to a failure of the heart, lungs, or both. A failure of oxygenation produces hypoxemia, which is defined as an arterial oxygen tension or pressure (PaO_2) that is below normal range. A failure to ventilate produces the clinical sign of hypercapnia. Acute respiratory failure happens quickly, over hours to days, and is not characterized by a gradual worsening of symptoms that would portray chronic respiratory failure. Acute respiratory failure presents with no time for compensation by the renal system. The hallmark of ARF is respiratory difficulty with abnormal ABGs.

Critical Alert
The elderly are predisposed to developing respiratory failure due to physiologic effects of aging on the respiratory system.

Categories and Causes
Hypoxemic Respiratory Failure
- Acute lung injury
- Acute respiratory distress syndrome
- Pneumothorax

Hypercapneic Respiratory Failure
- Oversedation
- Obesity
- Diaphragmatic fatigue

Nervous System Causes of Respiratory Failure
- Cervical spinal cord injury
- Guillain-Barré syndrome
- Myasthenia gravis

Signs and Symptoms of Acute Respiratory Failure

System	Signs/Symptoms
Respiratory	Dyspnea Tachypnea Shortness of breath (SOB) Use of accessory muscles for breathing Adventitious lung sounds (crackles, rhonchi, wheezes) Decreased breath sounds Inspiratory/expiratory stridor Cough Increased secretions Orthopnea
Neurological	Agitation Confusion Disorientation Difficult to arouse, sleepiness (hypercarbic respiratory failure) Muscle twitching
Cardiac	Tachycardia Dysrhythmias (ventricular ectopy) Diaphoresis Hypertension or hypotension
Radiologic	Pulmonary infiltrates Atelectasis Pneumothorax Normal

Diagnostics Tests for Hypoxemia and Hypercapneic Respiratory Failure

Test	Expected Abnormalities and Rationale	
ABGs Normal	Hypoxemic: failure of oxygenation	Hypercapneic: failure of ventilation
pH 7.35–7.45	7.35–7.45	< 7.30

(*continued*)

Diagnostics Tests for Hypoxemia and Hypercapneic Respiratory Failure (*continued*)

Test	Expected Abnormalities and Rationale	
PaO$_2$ 80– 100 mmHg	<60 mmHg	80–100 mmHg
PaCO$_2$ 35–45 mmHg	35–45 mmHg	>50–55 mmHg
HCO$_3$ 22–27 mmHg	22–27 mmHg	Can be < 22 mmHg
SaO$_2$ 95–99	<90 %	>90 %

Patient Care Management

- Correct and treat the hypoxemia
- Determine and treat the cause
- Supplemental oxygen devices to reverse the hypoxemia (nasal cannula, simple face mask, venture mask, nonrebreather mask)
- Noninvasive positive pressure ventilation (NPPV)
- Intubation and mechanical ventilation

Critical Alert
To treat life-threatening hypoxemia that does not respond to supplemental oxygen, successful intubation is an important procedure that demands that the nurse know how to assist the health care provider, administer medications, demonstrate skill with suctioning and use of the air-mask-bag unit (AMBU).

(See Procedures and Therapies: Endotracheal Intubation.)

Nursing Management

Critical Alert
The nurse should assess the patient carefully when: PaO$_2$ < 60 mmHg from ABGs SpO$_2$ < 90%. Notify health care provider and increase oxygen delivery.

Alteration in oxygenation, impaired gas exchange

- Provide oxygenation to maximize effective gas exchange
  - Oxygenation per order
  - Encourage deep breathing and coughing
  - Incentive spirometry
  - Intubation with mechanical ventilation, if needed
  - Suctioning as needed
  - Noninvasive positive pressure ventilation (NPPV) (See Procedures and Therapies: Mechanical Ventilation; Noninvasive Positive Pressure Ventilation (NPPV); and Suctioning Procedure.)
- Monitor oxygen saturation and ABGs
- Assess breath sounds and work of breathing
- Promote activities of daily living with rest periods

Risk of Infection
- Frequent turning and positioning, monitoring oximetry
- Lung sound assessment

Knowledge Deficit
- Explain procedures, oxygen equipment, and medications
- Manage anxiety by encouraging patient/family to verbalize
- Instruct when to call the health care provider

Pulmonary Edema

Pulmonary edema is an abnormal accumulation of fluid in the lungs caused by dysfunction of the lungs and/or the heart. The fluid accumulation prevents adequate gas exchange across the alveolar-capillary membrane. Acute pulmonary edema refers to the time frame during which the fluid accumulation develops. In acute pulmonary edema, this occurs quickly over minutes to hours. Pulmonary edema is divided into cardiogenic and noncardiogenic based on the cause.

Cardiogenic Pulmonary Edema (CPE)

Pulmonary edema caused by changes in hydrostatic pressure. Results from heart failure, muscle dysfunction, valvular problems, and may be precipitated by tachydysrhythmias. Fluid overload and chronic hypoxemia contribute to this type of pulmonary edema. Pulmonary hypertension is a compensatory mechanism that develops as a result of hypoxemia and can lead to remodeling of the pulmonary vasculature.

Causes

- Myocardial infarction
- Myocardial ischemia
- Hypertension
- Cardiomyopathies
- Viral myocarditis
- Acute dysrhythmias
- Valvular dysfunction
- Atrial myxomas
- Papillary muscle rupture
- Pericarditis
- Cardiac tamponade

Noncardiogenic Pulmonary Edema (NCPE)

Related to direct injury to the A-C membrane from sepsis, inflammation, inhaled toxins, and drugs. In NCPE usually there is no primary cardiac dysfunction. (See Acute Respiratory Distress Syndrome [ARDS] and Acute Lung Injury [ALI] for more information on NCPE.)

Signs and Symptoms

- Agitation
- Confusion
- Rapidly worsening dyspnea, shortness of breath, tachypnea
- Central cyanosis and circumoral pallor (bluish tinge to the lips and mucous membranes)

- Cough and production of pink frothy sputum
- Adventitious lung sounds—Crackles in the bases of the lungs bilaterally, wheezes and rhonchi
- Hypotension, tachycardia, and possibly S_3 or S_4 heart sounds, murmur
- Jugular venous distention
- Hypotension and cool diaphoretic skin (CPE)
- Respiratory distress progressing to respiratory failure

Diagnostics
- Chest x-ray—Increased pulmonary infiltrates, cardiac enlargement
- ABGs—Hypoxemia/hypercarbia with a respiratory acidosis
- Oximetry
- ABGs could reflect a respiratory acidosis with increased carbon dioxide levels
- Echocardiogram
- Serum testing for B-type natriuretic peptide to evaluate heart failure

Patient Care Management
- Optimize oxygenation
  - Airway management
  - Oxygen therapy
  - Intubation with mechanical ventilation if needed
  - Noninvasive positive pressure ventilation (NPPV)
- Medications for aggressive preload and afterload reduction

  (See Appendix #22, Summary of Medications to Treat Heart Failure.)

Nursing Management
Alteration in oxygenation, impaired gas exchange

- Provide oxygenation to maximize effective gas exchange

- Intubation with mechanical ventilation, if needed
- Noninvasive positive pressure ventilation (NPPV)
- Monitor oxygen saturation and ABGs
- Assess breath sounds and work of breathing
- Administer medications to decrease preload and afterload
- Monitor weight
- Monitor intake and output
- Promote activities of daily living with rest periods
- Monitor for deterioration
  - Labored respirations with retractions of the chest wall and use of accessory muscles
  - Diminished breath sounds, crackles, wheezing
  - Changes in heart sounds
  - Distended neck veins

Knowledge Deficit

- Teach management of oxygen equipment and medications
- Manage anxiety by encouraging patient to verbalize
- Instruct when to call the health care provider

Neurogenic Pulmonary Edema (NPE)

Associated with direct insult to the CNS. Seizures, cerebral hemorrhage, and head injury are common precipitating factors to the development of pulmonary edema.

Negative Pressure Pulmonary Edema (NPPE)

Caused by attempting to ventilate with an apparent airway obstruction. Develops because of the extreme pressures that are used to attempt to ventilate during the obstruction. Treatment consists of positive pressure ventilation with positive end-expiratory pressure (PEEP).

High-Altitude Pulmonary Edema (HAPE)

Listed as a cause of pulmonary edema in a specific population: skiers and climbers. This type of pulmonary edema develops in persons who rapidly ascend to heights greater than 2,500 to 3,000 meters (8,202 to 9,842 feet). Treatment is removal from high altitudes steroids and oxygen therapy.

Heroin-Related Pulmonary Edema (HRPE)

Develops within 24 hours of the administration of heroin and has been reported in users of cocaine and methadone. Treatment is mechanical ventilation.

Excessive Intravenous Fluid Administration

Any patient who has a continuous intravenous infusion and receives a large amount of fluid over a short period of time can develop pulmonary edema. If the patient has any comorbidities such as cardiac, pulmonary, or renal disease the risk of developing pulmonary edema increases.

Transfusion-Related Acute Lung Injury (TRALI)

Transfusions that can cause this syndrome include packed red blood cells, platelets, granulocytes, and fresh frozen plasma. The classic symptoms of dyspnea, hypoxemia, and bilateral pulmonary edema occur within 4 to 6 hours of administration of blood products. Treatment: intubation or noninvasive ventilation. An impressive feature of this type of NCPE is the speed of development and onset of pulmonary edema.

Hyperbaric oxygen therapy and SCUBA diving can predispose this special population to pulmonary edema related to the increased pressure of oxygen. Treatment is removal from the increased pressure setting.

Toxic Chemical or Bioterrorism Agents

Inhalation of bacteria, viruses, or biotoxins, such as anthrax, plague, smallpox, botulism, viral hemorrhagic fever, tularemia.

CORONARY ARTERY DISEASE (CAD)

CAD is defined as a progressive atherosclerotic disorder of the coronary arteries that results in narrowing or complete occlusion of the vessel lumen. CAD is not an acute process, but one that progresses over time and can begin as early in life as infancy. The rate of progression is related to risk factors such as genetic predisposition, gender, diet, sedentary lifestyle, and smoking. CAD presents as clinical conditions of stable angina pectoris, unstable angina pectoris, myocardial infarction, and sudden cardiac death. These conditions depict a continuum of progressively worsening imbalances between the amount of oxygen delivered to and required by myocardial tissues. The underlying pathophysiology is atherosclerosis caused by plaque buildup of cholesterol, lipids, and cellular debris infiltrating the intimal lining of the arterial wall, causing a reduced blood flow to the myocardium.

As vessel stenosis intensifies, signs and symptoms occur as a result of myocardial oxygen imbalance. Reductions in myocardial blood supply, especially in times of increased demand, are the cause of coronary syndromes, which include stable angina, unstable angina (UA), myocardial infarction (AMI), and sudden cardiac death (SCD). These conditions depict a continuum of progressively worsening imbalances between the amount of oxygenated blood delivered and that which is required by myocardial tissues.

Common Factors That Increase Oxygen Demand

- Exercise, eating, emotions, exposure to cold, hypertension, sexual activity

Common Factors That Decrease Oxygen Supply

- Coronary artery spasm, coronary artery disease, hypotension, dysrhythmias, anemia, smoking

Modifiable Risk Factors

- Hyperlipidemia
    - ↑ LDL-C—Goal < 100 mg/dL
    - ↓ HDL-C—Goal > 40 mg/dL
    - ↑ Triglycerides—Goal < 150 mg/dL
    - ↑ Total cholesterol—Goal < 200 mg/dL (Total cholesterol/HDL-C ratio > 4)
- Hypertension
- Tobacco smoke
- Diabetes
- Physical inactivity
- Overweight and obesity

Angina Pectoris

Angina is transient sudden onset of discomfort caused by an inadequate supply of oxygen and nutrients for the myocardium (ischemia). CAD is the most common cause of angina. Angina also can occur with normal coronary arteries, as a result of vasospasm, endothelial dysfunction, valvular heart disease, hypertrophic cardiomyopathy, uncontrolled hypertension, exacerbations of heart failure, and noncardiac conditions of the esophagus, chest wall, or lungs.

Stable Angina

Least serious type is triggered by a predictable degree of exertion or emotions, and there is a pattern in relation to what brings it on, its duration, its intensity of symptoms, and how to relieve it. Stable angina subsides by taking away the precipitating factors and using sublingual nitroglycerin. Stable angina is differentiated from unstable angina pathologically by the absence of plaque disruption and thrombus formation in the lumen of the artery. The majority of patients with stable angina achieve symptom control by medical management alone.

Unstable Angina

(See Acute Coronary Syndrome.)

Variant, Prinzmetal, or Vasospastic Angina

Most serious type of angina. It occurs when single or multiple sites in major coronary arteries and their large branches have vasospasm. Most often the right coronary artery is involved. Sites of vasospasm generally occur over eccentric lesions. Causes of vasospasm are unknown but may be related to an imbalance of vasoactive agents derived from damaged coronary endothelial tissue, vessel segment hypersensitivity to sympathetic stimulation, allergy, or hypomagnesemia. Symptoms are usually episodic, may last several minutes, are often associated with exercise, and can occur frequently at night.

Signs and Symptoms

The clinician is faced with comparing data abstracted from the patient to a set of characteristics associated with diseases that have common presenting signs and symptoms.

(See Appendix #24, Differential Diagnosis of Chest Pain.)

Typical Angina

- Central/substernal chest or left arm pain, discomfort, pressure, tightness, heaviness
- Provoked by exertion or emotional stress
- Relieved by nitroglycerin

Atypical Angina or Ischemic Equivalents, any two of the characteristics for typical angina, common symptoms of women

- Jaw, neck, ear, arm, back
- Weakness, dizziness, light-headedness, loss of consciousness, unexplained fatigue, diaphoresis
- New or worsening dyspnea on exertion
- Nausea/vomiting unexplained indigestion, belching, epigastric pain or discomfort
- Burning, aching, cramping

Nocturnal Angina

- Occurs at night usually during sleep; may be relieved by sitting upright; commonly associated with left ventricular dysfunction

Decubitus Angina, Preinfarction, Postinfarction Angina

- Recurring/stuttering angina; angina while lying down
- Prior to or after infarction. Preinfarction angina may precondition the heart for episodes of subsequent infarction, resulting in a reduction in infarct size. Postinfarction angina denotes increased risk for death or recurrent myocardial infarction (MI).
- Angina that comes and goes; denotes instability, thrombus formation, and dissolution

> **Critical Alert**
> Women, patients with diabetes, and elderly patients may not experience pain with myocardial ischemia. In addition, the characterization of pain by women may be different from that of men, with women expressing pain in less severe terms, if at all, and often ascribing the pain to causes other than cardiac issues.

Diagnostics

(See Acute Coronary Syndrome.)

Patient Care Management

> **Critical Alert**
> Angina in the presence of heart disease is a warning sign and needs to be treated emergently in an attempt to prevent an acute cardiac event, such as myocardial infarction.

- Assessment of symptoms—new onset or change in angina symptoms (see Acute Coronary Syndrome)
- STAT ECG evaluation
- Cardiac monitoring
- Oxygen during periods of pain
- Physical examination

- Health history
  - Evaluation of risk factors
  - Risk stratification for USA

    (See Appendix #25, Risk Stratification for Unstable Angina.)
- Activity restriction, removal of precipitating factors
- Medication Therapy
  - Nitrates
  - Calcium channel blockers
  - Beta-adrenergic blocking agents
  - ASA in daily doses of 81 to 325 milligrams

    (See Appendix #27, Summary of Medications to Treat Coronary Artery Disease.)

Nursing Management

Critical Alert

The nurse must stay with the patient who is experiencing angina and continue an ongoing assessment until the pain is gone or it is determined that the interventions are not effective and the health care provider needs to be notified.

Pain, Acute

- Pain/symptoms assessment
  - New or recurrent
  - Change in intensity or frequency
  - Description of sensation, location, radiation, duration, precipitating factors
  - Associated symptoms
  - Use numeric scale (0–10) to quantify pain—Goal is 0 pain
  - Evaluate for differential chest pains

    (See Appendix #24.)
- Provide therapy to reach goal of 0 pain (MONA)
  - Limit activity, which may eliminate symptoms

- Oxygen
- Nitroglycerine sublingually
- Morphine
- Administer ASA as ordered

Alteration in Cardiac Output and Tissue Perfusion

- Assess
  - Vital signs
  - Dysrhythmias
  - Fluid status
  - Lung sounds
  - Anxiety
  - Diaphoresis, pallor
- ECG
  - Evaluate for ischemic, injury changes
  - Immediate health care provider notification of ST and T wave changes
  - Repeat ECG for recurrent symptoms

Knowledge Deficit

- Teaching plan includes
  - Symptoms of ischemia, disease process and avoidance of precipitating factors
  - Importance of notifying nurse for any symptoms during hospitalization
  - Notification of health care provider for changes in intensity, frequency, and character of symptoms
  - Review of medication regimens and side effects
  - Lifestyle changes to prevent a progression of the disease

Acute Coronary Syndrome (ACS)

Acute coronary syndrome results when the plaque buildup in the artery becomes significant enough to cause ischemia that results in clinical manifestations. ACS involves fibrous plaque disruption and thrombosis formation, and can result in either a partial or a total occlusion of the lumen of the coronary artery. This process will either markedly decrease or completely cut off blood flow to the myocardium.

Diagnosis of ACS just means there is a cardiac event going on, and after admission and further testing, a more definitive diagnosis is made. Included under the umbrella of acute coronary syndrome (ACS) are the diagnoses of unstable angina (UA), non-ST segment elevation myocardial infarction (MI) (NSTEMI), and ST segment elevation MI (STEMI).

Unstable Angina

A transitory syndrome falling between stable angina and acute myocardial infarction (AMI) wherein thrombus forms in an area of arterial stenosis but is subsequently fully or partially lysed by endogenous antithrombotic mechanisms. Symptoms worsen such that the patient presents with the development of new onset exertion angina, angina present at rest for longer than 20 minutes, or symptoms that have accelerated in frequency, duration, or intensity.

- Cardiac enzymes indicating myocardial damage are normal.

- ECG changes, if present, are transitory and will return to normal.

- Based on the assessment and physical findings, patients are categorized as low, intermediate, or high risk and triaged appropriately.

  (See Appendix #25.)

Non-ST Elevation Myocardial Infarction (NSTEMI)

The term *myocardial infarction* (MI) denotes myocardial cell death as a result of prolonged muscle ischemia. Cell death results in a permanent loss of myocardial muscle function. NSTEMI is a correlate syndrome to UA with a common pathogenesis and clinical presentation. Both usually occur as a result of transient subtotal occlusion of a coronary artery with reduced coronary blood flow resulting from plaque disruption and ensuing pathophysiological processes.

- Cardiac enzymes indicating myocardial damage are positive.
- ECG changes are persistent distinguishing a more severe myocardial injury.

ST Segment Elevation Myocardial Infarction (STEMI)

The presence of ST segment elevation means that myocardial tissue is undergoing severe anoxia and cellular damage. In most cases this is a result of complete coronary artery blockage from thrombotic occlusion over an underlying plaque lesion. Unlike NSTEMI, the blockage is sustained. If blood flow is not reestablished in 20 minutes, cell death occurs. Ischemic damage traverses the myocardium vertically outward, starting with the subendocardial layer through to the epicardium. If the occlusion is treated early, a patient presenting with STEMI may suffer only subendocardial cell damage without subsequent Q waves, which would represent full thickness damage.

- Cardiac enzymes indicating myocardial damage are positive.
- ECG changes—ST elevation

Both STEMI and NSTEMI are classified according to the coronary artery occluded and area supplied by that vessel that can be affected. Most MIs affect the left ventricle.

- Left Main Coronary (LMC)
  - Referred to as a massive MI (LMC supplies blood to over 70% of the left ventricle). Myocardial infarctions involving the LMC, often referred to as "widow makers," typically are associated with complications such as heart failure.
- Anterior Wall MI
  - Left anterior descending (LAD) artery (supplies anterior left ventricle, anterior septum, papillary muscle, apex, bundle of His, and bundle branches)

- Inferior Wall MI
  - Right coronary artery (RCA) (supplies inferior left ventricle, inferior septum, papillary muscle, and right ventricle; SA node 60% of population; AV node 90% of population)
- Lateral Wall MI
  - Circumflex artery (supplies lateral wall of the left ventricle; SA node 40% of population; AV node 10% of population)

Silent Ischemia

Nearly 70% to 90% of daily life ischemic episodes are asymptomatic, and 25% of patients who experience an AMI have either no or atypical symptoms. The presence of silent ischemia predicts greater risk of adverse outcomes in patients with stable and unstable angina, and in patients following an AMI or revascularization therapies. Silent ischemia is more prevalent in the elderly, women, patients with diabetes, and patients with three-vessel disease.

Sudden Cardiac Death (SCD)

Cardiac arrest most often associated with abrupt coronary artery occlusion from plaque disruption over severely stenotic lesions in the setting of poorly developed collateral circulation. The abrupt occlusion triggers pulseless ventricular tachycardia, ventricular fibrillation, or asystole, which if not treated immediately is almost always fatal.

Signs and Symptoms

Pain/symptoms same as angina pectoris only usually more intense and longer in duration

- Chest pain lasting longer than 20 minutes may indicate cardiac damage.
- Pain is not relieved by rest and requires treatment with medications or interventions to open the occluded coronary artery.
- Men report the mid- to lower-sternal chest pain more often than women.

- Women more typically report shortness of breath (57.9%), weakness (54.8%), and fatigue (40.9%). Prodromal symptoms experienced 1 month prior to AMI include unusual fatigue (70.7%), sleep disturbance (47.8%), and shortness of breath (40.1%).

- Nausea, vomiting, dyspnea, syncope, anxiety, and a feeling of impending doom

- Approximately one-third of patients experiencing an AMI do not experience chest pain and initially exhibit other symptoms of decreased cardiac output such as shortness of breath and changes in sensorium, or syncope.

Critical Alert

Some patients are able to sense when a major cardiac event is occurring; and therefore, it is essential that the nurse pay close attention to patients who report impending doom.

Physical Assessment

- Blood Pressure
    - ↑ due to catecholamine release, anxiety
    - ↓ due to cardiac output decrease
- Heart Rate
    - ↑ due to catecholamine release, anxiety
    - ↓ due to ischemia of the electrical system
- Heart Sounds
    - Presence/absence of S3, S4, murmur
- Lung Sounds
    - Clear or rales/crackles due to heart failure with ↓ oxygen saturation

ECG Changes

(See Appendix #26, ECG Changes During an MI, Correlated with Coronary Anatomy.)

Diagnostics

- ECG
    - For ST segment and T wave changes to be considered diagnostic, they must appear in two or

more leads that correspond to a given area of myocardium damage.

(See Appendix #26.)

- Cardiac monitoring
- Stress test (exercise or pharmacologic)
- Nuclear myocardial perfusion imaging
- Echocardiography (thoracic or transesophageal)
- Stress echocardiography
- Electron beam computed tomography/multislice CT
- MRI
- Cardiac catheterization / Intravascular ultrasound
- Chest x-ray
- Laboratory
  - Hs-C-reactive protein—marker for inflammation
  - Cardiac enzymes

    (See Appendix #28, Cardiac Laboratory Markers' Pattern Consistent with Acute Myocardial Infarction.)

  - Electrolytes (magnesium, potassium)

Patient Care Management

Management of ACS is aimed at increasing oxygen supply to ischemic myocardium using these strategies:

- Raise the amount of oxygenated blood delivered to the tissues with supplemental oxygen and blood transfusions
- Relieve coronary smooth muscle vasoconstriction or spasm with vasodilators
- Reprofuse ischemic tissue by dissolving thrombus with thrombolytic agents or percutaneous coronary intervention (PCI)
- Prevent thrombus formation with anticoagulant therapy

- Reestablish blood flow through invasive revascularization procedures such as coronary artery bypass graft surgery (CABG) and percutaneous coronary intervention (PCI). (See Procedures and Therapies: Percutaneous Coronary Interventions (PCI); and Coronary Artery Bypass Graft Surgery.)

During Acute Diagnostic Phase

- Assessment of symptoms—new onset or changing in angina symptoms
- Stat ECG evaluation
- Cardiac monitoring
- Oxygen
- Physical examination
- Health history
  - Evaluation of risk factors
  - Risk stratification for USA
    (See Appendix #25.)
- Activity restriction, removal of precipitating factors
- Drug Therapy
  - Nitroglycerine
  - Morphine
  - Antiplatelet agents
    - ASA—chewable
    - ADP receptor blockers
    - Glycoprotein IIb/IIIa blockers
  - Fibrinolytic (thrombolytic therapy)
  - Calcium channel blockers
  - Beta-adrenegic blockers
  - ACE inhibitors
  - ARBs
  - Lipid lowering therapy
  (See Appendix #27.)

After AMI Diagnosis and Treatment
Manage and minimize complications

- Reduce Autonomic Stress Responses
  - Manage abnormal electrolyte levels, hypoxemia, acidosis, hyper/hypotension, tachy/bradycardia, fever, anemia, volume depletion, immobility, discomfort, pain, or psychoemotional stress
- Infarct Expansion, Ventricular Remodeling
  - Recurrent chest pain from ischemia
  - Serial enzymes, ECGs
  - Medication therapy
- Pericarditis—Dressler's syndrome
- Heart failure
- Dysrhythmias
- Left ventricular aneurysm and thrombus formation
- Mitral valve disruption
- Ventricular free wall rupture
- Ventricular septal defect (VSD)
- Cardiogenic shock

Patients with suspected cardiac ischemia, but without AMI confirmation:

- Cardiac workup is indicated.
- Serial ECGs, cardiac blood marker determinations, and possibly stress testing, echocardiography, perfusion tests, or cardiac catheterization

Nursing Management
Alteration in Cardiac Output and Tissue Perfusion

- Assess and observe for indications
  - Vital signs
  - Dysrhythmias
  - Fluid status
  - Lung sounds
  - Anxiety
  - Skin color, temp

> **Critical Alert**
> Dysrhythmias that accompany an MI are common and varied; it is essential that the nurse understand the impact of each type on the cardiac output and the necessary interventions to terminate the abnormal rhythm.

- Stat ECG
    - Evaluate for ischemic, injury changes
    - Immediate health care provider notification of ST and T waves changes
    - Repeat ECG for recurrent symptoms

Pain, Acute

- Pain/symptoms assessment
    - New or recurrent
    - Change in intensity or frequency
    - Description of sensation, location, radiation, duration, precipitating factors
    - Associated symptoms
    - Use numeric scale (0–10) to quantify pain—Goal is 0 pain
    - Evaluate for differential chest pains
    (See Appendix #24.)

> **Critical Alert**
> The nurse must stay with the patient who is experiencing angina and continue an ongoing assessment until the pain is gone or it is determined that the interventions are not effective and the health care provider needs to be notified.

- Provide therapy to reach goal of 0 pain (MONA)
    - Limit activity, which may eliminate symptoms
    - Oxygen
    - Nitroglycerine sublingually
    - Morphine
    - Administer ASA as ordered

- Imbalance of oxygen supply and myocardial demand
  - Provide oxygenation
    - Evaluate O_2 saturation
  - Reduce myocardial oxygen demand
    - Provide adequate rest
  - Avoidance of caffeinated and extreme hot or cold beverages
  - Limit pain from procedures such as chest tube insertion or sheath pulling from angiography that can cause local excitation of the vagus nerve and bradycardia
  - Monitor serum cardiac enzymes

Potential for Recurrent Pain/Ischemia or Complication

- Pain/symptoms assessment
  - Report recurrent pain/symptoms
  - Use numeric scale (0–10) to quantify pain—Goal is 0 pain
  - Evaluate for differential chest pains

  (See Appendix #24.)

Knowledge Deficit

- Teaching plan includes
  - Symptoms of ischemia, disease process, and avoidance of precipitating factors
  - Importance of notifying health care providers for recurrent symptoms
  - Review of medication regimens and side effects
  - Lifestyle changes to prevent a progression of the disease
  - Importance of cardiac rehabilitation that combines exercise training, lifestyle modification, and nutrition

  (See Appendix #29, Patient Care Plan for Acute Coronary Syndrome.)

Critical Alert

Silent heart attacks are not uncommon in the elderly. Physiological changes of aging include stiffer ventricles due to the lack of the ability for the muscle to relax completely, decreased pumping function, decreased response to adrenaline, and decreased elasticity of the arteries. In an older individual, AMI may result in more complications and a longer hospital stay. Should these patients choose a more invasive treatment strategy, they may have a more complicated recovery from procedures or surgery due to renal impairment, mobility limitations, mental status changes, and poor nutrition.

Diabetes Mellitus

Diabetes Mellitus (DM) is a disorder of carbohydrate, protein, and fat metabolism resulting from an imbalance between insulin availability and insulin need. It is not a single disease but a group of metabolic disorders characterized by hyperglycemia (high blood glucose) resulting from defects in insulin secretion, insulin action, or both.

Classifications

Pre-Diabetes

- A term used to identify people who are at increased risk for developing diabetes.

- Patients may have fasting plasma glucose levels above normal or they may have abnormal results on an oral glucose tolerance test.

- Individuals are at increased risk for developing type 2 diabetes.

Type 1 Diabetes Mellitus

- Catabolic, autoimmune disorder in which pancreatic cells are destroyed resulting in circulating insulin being very low or absent and plasma glucagon is elevated

- Individuals with type 1 diabetes produce no insulin; they require pharmacologic insulin therapy for survival.

- Type 1 diabetes can occur at any age, but is frequently diagnosed before 30 years of age.

Type 2 Diabetes Mellitus

- A condition of hyperglycemia that occurs despite the availability of insulin (referred to as relative insulin deficiency). Individuals with type 2 diabetes are not dependent on exogenous insulin to sustain life; however, insulin therapy and/or oral medications may be needed to control hyperglycemia.

- Typically it is diagnosed after the age of 30 years, but is beginning to occur more frequently at younger ages.

- These individuals are often obese and have a strong family history of type 2 diabetes.

Gestational Diabetes Mellitus (GDM)

- A condition in which the onset of diabetes is first diagnosed during pregnancy. Those diagnosed with GDM require dietary treatment and possibly insulin therapy to control hyperglycemia. Gestational diabetes mellitus poses an increased risk for the development of type 2 diabetes later in life.

Metabolic Syndrome

- A group of metabolic abnormalities that predisposes individuals to CVD and type 2 diabetes.

- Three or more of the following abnormalities must be present:
  - High blood pressure ≥ 130/85 mmHg
  - Hypertriglyceridemia ≥ 150 mg/dL
  - Low high density lipoprotein cholesterol: ≤40 mg/dL in men; ≤50 mg/dL in women
  - Abdominal obesity: waist circumference ≥ 102 cm in men; ≥88 cm in women
  - Elevated fasting glucose ≥ 100 mg/dL
  - Weight loss, exercise, and healthy eating can help prevent or delay the onset of type 2 diabetes.

Complications

- Cardiovascular

  - Heart disease death rates in adults with diabetes are 2–4 times higher than those without the disease.

  - CHD, PVD, and cerebrovascular disease are more common, occur earlier, and are more severe in people with diabetes.

  - CHD is the leading cause of diabetes-related deaths. In the United States, more than 60% of nontraumatic amputations are in patients with diabetes and usually result from the combination of PVD and neuropathy.

- Kidney Disease

  - Diabetes is the leading cause of chronic kidney disease (CKD).

- Blindness and Other Visual Disorders

  - Diabetes remains the leading cause of new cases of blindness among adults 20 to 74 years old.

  - The primary causes of visual impairment and blindness among patients with diabetes include diabetic retinopathy, cataracts, macular degeneration, and glaucoma.

- Neuropathy

  - About 60% to 70% of people with diabetes have mild to severe forms of nervous system damage.

  - The results of such damage include, but are not limited to, peripheral neuropathy (e.g., impaired sensation or pain in the hands, legs, and feet) and autonomic neuropathy (e.g., delayed gastric emptying, bladder dysfunction, impotence, orthostatic hypotension, and cardiac abnormalities).

- Complications of Pregnancy

  - Elevated glucose levels prior to conception and during the first trimester of pregnancy can cause major birth defects in 5% to 10% of pregnancies and spontaneous abortions in 15% to 20% of pregnancies.

- Chronic hyperglycemia diabetes during the second and third trimesters of pregnancy can result in macrosomia (excessively large babies), resulting in neonatal and obstetrical risks.

Diabetic Ketoacidosis (DKA)

- One of the most serious complications of diabetes and is most commonly associated with type 1 diabetes
- DKA is a state of absolute or relative insulin deficiency aggravated by ensuing hyperglycemia, dehydration, and acidosis-producing derangements (e.g., infection, surgery, trauma)
- The most common causes are underlying infection, disruption of insulin treatment, and new onset of diabetes
- Characterized by: hyperglycemia greater than 300 mg/dL, low bicarbonate level (<15 mEq/L), and acidosis (pH <7.30) with ketonemia and ketonuria

Hyperosmolar Hyperglycemic Syndrome (HHS)

- Decrease circulating insulin with severe hyperglycemia and dehydration
- Protein is not used for energy resulting in normal ketones and absence of acidosis.
- Characteristically found in the elderly infirm who are unable to meet their fluid needs
- Symptoms mimic those of a stroke.

Hypoglycemia (low blood glucose)

- Results from pharmacologic treatment with insulin or oral hypoglycemic medications

Signs and Symptoms

Signs and symptoms of type 1 diabetes originate from hyperglycemia and ketosis whereas the signs and symptoms of type 2 diabetes originate from hyper-glycemia only.

- Glucosuria (glucose in the urine resulting in osmotic diuresis)
- Polyuria (increased urination)
- Nocturia (frequent urination at night)
- Osmotic diuresis (results in dehydration)
- Hypotension
- Tachycardia
- Polydipsia (increased thirst)
- Polyphagia (increased appetite)
- Fatigue

Diagnostics

Diabetes Diagnosis

Any one of the following three criteria may be used to establish a diagnosis of diabetes:

- A random blood glucose of > 200 mg/dL with symptoms of hyperglycemia (e.g., polydipsia and polyuria)
- A fasting blood glucose of > 126 mg/dL on more than one occasion with or without symptoms of hyperglycemia
- An elevated blood glucose (>200 mg/dL) at 2 hours following consumption of 75 grams of glucose during an oral glucose tolerance test (OGTT)

Pre-Diabetes Diagnosis

Pre-diabetes includes two categories: impaired fasting glucose (IFG) and impaired glucose tolerance (IGT). The criteria for each are as follows:

- Impaired fasting glucose: FPG ≥ 100 and < 126 mg/dL on two occasions
- Impaired glucose tolerance: a 2-hour plasma blood glucose level ≥ 140 and < 200 mg/dL following 75 grams of oral glucose

Patient Care Management

Management of hyperglycemia in both type 1 and type 2 diabetes is associated with reductions of the development of diabetes-related complications (e.g., neuropathy, nephropathy, and retinopathy). Current management strategies for the treatment of diabetes include a combination of exercise, nutrition, miscellaneous lifestyle changes (e.g., smoking cessation), and pharmacologic therapy directed toward normalization of blood glucose, blood pressure, and blood lipid levels.

- Medical
  - Insulin (See Appendix #31, Comparative Effects of Common Insulin Preparations.)
    - Subcutaneous injection (via syringes, pens, or cartridges)
    - Continuous subcutaneous infusion pumps
    - Continuous intravenous infusions
  - Incretin mimetics (Exenatide)
    - Injectable medication used as adjunctive mealtime therapy for patients with type 2 diabetes mellitus who are taking oral agents
  - Oral hyperglycemic agents (See Appendix #32, Summary of Medications to Treat Type 2 Diabetes.)
  - Intravenous hydration (for DKA)
  - Hyperglycemia control monitoring
    - Blood glucose (random, preprandial, postprandial)
    - Glycosylated hemoglobin (HgA_1C)
  - Dietary and lifestyle modifications
    - Clinical nutritionist
    - Physical and occupational therapy (promote mobility and self-care)
  - Psychosocial support for issues related to coping with chronic illness
    - Social worker

- Psychologist
- Psychiatrist
- Clergy

Nursing Management

- Unstable Blood Glucose, Risk for
  - Hyperglycemia:
    - Administer insulin, incretin, mimetics, or oral diabetic medications administer medications to reduce blood glucose as ordered
  - Hypoglycemia:
    - If unconscious: administer dextrose 50% intravenously or glucagon
    - If awake and able to safely swallow: provide 3–4 glucose tablets, 1/2 cup of fruit juice, 5–6 pieces of hard candy
  - Monitor for signs of hyperglycemia (polydipsia, polyphagia, polyuria, fatigue, blurred vision, confusion)
  - Monitor for signs of hypoglycemia ($\uparrow$ HR, tremors, diaphoresis, ataxia, seizures, coma)

Critical Alert

Because the onset of action of rapid-acting insulin is so quick, it should be injected as close to the meal or snack as possible to avoid hypoglycemia. A critical role of the nurse is to be alert for signs and symptoms of hypoglycemia and educate patients and family about how to prevent and treat hypoglycemic reactions.

  - Reevaluate blood glucose levels and patient signs and symptoms at regular intervals after interventions to assess response to therapy and determine need for further treatment
- Fluid Volume, Risk for Deficient
  - Monitor for signs of dehydration ($\uparrow$ HR, $\downarrow$ BP, $\uparrow$ RR, $\downarrow$ urine output, poor skin turgor, dry mucous membranes, and confusion)

- Encourage fluid intake (in awake and alert patients)
- Intravenous hydration (0.9% normal saline or 0.45% normal saline)
- Accurate I&O
- Acute Confusion, Risk for
    - Assess for signs of metabolic acidosis (e.g. ↑ HR, ↑ RR, Kussmaul's respirations, fruity odor to breath, mental status changes)
    - Monitor laboratory tests the results closely: ABGs, anion gap, serum ketones, urinary ketones, and serum bicarbonate
    - Initiate safety precautions as appropriate
- Cardiac output, decreased
    - Monitor serum electrolytes (potassium, sodium, calcium, magnesium)
    - Intravenous electrolyte replacement as needed
    - Monitor signs of electrolyte imbalance (See Fluid and Electrolyte section.)
    - Monitor for ↑ HR, ↓ BP, cool, pale, and moist skin, ↓ UO, changes in mentation.

Critical Alert

Metformin is contraindicated in patients with acute or chronic metabolic acidosis, who have, heart failure requiring pharmacologic management, renal disease or dysfunction as evidenced by serum creatinine levels ≥ 1.5 mg/dL (males) and ≥ 1.4 mg/dL (females) or abnormal creatinine clearance, and age > 80 years with an abnormal creatinine clearance. It is important for the nurse to determine the patient's comorbidities and laboratory data in order to effectively collaborate with the health care provider in developing a plan of care.

- Knowledge Deficit
    - Instruct regarding disease and potential complications
    - Educate regarding medication names, dosages, timing, side effects, and refill information

- Demonstrate appropriate technique for preparation and administration of insulin injection (if required)
- Demonstrate appropriate technique for monitoring capillary blood glucose levels, including information related to necessary frequency
- Educate regarding importance of healthy eating concepts and timing of meals when taking insulin
- Educate regarding target blood glucose goals and when to call the health care provider
- Explain the signs, symptoms, and treatment for hypoglycemia and hyperglycemia
- Instruct regarding dietary modifications necessary to control blood glucose (e.g., 45–65% CHO, 15–20% protein, limit saturated fat and cholesterol)
- Explain the importance of regular exercise (30 minutes per day).

Critical Alert

In general, patients with diabetes using pharmacologic therapy are at greater risk for hypoglycemia during and following exercise. The hypoglycemic effect of exercise can persist for several hours; therefore, patient education about preventing and treating exercise-related hypoglycemia is essential.

- Educate regarding appropriate foot care (inspect daily with mirror, wash daily with mild soap and water, trim nails, wear correct fitting shoes, and routine inspection by health care provider)
- Instruct regarding appropriate eye care (routine eye examinations, if visual changes noted, contact health care provider)
- Instruct regarding managing diabetes during illness, stress, and trauma

FEMALE REPRODUCTIVE DISORDERS

Breast Disorders
Fibrocystic Breast Disease

Fibrocystic breast changes most often occur as a result of hormone shifts associated with menses but can be exacerbated by stress or anxiety, nutritional factors, and physical or environmental stimuli. Changes are characterized by an increase in glandular and fibrous tissues in the breast.

Signs and Symptoms
- Smooth, mobile, well-defined, tender lump located in the upper outer quadrant of the breast
- Breast pain prior to menstruation beginning
- Coffee, tea, cola soft drinks, and chocolate aggravate the masses and cause increased tenderness

Diagnostics
- Health history and physical examination
  - Increase in fibrous tissue is palpable on examination
- Imaging
  - Mammogram

Patient Care Management

Fibrocystic changes are not precancerous and do not increase the woman's risk of developing breast cancer, but they can cause pain and anxiety.

- Medical
  - Decreasing the estrogen level using Danazol for pain control

Nursing Management

Nursing care should include obtaining a focused history of the patient with a breast mass to determine the risk of breast cancer. Relevant history includes family history, age of menarche and menopause, history of breast-feeding, and number of pregnancies and live births. Documentation of oral or transcutaneous contraceptives or hormone replacement therapy is also pertinent.

Mastitis

Mastitis is an inflammation of the breast tissue, occurs most frequently in women who are breast-feeding. Microorganisms invade the tissue through a portal of entry such as a crack or a fissure in the nipple, or through a duct.

Signs and Symptoms

- Breast tenderness
- Redness inflammation
- Edema
- Fatigue, malaise, fever, or chills

Patient Care Management

- Medical
  - Rest and fluids
  - Antibiotics
  - Alternating warm and cold compresses (aids in pain relief and increases circulation to the area)
  - Continued breast-feeding

Nursing Management

Nursing care is aimed at prevention of breast tissue damage from engorgement by encouraging breast-feeding, relieving discomfort (use of a support bra), treating the infection causing the inflammation, and prevention of recurrence. Women who are nursing infants should use lanolin creams to the nipples regularly to avoid cracking of the nipples and thus preventing invasion of bacteria into the breast tissue.

Ectopic Pregnancy

An ectopic pregnancy is implantation of the products of conception outside the uterine endometrium. The most common location for an ectopic pregnancy is the fallopian tube. The other 5% may occur in such places as the cervix, ovary, or abdomen.

Causes
- Pelvic inflammatory disease (PID)
- Previous ectopic pregnancy
- Endometriosis
- Tubal surgery
- Intrauterine device (IUD) for birth control

Signs and Symptoms
- Acute lower abdominal pain
  - Intense, sharp, unilateral pain referred to the shoulder as a result of irritation of the diaphragm by blood in the abdominal cavity (with fallopian tube rupture)
- Internal bleeding and hypovolemic shock
- Elevated quantitative human chorionic gonadotropin (HCG)
- Amenorrhea, nausea, and light vaginal bleeding

Diagnostics
- Health history and physical examination
  - Prime time for ectopic pregnancy is at approximately 7 weeks after a missed period
- Laboratory
  - Urine pregnancy test
  - HCG
- Imaging
  - Transvaginal ultrasound (examines ovaries, uterus, and fallopian tubes)

Patient Care Management
- Medical
  - Methotrexate (destroys ectopic cells)
    - Given only if the ectopic is unruptured
- Surgery
  - Repair or removal of the tube

Nursing Management

Nursing responsibilities include an understanding of the care of the postoperative patient. (See Appendix #1, Nursing Process: Patient Care Plan for the Postoperative Patient Following General Surgery.)

Endometriosis

Endometriosis is a condition in which endometrial-like cells that are normally found only in the uterus are found outside of the uterus attached to ovaries, fallopian tubes, the bowels, or abdominal organs. During the menstrual cycle, these cells respond to hormone production and may swell and bleed. In response, the body will surround these lesions with scar tissue, which can form adhesions on the area of attachment. These adhesions respond to the hormones that stimulate the monthly period with the proliferation of blood and tissue. Tissue and blood that are shed into the body cause inflammation, scar tissue, and subsequently pain. As the misplaced tissue grows, it can cover and grow into the ovaries and block the fallopian tubes, causing problems of infertility.

Risk Factors
- Family history
- Menstrual flow of greater than 6 days
- Menstrual cycle of less than 28 days
- Menarche at an early age
- Very heavy menses and periods that last more than 7 days

Signs and Symptoms
- Pain (mild to severe)
  - Lower abdomen and pelvis radiating down the thighs and to the lower back
  - Feeling of rectal pressure and discomfort when defecating
  - Dysmenorrhea and pain with sexual intercourse (dyspareunia)
- Abnormal uterine bleeding
- Difficulty becoming pregnant
- Infertility

Diagnostics
- Health history and physical examination
- Imaging
  - Pelvic ultrasound
- Other
  - Laparoscopy

Patient Care Management
- Medical
  - Oral contraceptives
  - High dose progesterone (Danazol)
- Surgical
  - Laparoscopy
    - Examine reproductive organs
    - Obliterate or remove endometrial tissue
  - Hysterectomy

Nursing Management
- Potential for Tissue Perfusion
  - Monitor complete blood count (CBC) to determine changes in hemoglobin and hematocrit. Report a drop of 1 gram or more in the hemoglobin or a drop of 3% or more in the hematocrit.

- Fatigue
  - Encourage the patient to pace activities to avoid fatigue
- Chronic Pain and Acute Pain
  - Instruct patient in pain management techniques, including use of NSAIDs and heat, along with relaxation techniques and diversion
- Knowledge Deficit
  - Provide a nonjudgmental environment in which to discuss problems with dyspareunia and sexual dysfunction
  - Provide resources for further counseling
- Ineffective Sexuality Pattern, Anxiety and Grieving related to decreased fertility
  - Provide resources for infertility counseling as indicated

Female Reproductive System Disorders: Cystocele, Rectocele, Uterine Prolapse

Cystocele

A cystocele occurs when the wall between the bladder and the anterior vagina weakens and the bladder protrudes into the vaginal vault. This frequently occurs following multiple vaginal deliveries.

Signs and Symptoms

- Urine leakage with sneezing, coughing or laughing
- Incomplete emptying of the bladder
- Feeling of pelvic pressure
- UTIs

Rectocele

A rectocele occurs when the posterior vaginal wall is weakened and the rectum bulges into the vagina. This can occur in women who have had conditions that involve repetitive bearing down, such as chronic constipation, chronic coughing, or repetitive heavy lifting.

Signs and Symptoms

- Difficulty initiating a bowel movement
- Constipation
- Rectal pressure

Uterine Prolapse

A uterine prolapse is another common structural disorder that occurs as a result of weakening of the pelvic floor musculature. The uterus is displaced downwardly into the vaginal canal and can be seen outside the vagina. The structures supporting the uterus are sometimes weakened during pregnancy and childbirth. There is an increased risk for uterine prolapse with obesity, chronic coughing, and straining during bowel movements. In addition, multiple pregnancies, congenital weakness, and loss of elasticity and muscle tone due to the aging process can contribute to the problem.

Signs and Symptoms

- Incontinence or retention
  - Aggravated by coughing or lifting heavy objects

Patient Care Management

- Surgery
  - Insertion of Pessary
    - Device to help support the vaginal walls reducing the bulging into the vagina
    - Used before and after pelvic hysterectomy to support the pelvic floor muscles
    - Complications
      - Vaginal irritation, infection, discharge, pressure sores, or allergy to the components of the pessary
  - Colporrhaphy (anterior/posterior (A&P) repair)
    - Anterior wall repair (done for a cystocele shortening of pelvic muscles providing greater support for the bladder or suspending the urinary bladder in the proper position)

- Posterior repair (done for rectocele and tightens the pelvic floor muscles to provide greater support for the rectum)
- Risks are minimal but can include bleeding and infection.

Nursing Management

- Deficient Fluid Volume
  - Monitor vital signs for dehydration ($\uparrow$ HR, $\downarrow$ BP)
  - Accurate intake and output
  - Assess for vaginal bleeding
  - Encourage fluids as tolerated
  - Indwelling urinary catheter
- Risk for Infection
  - Monitor for signs of infection ($\uparrow$ HR, $\uparrow$ T, foul-smelling vaginal drainage)
  - Antibiotics as prescribed
  - Monitor WBC
- Pain, Acute
  - Assess pain using numeric scale 0–10 and self-report descriptors
  - Administer analgesics and reassess accordingly
- Knowledge Deficit
  - Encourage use of stool softeners
  - Instruct regarding the importance of a well-balanced, high-fiber diet
  - Encourage patient to avoid activities that might stress the incision, including intercourse or placing anything in the vagina
  - Encourage patient to avoid long periods of standing, coughing, and sneezing, which also decrease strain on the surgical site
  - Instruct patient the pessary does not provide any method of birth control or protection against sexually transmitted infections

- Instruct regarding the effective placement and removal of the pessary and how to care for and clean it

Toxic Shock Syndrome

Toxic shock syndrome (TSS) is caused by the *Staphylococcus aureus* (*S. aureus*) bacterium, which is thought to be found in tampons and intravaginal contraceptive devices. Although *S. aureus* is colonized commonly on skin surfaces, it can cause multisystem problems when it invades the body through a break in the skin.

Signs and Symptoms
- Sudden onset of high fever and chills
- Vomiting and diarrhea
- Intense muscle pain
- Diffuse red rash
  - Similar to a sunburn
  - Located on the palms of hands and soles of feet
  - Some peeling may be seen
- Low blood pressure
- Confusion/delirium
- Redness of eyes, mouth, and throat
- Seizures
- Headache

Diagnostics
- Health history and physical examination
  - Based on $\uparrow$ T, $\downarrow$ BP, peeling rash, and 3 organs with signs of dysfunction
- Laboratory
  - Blood cultures
  - Electrolytes, liver function tests, coagulation studies (to determine organ dysfunction)

Patient Care Management

- Medical
  - Intravenous fluids
  - Vasopressors
  - Antibiotics
  - Dialysis (for acute renal failure)

Nursing Management

- Ineffective Tissue Perfusion
  - Cerebral perfusion
    - Monitor changes in mentation
  - Cardiopulmonary perfusion
    - Monitor for $\uparrow$ HR, $\downarrow$ BP,
    - Monitor for $\uparrow$ RR, $\downarrow$ O_2 sats, increased respiratory effort
    - Assess skin for warmth, color, and moisture
    - Monitor ECG
  - Renal perfusion
    - Accurate I&O
  - GI perfusion
    - Assess bowel sounds and presence of jaundice
- Infection
  - Monitor WBC
  - Monitor temperature
  - Administer antibiotics
- Fluid Volume Deficit
  - Maintain two intravenous lines
  - Provide intravenous hydration
  - Note signs of dehydration ($\downarrow$ urine output, poor skin turgor, $\downarrow$ BP, $\uparrow$ HR)
- Knowledge Deficit
  - Instruct patient regarding signs and symptoms to report to health care provider
  - Instruct patient to avoid use of tampons

- Encourage patient to avoid using diaphragm or contraceptive sponge (can cause TSS)

Uterine Fibroid Tumors

Fibroid tumors of the uterus, also known as leiomyomas and myomas, occur in more than 30% of women 40 to 60 years of age but are almost always benign. They develop slowly in women ages 25 through 40, and tend to enlarge during pregnancy and after menopause; fibroids often decrease on their own, due to decreased estrogen production.

Risk Factors
- Female age 40 or older
- Nulliparity (female who has never given birth)
- Obesity
- Family history
- Race (African American)
- Hypertension

Signs and Symptoms

Fibroids often cause no symptoms, so many are undiscovered unless the patient has dysfunctional uterine bleeding, pelvic pain, and infertility or pregnancy loss. Uterine tumors can add pressure to surrounding organs, causing pain, constipation, urinary problems, menorrhagia (heavy bleeding), and metrorrhagia (irregular bleeding).

Diagnostics
- Imaging
  - Transvaginal ultrasonography
  - Hysteroscopy

Patient Care Management
- Medical
  - Observational management (for women with asymptomatic tumors)

- Pain control (nonsteroidal anti-inflammatory drugs [NSAIDs])
- Decrease the size of the fibroids and the associated discomfort (birth control pill and hormone therapy)

- Surgical/Procedural
  - Uterine fibroid embolization
    - Nonsurgical treatment done under intravenous sedation that shrinks the fibroid
  - Myomectomy
    - Laser surgery for large tumors or severe symptoms
    - Preserves fertility
  - Hysterectomy
    - Indicated for situations where the tumors potentially could mask other pathology and increase operative complication rates

FLUID AND ELECTROLYTES

Calcium Abnormalities: Calcium is found primarily in the bones and teeth, where only 2% is found in the blood. Regulation of calcium serum levels is controlled by vitamin D, calcitonin from the thyroid gland, and parathyroid hormone (PTH) from the parathyroid glands. Calcium is important for neuromuscular transmission, contraction of muscles, blood clotting, bone and tooth construction, cellular membrane function, and energy conversion.

Hypercalcemia

(serum calcium $>$ 10.5 mg/dL or ionized calcium $>$ 5.5 mg/dL)

Causes

- Primary hyperparathyroidism (dysfunction of the parathyroid gland)
- Bone malignancy
- Drug toxicity (e.g., thiazide diuretics, lithium carbonate, and vitamins A and D)
- Prolonged bed rest (causes mobilization of bone calcium)
- Adrenal insufficiency
- Hyperthyroidism
- Rhabdomyolysis (massive muscle destruction resulting in release of myoglobin into the blood with subsequent obstruction of the renal glomeruli)

Signs and Symptoms

- Central nervous system: Fatigue, weakness, decreased deep tendon reflexes, headache, impaired concentration, memory defects, personality changes, confusion, lethargy, and depression

- Renal system: polyuria, kidney stones, acute or chronic renal failure with decreasing urine concentrating ability
- Gastrointestinal system: anorexia, nausea, vomiting, pain, constipation; in severe cases, pancreatitis
- Cardiovascular system: cardiac dysrhythmias with shortening of the ST segment and QT interval and a prolonged PR interval that can lead to heart block and possible cardiac arrest
- Musculoskeletal system: muscle weakness, acute arthritis, painful joints, itching, and bony cysts
- Eyes and skin: Conjunctival calcifications leading to conjunctivitis. Calciphylaxis occurs when excess calcium deposits in the skin, causing lesions primarily in the lower extremities as irregular violet plaques or nodules. These lesions are painful, pruritic, and may progress to necrosis and gangrene.

Patient Care Management

- Medical
  - Intravenous normal saline with Lasix
    - Rapidly infused to dilute the blood and result in increased calcium secretion
  - Chemotherapy for malignancy
  - Bisphosphonates (reduces decalcification of the bone in the presence of malignancy)
  - Gallium nitrate may be given to inhibit malignancy-related bone reabsorption.
  - Discontinuation of vitamins A, D, and calcium supplements
  - Cortisone (decrease calcium absorption)
  - Weight-bearing activity will reduce bone reabsorption.
  - Calcitonin (promotes calcium deposition in the bone and increase calcium excretion)

- Low-calcium diet
- Discontinuation of thiazide diuretics
- Surgical
  - Partial parathyroidectomy (due to excess PTH)

Nursing Management
- Cardiac Output, Decreased
  - Assess ECG for changes in QT interval and development of heart block
  - Assess heart sounds (for an S_3 heart sound)
  - Monitor serum digitalis levels (for toxicity)
  - Assess for fluid overload
    - Auscultate breath sounds for "crackles" and rhonchi
    - Monitor I&O (to prevent overload and ensure adequate kidney function)
    - Note RR, depth of respiration, and work of breathing
- Injury, Risk for
  - Turn carefully (prevents pathologic fractures)
  - Provide meticulous skin care
  - Monitor level of confusion and muscle strength

Hypocalcemia
(serum calcium level < 8.5 mg/dL and ionized levels < 4.0 mg/dL)

Causes
- ↓ Calcium intake or absorption (vitamin D deficiency or excessive phosphorous intake)
- ↓ PTH (during thyroid surgery, temporary in nature)
- ↑ Serum phosphorus, ↓ magnesium levels, hypoalbuminemia, and alkalosis
- Gastrointestinal surgery, chronic pancreatitis, and small-bowel disease

- Renal failure
- Loop diuretics
- Blood transfusions (with citrated blood)

Signs and Symptoms
- ECG
  - Bradycardia, prolonged QT intervals, dysrhythmias
- Hypotension, ↓ cardiac contractility
- Numbness and tingling of the fingers and circumoral area
- Hyperactive reflexes, muscle cramps
- Laryngeal spasm, bronchospasm
- Muscle tetany
- Confusion, hallucinations, tonic clonic seizures
- Pathologic fractures
- Trousseau's sign (carpopedal spasm)
  - Induced by inflating a blood pressure cuff on the upper arm 20 mm above the systolic blood pressure and maintaining the inflation for 3 minutes, resulting in wrist and fingers contracting inward
- Chvostek's sign
  - Twitching of the facial muscles obtained by tapping the facial nerve just below the temple on the zygomatic arch

Patient Care Management
- Medical
  - Intravenous or oral administration of calcium
  - Intravenous vitamin D
  - Magnesium (prevents hypomagnesemia-induced hypocalcemia)
  - Laboratory
    - Phosphorous levels (evaluate for hyperphosphatemia)

Nursing Management

- Ventilation, Impaired
  - Monitor RR, O_2 sat, work of breathing
  - Position for optimal ventilation
- Cardiac Output, Decreased
  - Assess changes in ECG for bradycardia, prolonged QT intervals, and dysrhythmias
  - Monitor for ↓ BP and presence of heart failure (e.g., edema, weight gain, dyspnea)
  - Accurate I&O
  - Administer calcium replacement and monitor serum calcium

Critical Alert

Sudden drop in blood pressure may occur because of vasodilation and decreased cardiac contractility with rapid administration of IV calcium. Infuse calcium at a rate less than 0.5 to 1 mL/min to avoid hypotension.

- Injury, Risk for
  - Assist with activity to conserve energy
  - Monitor for gait disturbances due to changes in sensation and cramping
  - Assess mentation, reoriented as needed
- Knowledge Deficit
  - Instruct patient and family regarding causes of hypocalcemia and strategies to prevent reoccurrence
  - Encourage patient to take oral calcium before meals or at bedtime for maximum absorption
  - Remind patient that phosphorous-binding antacids should be taken with meals

Magnesium Abnormalities: Magnesium is an intracellular cation primarily stored in muscle and bone. Two-thirds of serum magnesium exists in ionized form and one-third is bound to plasma proteins. It is involved in carbohydrate metabolism, protein synthesis, and muscular contraction.

Hypermagnesemia

(serum levels > 2.1 mg/dL)

Causes
- Renal failure
- Adrenal insufficiency
- Pregnancy

Signs and Symptoms
- Cardiovascular
  - ↓ BP and HR
  - Flushing and sense of warmth
  - Respiratory or cardiac arrest
- Gastrointestinal
  - Nausea and vomiting
- Neurological
  - Drowsiness
  - ↓ deep tendon reflex
  - Respiratory depression
  - Coma

Patient Care Management
- Medical
  - Cessation of magnesium-containing products
  - Intravenous administration of normal saline
  - Intravenous administration of 10 mL of 10% calcium gluconate
  - Dialysis

Nursing Management
- Cardiac Output, Decreased
  - Monitor ECG for bradycardia

> **Critical Alert**
> Complete heart block may occur at levels of more than 15 mEq/L. If this occurs stop magnesium-containing products and provide IV push administration of 10 mL of 10% calcium gluconate or dialysis.

- Monitor for ↓ BP
- Assess skin for temperature and color
- Accurate I&O
- Injury, Risk for
  - Assess deep tendon reflexes
  - Monitor respiratory status for ↓ O_2 sats, ↑ RR, ↑ work of breathing (indicates possible respiratory failure)

> **Critical Alert**
> In hypermagnesemia, the deep tendon reflex is lost at 8 mEq/L and respiratory failure is likely if the serum level exceeds 10 mEq/L.

- Assess IV site frequently when infusing calcium because infiltration can cause tissue sloughing
- Knowledge Deficit
  - Instruct patients in renal failure to avoid medications with magnesium (e.g., MOM)
  - Instruct patient and family regarding effects of hypermagnesemia and rationale of treatment

Hypomagnesemia

(serum magnesium of < 1.4 mg/dL)

Causes

- Malnutrition (inadequate intake of magnesium-containing foods)
- Increased urinary excretion
  - Alcoholism
  - Osmotic diuresis in diabetes
  - Loop diuretics

- GI loss
  - Vomiting and diarrhea
  - Malabsorption syndromes

Signs and Symptoms
- Cardiac
  - HTN
  - Cardiac dysrhythmias
    - Supraventricular tachycardia
  - Coronary artery spasms
  - Sudden cardiac death
  - Digitalis toxicity
- Neurologic
  - Confusion and lethargy
  - Seizures
  - ↑ deep tendon reflexes
  - Tetany
  - Hallucinations
- GI
  - Nausea and vomiting

Patient Care Management
- Medical
  - Intravenous administration of magnesium
  - Oral magnesium salts, magnesium-containing antacids, and foods high in magnesium

Nursing Management
- Cardiac Output, Decreased
  - Monitor ECG for tachycardia
  - Monitor for HTN and associated symptoms (headache, blurred vision)
  - Monitor for signs of digitalis toxicity (halo vision, nausea, vomiting)

- Assess skin for temperature and color
- Accurate I&O
- Injury, Risk for
  - Assess deep tendon reflexes
  - Seizure precautions
- Knowledge Deficit
  - Instruct patient and family regarding dietary sources of magnesium
  - Instruct patient and family regarding rationale for treatment

Potassium Abnormalities: Potassium is an intracellular cation that is found primarily within the cells, although small amounts are found in blood and bone. The function of potassium is to maintain intracellular osmolality and participate in the sodium-potassium exchange that causes cellular depolarization and repolarization. Potassium is essential for cellular integrity, transmission of neuromuscular impulses, acid–base balance, conversion of carbohydrates into energy, and the formation of amino acids into proteins. Serum potassium affects the strength and rate of cardiac contraction.

Hyperkalemia

(serum potassium > 5.0 mEq/L)

Causes

- ↑ potassium intake
- ↓ urinary excretion (due to renal failure)
- Cellular damage that releases a lot of potassium into the blood (e.g., surgery, fever, sepsis, or trauma)

Signs and Symptoms

- Muscular weakness and paresthesia
- Irritability
- Abdominal distention and cramping, diarrhea
- Metabolic acidosis per arterial blood gases (ABGs)

- Irregular pulse
- ECG: progressively widening PR and QRS intervals, peaked T waves

Patient Care Management
- Medical
  - Kayexalate enema
  - Kayexalate with sorbitol oral
  - Intravenous 10% calcium gluconate with glucose (dextrose 50%) and IV insulin
  - Beta-adrenergic agonists (albuterol)
  - Sodium bicarbonate (if the hyperkalemia is due to metabolic acidosis)
  - Dialysis

Nursing Management
- Cardiac output, decreased
  - Monitor ECG for widened QRS, peaked T waves
  - Monitor quality of pulses, skin color, and temperature
  - Monitor for changes in mentation and urine output
  - Assess serum potassium levels to determine trend
- Injury, Risk for

Critical Alert
If potassium > 6.0 mEq/L immediately stop all potassium supplements (intravenous and oral) and notify health care provider. This is a potentially life-threatening situation due to the effects of hyperkalemia on the cardiac muscle.

  - Assist with ambulation
  - Provide rest periods to conserve energy and prevent falls

- Knowledge Deficit
  - Instruct patient and family regarding importance of recognizing early signs of hyperkalemia and when to report signs to health care provider
  - Instruct patient regarding appropriate use of potassium supplements and medications

Hypokalemia
(serum potassium level < 3.5 mEq/L)

Causes
- Diuretics (Lasix, Bumex)
- Hypomagnesaemia
- ↓ potassium intake
- GI and renal disorders
- Cushing's disease
- ↑ serum insulin
- Diarrhea, vomiting, or nasogastric suction
- Draining wounds
- Corrected acidosis

Signs and Symptoms
- Muscle weakness, paresthesia, lethargy, confusion
- Abdominal cramps, nausea, and vomiting
- ↓ bowel sounds with possible ileus
- Weak, irregular pulse
- ECG: flattened T wave, ventricular ectopy

Patient Care Management
- Medical
  - Dietary supplements
  - Oral or intravenous supplements

Nursing Management
- Cardiac output, decreased
  - Monitor ECG for flattened T waves and ventricular ectopy

- Monitor quality of pulses, skin color and temperature
- Monitor for changes in mentation and urine output
- Assess serum potassium levels to determine trend
- Monitor serum digitalis levels ($\downarrow$ potassium can result in digitalis toxicity)

- Injury, Risk for

> **Critical Alert**
> Potassium is never administered IV push! Too rapid administration of potassium can result in life-threatening dysrhythmias.

- Assist with ambulation
- Provide rest periods to conserve energy and prevent falls
- Provide antiemetic for nausea
- Provide anti-diarrhea medication

- Knowledge Deficit
  - Instruct patient and family regarding importance of recognizing early signs of hypokalemia and when to report signs to health care provider
  - Instruct patient regarding appropriate use of potassium supplements and medications

Sodium Abnormalities: Sodium is the most numerous cation in the ECF. It maintains ECF volume through osmotic pressure, regulates acid–base balance by combining with chloride or bicarbonate ions, and conducts nerve impulses via the sodium channels of cells.

Hypernatremia

(serum sodium > 145 mEq/L)

Hypernatremia represents a deficit of water in relation to the body's sodium levels.

Causes

- Cushing's syndrome (aldosterone excess) due to excess sodium retention

- Diabetes insipidus (due to loss of ADH, head trauma)
- Excess sweating without adequate fluid replacement (e.g., heat stroke)

Signs and Symptoms
- Low-grade fever
- Thirst
- Peripheral and pulmonary edema
- Postural hypotension
- Altered mental status
- Neuromuscular irritability
- Coma or seizures
- ↑ serum osmolality
- ↑ urine specific gravity (due to the effect of ADH to conserve water)

Patient Care Management
- Medical
  - Drugs to decrease the activity of the adrenal glands (ketoconazole, metyrapone, aminoglutethimide, or mitotane)
  - Desmopressin acetate nasal spray (provides ADH in diabetes insipidus)
- Surgical
  - Removal of adrenal or pituitary gland tumors

Nursing Management
- Risk for Imbalanced Fluid Volume
  - Monitor fluids and electrolytes and acid–base balance
  - Monitor for ↑ BP, ↑ HR, and ↑ T
  - Assess postural vital signs while providing safety
- Administer IV fluids
  - Sodium needs to be slowly reduced at a rate of 0.5–1.0 mEq/L until it reaches 147 mEq/L.

- Assess level of consciousness every 4 hours
- Observe for ↑ cerebral edema (lethargy, headache, nausea, vomiting, increased blood pressure, or altered sensorium)
- Knowledge Deficit
  - Provide discharge instructions to patient and family member on causes and treatment of hypernatremia.
  - Provide reminders of adequate fluid intake and treatment adherence for Cushing's syndrome or diabetes insipidus.

Hyponatremia

(serum sodium < 135 mEq/L)

Hyponatremia develops with excessive retention of water, inadequate sodium intake, or loss of sodium-rich fluids that are replaced with water.

Causes

- Diuretics
- Congestive heart failure
- Lung cancer
- Vomiting and diarrhea
- GI suctioning
- Loss of wound fluids from very large wounds (e.g., burn wounds)
- Excessive use of dextrose 5% intravenous (IV) fluid
- Syndrome of inappropriate antidiuretic hormone (SIADH)

Signs and Symptoms
- Lethargy and muscle weakness
- Headache
- Confusion
- Personality changes and apprehension
- Seizures and coma
- Hypotension
- ↓ urine output

Patient Care Management
- Medical
  - Water restriction
  - Administration of electrolytes
  - Intravenous hypertonic saline

Nursing Management
- Risk for Fluid Imbalance
  - Monitor neurological status (orientation to person, place, time)
  - Accurate I&O
  - Monitor serum electrolytes and acid–base balance
  - Restrict fluids to < 1,000 mL/day to prevent further dilution of sodium
  - Assess for drop in blood pressure and associated dizziness
- Injury, Risk for
  - Assess for gait disturbances and assist as needed
  - Seizure precautions
  - Administer intravenous hypertonic saline (3% sodium) in the presence of severe symptoms

- Knowledge Deficit
    - Explain to patient and family that disorientation is temporary
    - Use clocks, calendars, and familiar personal items to reorient the patient and reduce confusion
    - Provide discharge instructions that identify cause, to teach adherence to treatment, and to prevent future occurrences of hyponatremia

Gastrointestinal Disorders

Appendicitis

Appendicitis is an inflammation of the appendix and accounts for the majority of emergency abdominal surgeries.

Simple Appendicitis

Appendix is inflamed but remains intact.

Gangrenous Appendicitis

Appendix is infected, necrotic, and microscopic areas of perforation.

Perforated Appendicitis

Appendix has large areas of perforation that allow contents to spill into the peritoneal cavity.

Signs and Symptoms

- Pain
  - Periumbilical radiating over lower abdomen
  - Right lower quadrant pain (RLQ)
  - Discomfort with pressure applied to RLQ
  - Pressure applied to left lower quadrant (LLQ) for 5 seconds is felt in the RLQ.
- Fever
- Peritonitis
  - Severe pain with knees pulled to chest
  - ↑ HR and T
  - Diaphoresis

Diagnostics

- Health history and physical examination
- Laboratory
  - Complete blood count (CBC) to determine presence of infection/inflammation by $\uparrow$ WBC
- Imaging
  - Abdominal x-rays
  - Abdominal ultrasound and CT scan

Patient Care Management

The main goals for a patient who is experiencing appendicitis are pain control and surgical intervention (appendectomy).

Nursing Management

- Pain, Acute
  - Assess pain using numeric scale 0–10
  - Using self-report assess for pain characteristics
  - Administer narcotic analgesics and reassess appropriately
- Infection, Risk for
  - Monitor for $\uparrow$ WBC, $\uparrow$ T, $\uparrow$ HR
  - Assess O_2 sat and lung sounds.
  - Encourage use of incentive spirometer, deep breathing, and coughing
  - Monitor for $\uparrow$ abdominal pain
  - Assess incision line for approximation, drainage, redness
- Knowledge Deficit
  - Instruct patient and family regarding postoperative routines

Cirrhosis

Cirrhosis is an irreversible, progressive deterioration of the liver that results from chronic liver disease. Long-term hepatocellular injury and inflammation result in damaged or dead liver cells that are replaced with fibrotic scarring. Liver cells continue to regenerate but in an abnormal pattern creating collateral vessels that connect the portal vein to the hepatic artery. This change in the vascular network causes an increased resistance to the flow of blood throughout the liver resulting in portal venous hypertension.

Causes
- Chronic hepatitis
- Alcoholism (most common within the United States)
- Prolonged and severe right-heart failure
- Long-term obstruction to biliary flow
- Sclerosing cholangitis
  - Inflammatory disorder of the biliary tract that leads to fibrosis and strictures in the biliary system
- Primary biliary cirrhosis
  - Autoimmune disease where there is inflammation and destruction of the intrahepatic biliary system that results in fibrosis

As cirrhosis progresses severe systemic complications occur, each having their own clinical manifestations and complications.

Hepatic Encephalopathy
Hepatic encephalopathy is the result of an increased level of circulating neurotoxins. The most abundant neurotoxin is ammonia, which forms as the end product of protein digestion.

- Asterixis (flapping tremor of the hands when the arms are outstretched)
- Agitation, restlessness, and changes in mentation

Hepatorenal Syndrome
Hepatorenal syndrome is characterized by the occurrence of azotemia in a patient with liver failure when other causes of renal failure have been excluded. The presence of oliguria, sodium and water retention, hypotension, and peripheral vasodilation indicates a poor prognosis.

Portal Hypertension

As structure of the liver changes as a result of scarring, venous blood flow through the portal venous system is impeded. This increases the portal venous blood pressure, from a normal of about 3 mmHg to at least 10 mmHg. Because the portal veins carry blood from the GI tract, spleen, and pancreas to the liver, the obstruction of this blood flow from cirrhosis causes increased pressure in the vessels in the aforementioned organs. The increased pressure causes increased blood flow in collateral vessels, which normally have lower pressure resulting in varices (distended, tortuous, collateral veins) to develop particularly in the esophagus and rectum.

- Esophageal varices
  - Thin-walled vein that is prone to rupture, causing massive, life-threatening hemorrhage
  - Bleeding can be slow and chronic leading to anemia and melena (black or maroon, sticky, foul-smelling feces resulting from the digestion of blood).
  - Rupture is seen with hemorrhage and vomiting of large volumes of dark-red blood.
- Splenomegaly (enlargement of the spleen)
  - Anemia
  - Impaired clot formation due to platelets being sequestered in the spleen
- Ascites (accumulation of protein-rich fluid in the abdominal cavity)
  - Due to hypoalbuminemia and extra aldosterone

Signs and Symptoms

Cirrhosis can be asymptomatic until liver function is severely affected and, even then, the onset of symptoms is gradual. The manifestations of cirrhosis can be nonspecific and are the result of the hepatocellular damage and portal hypertension. (See Appendix #6, Nursing Process: Patient Care Plan for the Patient with Cirrhosis for comprehensive list.)

- Fatigue and weakness
- Anorexia and weight loss

- Deficiency of vitamin K
  - Impaired blood clotting and fat malabsorption
- Hypoalbuminemia
- Edema
- Ascites
- Jaundice (skin and sclera)

Diagnostics
- Laboratory
  - ↑ Liver function tests (LFTs)
    - ALT, AST, alkaline phosphatase (ALP), and GGT
  - ↓ Serum albumin
  - ↓ Platelets
  - ↑ Prothrombin time (PT)
  - ↑ Partial thromboplastin time (PTT)
  - ↑ Clotting time
  - ↑ Bilirubin
  - ↑ Serum ammonia
- Other
  - Liver biopsy

Patient Care Management
- Medical
  - Spironalactone (Aldactone)
    - Potassium sparing diuretic used to treat edema and ascites
  - Furosemide (Lasix)
  - Intravenous albumin (for severe edema resulting in ↓ BP and ↑ respiratory effort)
  - Lactulose (to clear ammonia and improve mentation)
  - Oxazepam (Serax) (used cautiously to treat agitation)
  - Antibiotics

- Octreotide (decreases portal hypertension and improves varices)
- Vitamin K (improves clotting)
- Fluid sodium restrictions
- Protein restriction (during acute phase of hepatic encephalopathy)
- Surgical
  - Transplantation (considered for non-alcohol induced cirrhosis)
- Other
  - Paracentesis (See Procedures & Therapies, Paracentesis.)
  - Transjugular intrahepatic portosystemic shunt (TIPS)
    - Used to relieve refractory ascites
    - Stent is placed between the hepatic vein and the portal vein, which allows blood to bypass the liver and effectively reducing portal pressure.
  - Dialysis (for hepatorenal syndrome)
  - Endoscopy with sclerotherapy and banding (See Procedure & Therapies, Endoscopy.)
  - Balloon tamponade using Sengstaken-Blakemore or Minnesota tube

Nursing Management

Because alcoholism is a major cause of cirrhosis in the United States, efforts at alcohol abstinence are encouraged. This requires the involvement of the family as well as other forms of support. Comprehensive treatment of cirrhosis includes medications, surgical intervention, diet, and counseling. (See Appendix #7, Nursing Process: Patient Care Plan for Pancreatitis for detailed plan of care for patient with end stage liver disease.)

Diverticular Disease

Diverticular disease results from the occurrence of abnormal saclike outpouchings of the intestinal wall called diverticula. Diverticula can occur anywhere in the gastrointestinal tract except the rectum, but usually occur in the distal large intestine. Diverticula themselves cause few problems; however, if undigested food or bacteria becomes trapped in the diverticula, they form a hard mass called a fecalith and intraluminal pressure increases, resulting in compromise of the blood supply. This results in ischemia of the diverticula and may lead to perforation.

Diverticulitis

Inflammation of the diverticula with possible rupture into the colonic lumen

Diverticulosis

The presence of one or more diverticula

Risk Factors

- Dietary intake high in refined foods
- More common in those over 60 years of age
- Constipation

Complications of diverticular disease are relatively rare but can include hemorrhage, peritonitis, bowel obstruction, and fistula formation.

Signs and Symptoms

- Left lower quadrant pain
  - Intermittent in nature
  - May progress to steady and mild to severe in quality.
- ↑ Temperature (with chills), ↑ HR
- Nausea, vomiting, and either diarrhea or constipation
- Abdominal distention and flatulence

Diagnostics

- Health history and physical examination
- Laboratory
  - Complete blood count (CBC) assess for infection and bleeding
  - Occult blood (stool)

- Imaging
  - Ultrasound (detects an abscess or bowel thickening)
  - Abdominal x-rays (detects free abdominal air, which is characteristic of perforation)
- Other
  - Colonoscopy

Patient Care Management

- Medical
  - Rest: Avoid activities that increase intra-abdominal pressure (lifting, straining, coughing, sneezing, and bending)
  - Dietary modifications
    - Clear liquid diet
    - Diet high in both soluble and insoluble fiber (introduced as tolerated)
  - Drug therapy
    - Analgesics for pain control
    - Antibiotics
    - Metamucil (bulk-forming agent)
    - Colace (stool softener)
  - Hydration
  - Nasogastric suction (NGT) to allow for bowel rest
- Surgical
  - For presence of peritonitis from ruptured diverticulum, abscess, bowel obstruction, fistula, or uncontrolled bleeding
  - Bowel resection with anastomosis
  - Temporary colostomy (usually closed in 2 to 3 months)

Nursing Management

Nursing care for a patient with diverticular disease will require an understanding of routine NGT, colostomy, and postoperative care. (See Appendices #1 and #3, and Procedures & Therapies.)

- Pain, Acute
  - Assess pain using numeric scale 0–10 and self-reported characteristics
  - Provide analgesics and reassess accordingly
  - Instruct the patient to inform the nurse if pain gets worse or is not relieved.
- Tissue Perfusion, Ineffective
  - Monitor for $\uparrow$ HR and $\uparrow$ RR (indicates $\uparrow$ inflammation with vascular leaking)
  - Monitor for $\uparrow$ T (indicates perforation and peritonitis)
  - Assess bowel sounds ($\downarrow$ sounds indicate obstruction or peritonitis)
  - Assess abdomen for guarding and tenderness
  - Measure abdominal girth
  - Examine stools for blood
  - Notify health care provider for $\uparrow$ pain, nausea, vomiting, or abdominal distention
- Knowledge Deficit
  - Instruct patient and family regarding importance of high-fiber diet
  - Instruct patient and family regarding purpose of treatment regime
  - Encourage patient to notify health care provider if signs of worsening condition exist

Gallbladder Disease

The gallbladder is a saclike structure that concentrates and stores bile. Bile is produced by the liver and is necessary for the absorption of dietary fat and fat-soluble vitamins. Most gallbladder disorders result in obstructed bile flow from the liver to the gallbladder or from the gallbladder to the duodenum.

Cholelithiasis (Gallstones)

Gallstones result from a combination of factors, including biliary stasis, inflammation of the gallbladder, and abnormal bile composition and reabsorption. There are two types of gallstones: those predominantly composed of cholesterol and those composed of calcium bilirubinate.

Risk Factors

- Female
- Obesity
- High estrogen states
- Diabetes
- Hyperlipidemia
- Cirrhosis
- Crohn's disease
- Medications (clofibrate, ceftriaxone, oral contraceptives, and hormonal replacement therapy)

Signs and Symptoms

- Pain
  - Epigastric and/or right upper quadrant
  - Steady and severe with radiation to the mid-upper back, right scapula, and shoulder
  - May last for 4 to 5 hours
- Intolerance to fatty foods
- Nausea, vomiting, diarrhea
- Flatulence, bloating, and abdominal distention
- Chest pain
- Jaundice (if stone is lodged in common bile duct)

Cholecystitis

Cholecystitis is simply inflammation of the gallbladder and can be an acute or chronic problem. The most common cause of both acute and chronic cholecystitis is a gallstone lodged in the cystic duct. When the flow of bile out of the gallbladder is obstructed, the gallbladder becomes distended and an inflammatory response is initiated. In at least 90% of the patients with cholecystitis, cholelithiasis is the cause. If the gallstones are in the cystic duct, pressure in the gallbladder increases, causing ischemia of the mucosal wall and inflammation. Prolonged ischemia leads to necrosis and in severe cases gangrene can result.

Signs and Symptoms

- Similar to those of cholelithiasis
- Fever and chills
- Gallbladder may be palpable on abdominal exam. There may be tenderness with possible guarding on palpation of the RUQ.
- Jaundice

Diagnostics

- Health History and Physical Examination
- Laboratory
  - Serum bilirubin
    - Direct (conjugated)
      - Elevated indicates obstructive process within liver or biliary system
    - Indirect (unconjugated)
      - Elevated indicates RBC hemolysis or cellular damage
  - Amylase and lipase
    - Determines pancreatic involvement, common bile duct obstruction, or presence of pancreatitis
  - AST and ALT
    - Determines whether any liver injury has occurred as a result of a stone in the common bile duct
  - CBC
    - Determines presence of infectious process of elevated WBC
- Imaging
  - Ultrasound of the gallbladder

Patient Care Management

- Dietary and Lifestyle Management
  - Low-fat diet (for mild cases)

- Vitamins
  - Fat soluble vitamins A, D, E, and K
- Weight loss
- Exercise
- Medication
  - Ursodiol (Actigall) or chenodiol (Chenix) used to dissolve the gallstones by reducing the cholesterol content of the stone
  - Antibiotics
  - Cholestyramine (Questran) binds bile salts, which are then excreted in the stool.
  - Narcotic analgesics
- Surgery
  - Indicated for presence of frequent, severe symptoms, or cholecystitis
  - Laparoscopic cholecystectomy
  - Open cholecystectomy
    - Indicated for a very large or infected gallbladder
  - T-tube
    - Placed if stones are located in the common bile duct
    - Allows bile to pass from the liver into the duodenum until the edema from surgery diminishes
    - Procedures
      - Ultrasound Therapy
      - Extracorporeal shock wave lithotripsy (ESWL)
      - Breaks up large gallstones by using ultrasound waves
      - Requires oral dissolution therapy to help dissolve the stone fragments

Nursing Management

In addition to monitoring for pain and infection, the nursing responsibilities for patients with cholelithiasis or cholecystitis include understanding routine postoperative care and care of a T-tube. (See Procedures & Therapies, T-Tubes, and Appendix #1, Patient Care Plan for the Postoperative Patient Following General Surgery.)

- Pain, Acute
  - Assess pain using numeric scale 0–10
  - Using self-report assess for pain characteristics
  - Administer analgesics and reassess appropriately
- Infection, Risk for
  - Monitor for ↑ WBC, ↑ T, ↑ HR
  - Monitor for ↑ abdominal pain
- Knowledge Deficit
  - Instruct patient regarding purpose for dietary modifications to decrease or prevent episodes
  - Encourage patient to participate in exercise and weight-loss program
  - Instruct patient and family regarding routine postoperative care, including how to care for T-tube

Gastroesophageal Reflux Disease (GERD)

Gastroesophageal reflux is the backward flow of stomach contents (chyme) into the esophagus without associated vomiting. It is caused by relaxation of the lower esophageal sphincter, which allows for reflux of stomach contents into the esophagus, particularly during activity that increases intra-abdominal pressure, such as lifting, bending, straining, or recumbency. The esophageal mucosa does not contain the same protective mechanism against the acidic stomach contents as does the stomach, and mucosal damage and erosion result.

Risk Factors
- Obesity
- Pregnancy
- Hiatal hernia
- Alcohol and nicotine

- Caffeine, chocolate
- Fatty foods
- Citrus fruit
- Onions
- Tomatoes
- Beta-adrenergic blockers (Inderal)
- Calcium channel blockers (Verapamil)

Complications
- Barrett's esophagus (premalignant tissue caused by chronic inflammation)
  - Increases the risk for esophageal cancer
- Esophageal strictures

Signs and Symptoms
- Heartburn (mild to severe)
- Sour taste in the morning on arising
- Regurgitation
- Dysphagia
- Coughing
- Belching
- Chest pain

Diagnostics
- Health History and Physical Examination (severity of symptoms may not correlate with the severity of disease)
- Imaging
  - Barium swallow (evaluates for hiatal hernia)
- Other
  - Endoscopy with tissue sampling (See Procedures & Therapies, Endoscopy.)

Patient Care Management
- Medical
  - Dietary Modifications

- Avoid spicy foods
- Eat small, frequent meals with the largest meal at midday
- Avoid eating anything within 4 hours of bedtime
- Elevate the head of the bed
- Avoid caffeine, tobacco, and alcohol
- Weight loss
- Medications
  - Antacids
  - Histamine$_2$-receptor blockers (cimetidine (Tagamet), ranitidine (Zantac), nizatidine (Axid), and famotidine (Pepcid)
  - Proton pump inhibitors (omeprazole (Prilosec), lansoprazole (Previcid), or pantoprazole (Protonix)
  - Metoclopramide (Reglan) (promotes gastric motility and speeds gastric emptying, but does not affect acid secretion)
- Surgery
  - Nissen fundoplication

Nursing Management

- Pain, Acute
  - Use pain scale (0–10) to quantify pain and discomfort
  - Provide antacids, histamine$_2$-receptor blockers, proton pump inhibitors
- Knowledge Deficit
  - Teach the importance of eating 4–6 small meals a day and to eliminate foods known to decrease lower esophageal sphincter (LES) pressure or cause irritation
  - Instruct the patient to avoid lying down after eating
  - Educate the patient about medication regimen and possible side effects

- Assess cultural and religious dietary practices
- Explain the possibility of developing cancer if reflux goes untreated over time

Hepatitis

Hepatitis is defined as inflammation of the liver most often due to exposure to viral agents. It can be an acute or chronic infection that may be mild or life threatening, depending on the infectious agent. Some of the many causes of liver inflammation include viruses, bacteria, metabolic and vascular disorders, drugs, alcohol, and other toxic substances such as cleaning fluids, industrial toxins, and plant poisons.

Hepatitis A

The hepatitis A virus (HAV) is transmitted through the fecal–oral route, meaning persons contract the virus by drinking water contaminated with sewage, eating uncooked food washed in this water, eating shellfish harvested from contaminated water, or eating food contaminated by a person who is infected and did not use hand washing after using the toilet. It is also considered a sexually transmitted disease, mainly through oral sex. The incubation period (time between exposure and onset of symptoms) for HAV is anywhere from 2 to 6 weeks. The onset of symptoms is mild and resembles the flu.

Hepatitis B

The hepatitis B virus (HBV) is transmitted through the blood, semen, cervical secretions, saliva, and wound drainage with the highest concentration occurring in blood and blood products. High-risk groups include health care workers, IV drug users, homosexual men, those who have multiple sex partners, and from mother to fetus. The incubation period for HBV is longer than that of other hepatic viruses, lasting anywhere from 2 to 6 months, during which time transmission is possible even when symptoms are absent. HBV can exist as a carrier state, and/or it can create a chronic active state of infection, which can progress to cirrhosis and liver failure, thus requiring liver transplantation.

Hepatitis C

The hepatitis C virus (HCV) is found predominantly in blood, blood products, and transplanted tissue. Additionally, the disease can be transmitted through multiple sex partners, IV drug abuse, and percutaneous (tattooing, body piercing). The HCV replicates at a very high rate, which causes the host immune system to have difficulty building a response. This in turn leads to a high rate of chronic infections.

Hepatitis D

The hepatitis D virus (HDV) transmission occurs in the same manner as for HBV. IV drug users have a high rate of HDV with a mortality rate of about 3%. Symptoms occur between 1 to 6 months after exposure and frequently lead to a chronic state.

Hepatitis E

The hepatitis E virus (HEV) is transmitted via the fecal–oral route and is similar to hepatitis A in clinical manifestations. Unlike HAV, however, the mortality rate for pregnant women who contract HEV is higher at 10% to 20%. The virus has an incubation period of 15 to 60 days and remains uncommon in the United States.

Hepatitis G

The hepatitis G virus (HGV) is transmitted via the percutaneous route or through sexual contact. The virus has been detected in at least 50% of IV drug users, 30% of patients undergoing hemodialysis, and 15% of patients with chronic HBV or HCV.

Signs and Symptoms

Regardless of the cause, the clinical manifestations of hepatitis are frequently very similar. The severity of the symptoms can range from almost none or asymptomatic, to fulminating hepatitis, progressing to liver failure and death.

- Prodromal Phase
  - The phase of acute hepatitis that occurs between exposure to the virus and the appearance of jaundice
  - Either an insidious or a rapid onset

- Anorexia, nausea, and vomiting
- Malaise, myalgia, arthralgia, and easy fatigue
- Abdominal pain (mild, constant, in the right upper quadrant [RUQ] or epigastrium)
- Fever $< 103°F$ (39.4°C)
- Icteric Phase
  - Onset of jaundice
  - Prodromal symptoms become worse with the onset of jaundice
  - Dark amber urine
- Convalescent Phase
  - Increased sense of well-being
  - Increased appetite and energy level
  - Jaundice and abdominal pain disappear
  - Complete clinical recovery may take 9–16 weeks

Diagnostics

- Health history and physical examination
- Laboratory (elevations throughout the various phases of the disease)
  - Alanine aminotransferase (ALT)
  - Aspartate aminotransferase (AST)
  - Alkaline phosphatase (ALP)
  - Gamma-glutamyltransferase (GGT)
  - Lactic dehydrogenase (LDH)
  - Serum bilirubin
  - Serological tests for viral antigens, antibodies, or the virus itself
- Other
  - Liver biopsy (to evaluate chronic hepatitis due to HBV or HCV)

Patient Care Management

The goals of medical treatment for hepatitis are to identify the cause of the inflammation, either infectious or chemical, provide symptomatic treatment, monitor the damage to the liver, and support the liver's ability to regenerate and heal itself. Patients with fulminating liver failure will require hospitalization and more aggressive treatment (See Cirrhosis section.)

- Medical
  - Preventive Drug Treatment
    - HAV and HBV vaccines
    - Immune globulin (IG) for HAV and HBV post exposure prophylaxis.
    - PEG-Intron (pegylated interferon alfa-2b) subcutaneously and Ribavirin oral (prevention for chronic HCV)
  - Supportive Treatment
    - Dietary Modifications
      - Low-fat, high-calorie diet, increased protein intake
      - Alcohol and other agents toxic to the liver must be avoided.
    - Energy conservation

Nursing Management

Nursing care for the patients with hepatitis involves supportive measures and education. Those patients requiring hospitalization would be those with fulminating hepatitis, or chronic hepatitis that has progressed to cirrhosis, liver cancer, or liver failure.

- Activity Intolerance, Fatigue
  - Encourage frequent rest periods during the day
  - Facilitate the identification of essential activities and delegate tasks to others
  - Encourage increased activity as fatigue improves
- Nutrition, Readiness for Enhanced
  - Instruct the patient to eat foods rich in carbohydrates (for sufficient energy) and proteins (needed for healing)
  - Teach the patient to read food labels and choose foods that are low in fat and have adequate levels

of vitamins and minerals (e.g., instant breakfast drink)

- Explain the importance of avoiding substances that can be toxic to the liver, such as alcohol and acetaminophen

- Skin Integrity, Risk for Impaired
  - Instruct the patient to use cool, lightweight, non-restrictive clothing and avoid woolens
  - Explain that a cool environmental temperature and cool water for bathing may increase comfort related to pruritus
  - Instruct the patient to keep her fingernails trimmed and well cared for to decrease the likelihood of excoriating when scratching
  - Instruct the patient to take antihistamine medication as ordered to reduce pruritus

- Infection, Risk
  - Use standard or universal precautions when handling blood or body fluids
  - Explain that the time of highest infectivity is before symptoms appear, and that good hand hygiene can prevent the spread of the disease
  - Teach about safe sex practices
  - Encourage prophylactic treatment for close contacts and/or vaccination against HAV and HBV

Hernias
Hiatal Hernia

A hiatal hernia involves the herniation of the upper portion of the stomach into the thorax through the esophageal hiatus. This condition is more common in women and in those persons who are 70 years or greater.

Sliding (Direct) Hiatal Hernia

- Most common
- A portion of the fundus of the stomach moves upward through the esophageal hiatus into the thoracic cavity.
- Results in GERD

Rolling (Paraesophageal) Hernia

- Herniation of the greater curvature of the stomach through the esophageal hiatus
- Results in gastritis

Inguinal Hernia

(See Male Reproductive Disorders.)

Signs and Symptoms

- Reflux and heartburn
- Complaints of feeling full, belching, and indigestion
- Substernal chest pain

Diagnostics

- Health History and Physical Examination
- Imaging
  - Barium Swallow
  - Endoscopy (See Procedures & Therapies, Endoscopy.)

Patient Care Management

- Medical
  - Dietary and lifestyle changes (See GERD section.)
  - Histamine$_2$ (H$_2$)-receptor blocker (ranitidine, famotidine)
  - Proton pump inhibitor (PPI) (lansoprazole, omeprazole)
- Surgical
  - Nissen fundoplication

Nursing Management

- Pain, Acute
  - Use pain scale (0–10) to quantify pain and discomfort.
  - Provide antacids, histamine$_2$-receptor blockers, proton pump inhibitors

- Knowledge Deficit
  - Teach the importance of eating 4–6 small meals a day and to eliminate foods known to decrease lower esophageal sphincter (LES) pressure or cause irritation
  - Instruct the patient to avoid lying down after eating
  - Educate the patient about medication regimen and possible side effects
  - Assess cultural and religious dietary practices
  - Explain the possibility of developing cancer if reflux goes untreated over time

Inflammatory Bowel Disease (IBD)

IBD is an immunologic disease that results in idiopathic intestinal inflammation. It includes two distinct, yet similar conditions: ulcerative colitis (UC) and Crohn's disease. Both ulcerative colitis and Crohn's disease have common clinical manifestations as well as similar pathophysiology involving an inflammatory process.

Causes
- Genetic susceptibility
- Abnormal immune response
- Imbalance in beneficial and pathogenic bacteria in the intestines
- Intestinal epithelial defects

Ulcerative Colitis (UC)

Ulcerative colitis is a chronic inflammation of the mucosal and submucosal layers of the colon and the rectum. It usually begins in the rectum and advances proximally, involving only the large intestine and usually only the sigmoid colon and rectum. The ulcers bleed easily, causing bloody stools, a characteristic manifestation of UC.

Crohn's Disease

Crohn's occurs in any portion of the gastrointestinal tract from the mouth to the anus; however, it is usually limited to the ileum or ileocecal valve. The lesions are granulomatous with areas of inflamed tissue circumscribed by scar tissue, giving the intestinal lumen a cobblestone appearance. As the disease progresses, the chronic inflammation causes fibrosis and loss of intestinal flexibility, resulting in obstruction, abscess, and fistula formation.

Signs and Symptoms
- Abdominal pain
  - Cramping type
  - Continuous or intermittent
  - Localized, in either lower quadrant, or more diffuse
- Diarrhea
  - Frequent episodes daily
  - Loose and/or watery
  - Bloody diarrhea (common in UC)
- Rectal urgency
- Incontinence
- Tenesmus (feeling of incomplete defecation)
- Fever
- Fatigue
- Joint pain
- Mouth sores

Diagnostics
- Health history and physical examination
- Laboratory
  - CBC
    - Detects anemia
    - ↑ WBC (inflammatory process and abscess formation)

- Electrolytes, glucose, albumin, BUN, creatinine, and serum levels of vitamins (monitors the degree of malabsorption in Crohn's disease)
- Genetic testing
- Imaging
  - Colonoscopy (mucosal biopsy shows continuous inflammation of UC or patterned inflammation with Crohn's)
  - Barium swallow and barium enema

Patient Care Management

- Medical
  - Sulfasalazine (Azulfidine) for UC
  - Corticosteroids (for an acute exacerbation of IBD)
  - Immunomodulators (azathioprine [AZA] and 6-mercaptopurine [6-MP])
  - Biologic modifiers (infliximab, a tumor necrosis factor-α [TNF-α] inhibitor) for use in Crohn's disease.
  - Dietary modifications
    - Well balanced
    - Avoid foods that cause problems
    - High-fiber diet (lessens diarrhea)
      - Contraindicated in acute symptoms
    - NPO (during an acute exacerbation)
    - Total parenteral nutrition (TPN) (See Procedures & Therapies, Parenteral Nutrition.)
- Surgery
  - Total colectomy

Nursing Management

Nursing care involves preparing the patient for diagnostic tests, managing the medication regimen, educating the patient about drug treatments and stress reduction, assessing the effectiveness of the interventions, and caring for the patient during the surgical experience. Support networks (Crohn's & Colitis Foundation of America) are vitally important for this very life-disrupting disease. (See Appendix #8, Patient Care Plan for Inflammatory Bowel Disease and Ileostomy for a detailed nursing care plan for the patient with IBD and ileostomy.)

Intestinal Obstruction

- Complete or partial obstruction of any portion of the bowel. Most bowel obstructions occur in the small intestines with only about 15% occurring in the large bowel.

- Impairment of forward movement of intestinal contents due to:
  - Mechanical cause:
    - Adhesions
    - Crohn's disease
    - Diverticular disease
    - Foreign bodies
  - Functional cause:
    - Surgery
    - Anesthesia
    - Medications

- Functional bowel obstructions are also called ileus, paralytic ileus, or adynamic ileus.

- Mechanical obstructions include an increase in motility and secretions of the bowel, both proximal and distal to the obstruction.

Classifications

- Simple bowel obstructions:
  - No impairment of the vascular or neurologic innervation to the intestine
  - Gas and intestinal secretions accumulate proximal to the obstruction and the distal bowel collapses.
  - Bowel wall becomes edematous and congested due to inflammation.

- Possibility of ischemia, necrosis, perforation, and death
- Strangulated bowel obstructions:
  - Extremely serious
  - Most commonly caused by hernias, intussusception (telescoping of the bowel), volvulus (twisting of the bowel), or vascular occlusion. Additionally, can be due to surgical adhesions and tumors.
  - Interruptions of both arterial and venous blood flow
  - Possibility of ischemia, infarction progressing to gangrene, and perforation and death

Signs and Symptoms

The manifestations vary depending on the location, type of obstruction, and the rapidity of development. The most common symptom is pain that presents intermittently becoming constant with the progression of the obstruction. The pain is described as cramping or colicky in nature.

- Small Bowel Obstruction
  - Distension
  - Visible peristaltic waves
  - Nausea and vomiting (possibly may contain fecal material)
  - Bowel sounds are hyperactive and high-pitched tinkling.
  - Bowel sounds cease later in the course of the obstruction.
  - Bowel sounds may be diminished or absent with paralytic ileus.
  - Abdominal tenderness may be evident on palpation.
  - Tachycardia, hypotension, tachypnea (due to electrolyte and fluid loss)
- Large Bowel Obstruction
  - Colicky pain. Severe and continuous may indicate bowel ischemia or perforation.
  - Distention

- Constipation
- Large palpable mass
- Gangrene and perforation
- Vomiting later in the process

Diagnostics

- Health history and physical examination
- Laboratory
  - Complete blood count (CBC) with differential (determine presence of infection)
  - Serum amylase
  - Serum osmolality (determine dehydration)
  - Serum electrolytes
- Imaging
  - Abdominal x-rays
  - CT scan with contrast media
  - Barium swallow

Patient Care Management

- Medical
  - NPO (nothing by mouth)
  - Peripheral intravenous line (IV)
    - Isotonic fluids (NS, Ringer's lactate) to correct dehydration
  - Electrolyte replacement (potassium)
  - Blood products (for perforation or strangulation)
  - Antibiotics intravenous (for surgery)
  - Nasogastric tube (NGT) to intermittent suction (for gastric decompression)
  - Pain medication
- Surgery (if ineffective response to other treatments)
  - Bowel resection (except for adhesions)
    - Possible ileostomy or colostomy
  - Release of adhesions

Nursing Management

Nursing care of the patient with an intestinal obstruction will require an understanding of routine postoperative care. (See Appendix #1.)

- Fluid Volume, Risk for Deficient
  - Accurate I&O
  - Assess frequency and characteristics of emesis or diarrhea
  - Assess skin turgor
  - Assess orthostatic vital signs
  - Assess dizziness and lightheadedness
  - Assess abdominal girth every shift
  - Assess for indications of dehydration (tachycardia, tachypnea, hypotension)
  - Electrolytes
    - Monitor trends in laboratory data (potassium, hemoglobin, hematocrit)
    - Assess for signs of hypokalemia (muscle weakness, shallow respirations, dyspnea, anorexia, flattened T waves on ECG)
    - Assess for signs of anemia (pallor, palpitations, fatigue, lightheadedness)
- Pain, Acute
  - Nasogastric tube placement for gastric decompression

(See Procedures & Therapies, Nasogastric Tube.)

  - Assess amount and characteristics of returns
  - Assess placement per policy
  - Maintain NPO status
  - Assess with vital signs according to self-report scale of 0–10.
  - Provide comfort measures (oral care, medications, etc.)
- Knowledge Deficit

- Explain routine postoperatives care to patient and family
- Instruct patient and family regarding prescribed treatment plan

Pancreatitis

Pancreatitis, or inflammation of the pancreas, can be acute or chronic and is a potentially serious disease. Mortality is high if the patient develops cardiac, pulmonary, or renal complications.

Risk Factors

- Alcoholism
- Biliary obstruction
- Peptic ulcers
- Trauma
- Extreme hyperlipidemia and hypertriglyceridemia

Acute Pancreatitis

It is believed that activated pancreatic enzymes, particularly trypsin, leak into the pancreatic tissue and begin the process of autodigestion; the pancreas begins to digest itself. Tissue necrosis factor-alpha (TNF-α), substance P, and many interleukins and kinins enter the systemic circulation causing damage to tissue in the lungs, blood vessels, and kidneys, which results in increased mortality.

Signs and Symptoms

- Sudden, severe, steady epigastric pain
  - Worse when the patient is lying supine or when walking
  - Pain radiates to the right or left side of the back and is made better by sitting, leaning forward with the knees bent
  - Nausea and vomiting
  - Diaphoresis
  - Anxiety

- Abdominal distention, decreased bowel sounds, and rigidity
- Turner's sign (ecchymosis in the flanks) and Cullen's sign (bruising around the umbilicus) may appear as a result of retroperitoneal bleeding
- Pleural effusions, atelectasis, or pulmonary edema (tachypnea, tachycardia, and hypoxia)
- Hyperglycemia

Diagnostics

- Health History and Physical Examination
- Laboratory
  - ↑ Bilirubin, ↑ alkaline phosphatase, ↑ ALT
  - ↑ Amylase (within hours of onset, normalizes in 3–4 days)
  - ↑ Lipase (rise rapidly, remain elevated up to 14 days, and then normalize)
  - ↑ Alkaline phosphatase and ↑ Bilirubin (obstruction of bile duct)
  - ↓ Calcium
  - ↑ C-reactive protein (CRP) elevations after 48 hours indicate the possibility of pancreatic necrosis
  - ↑ WBC
- Imaging
  - Abdominal x-ray
  - A CT scan (evaluates for necrotizing pancreatitis)

Patient Care Management

- Medical
  - NPO (nothing by mouth) to rest pancreas
    - Clear liquids once pain has subsided; advance to low fat
  - Nasogastric tube (NGT) low intermittent suction. (See Procedures & Therapies, Nasogastric Tube.)
  - Intravenous hydration

- Medication
  - Pain control with narcotic analgesics
  - Antibiotics
  - Calcium gluconate
  - Total parenteral nutrition (TPN) if patient is NPO longer than 7 days
- Surgery
  - Debridement of the pancreas and surrounding tissue is indicated for patients that have infected necrotizing pancreatitis.
  - Percutaneous or open surgical drainage (for pancreatic abscesses)

Chronic Pancreatitis

Chronic pancreatitis is an irreversible process of gradual destruction of pancreatic tissue. Causes include chronic, cystic fibrosis, obesity, type II diabetes mellitus, and insulin resistance.

Signs and Symptoms

- Recurrent epigastric and left upper quadrant pain that may be referred to the left lumbar region
- Anorexia, nausea, vomiting, weight loss
- Flatulence and constipation
- Steatorrhea

Diagnostics

- Health History and Physical Examination
- Laboratory (similar to those of acute pancreatitis; however, the amylase and lipase may be normal)
  - Hyperglycemia
- Imaging
  - Endoscopic retrograde cholangiopancreatography (ERCP) locates the cause of a biliary obstruction.
  - Magnetic resonance cholangiopancreatography (MRCP) (noninvasive)
  - Endoscopic ultrasonography with tissue sampling

Patient Care Management

During an acute exacerbation of chronic pancreatitis, the patient will be treated in much the same way as a patient with acute pancreatitis.

- Medical
  - Dietary and lifestyle changes
    - Avoid alcohol
    - Low-fat diet
  - Medications
    - Narcotic analgesics used sparingly
    - Pancreatic enzymes
    - H_2-receptor antagonist (ranitidine) or a proton pump inhibitor (omeprazole)

Nursing Management (Acute and Chronic Pancreatitis)

The major focus of nursing care for the patient with pancreatitis is pain control, nutrition, and health teaching about alcohol abstinence. (See Appendix #7.)

Peptic Ulcer Disease

Peptic ulcer is a generic term used for any ulceration in the digestive surfaces of the upper GI tract, including gastric and duodenal ulcers. The ulcers are disruptions in the protective mucosal lining, thereby exposing the submucosal tissue to gastric secretions and digestion of the submucosa (autodigestion).

Gastric Ulcers

Most gastric ulcers develop in the antrum, adjacent to the body of the stomach where acid is produced. Gastric ulcers are not associated with increased acid secretion, but rather with a defect in the mucosal barrier to hydrogen ions, allowing the ions to permeate the mucosa.

Causes

- Chronic gastritis (prevents the mucosa's ability to produce a protective layer of mucus)

- *Helicobacter pylori* (*H. pylori*), a bacterium causing gastritis
- Aspirin and nonsteroidal anti-inflammatory drugs (NSAIDs) decrease prostaglandin secretion by the mucosa, therefore diminishing its protective ability.
- Duodenal reflux of bile

Duodenal Ulcers

Duodenal ulcers are the most common type of peptic ulcer in the United States and are found more often in younger people.

Causes

- *Helicobacter pylori* (*H. pylori*), a bacterium causing gastritis
- Hypersecretion of acid and pepsin
- Cigarette smoke (stimulates acid production)
- Aspirin and nonsteroidal anti-inflammatory drugs (NSAIDs) decrease prostaglandin secretion by the mucosa, therefore diminishing its protective ability.

Complications

- Hemorrhage (due to an erosion of a blood vessel)
  - Slow or severe bleeding
  - Anemia
  - Occult blood in stool
  - Bright red emesis
  - Coffee ground emesis (partially digested food)
  - Melena (dark, tarry stools)
- Pyloric or gastric outlet obstruction
  - Result of edema, inflammation, scarring of the pylorus, or a combination of these conditions
  - Begins with a feeling of epigastric fullness progressing to vomiting
  - Complete obstruction
    - Metabolic alkalosis and electrolyte imbalance

- Perforation (most serious)
  - Severe, sudden upper abdominal pain that radiates throughout the abdomen
    - Rigid board-like abdomen
    - Absence of bowel sounds
  - Peritonitis (due to gastroduodenal contents containing acid, pepsin, bile, and pancreatic juice entering the abdominal cavity)

Signs and Symptoms
- Pain (upper abdomen)
  - Intermittent, gnawing, burning, aching, or hunger-like
  - Occurs when the stomach is empty
  - Relieved by food or antacids
- Chest pain
- Dysphagia
- Anemia (especially in geriatrics)

Diagnostics
- Health history and physical examination
- Imaging
  - Barium swallow
  - Endoscopy
    - Tissue specimens to detect *H. pylori* and malignancy

Patient Care Management
- Medical
  - Antibiotics
  - Proton pump inhibitor
  - Antacids
  - Lifestyle modifications
    - Limit alcohol consumption
    - Avoid smoking
    - Hand washing (prevents spread of *H. pylori*)

- Surgical
  - Gastric resection may be required to treat the complications (e.g., perforation)

Nursing Management

- Pain, Acute
  - Assess pain using scale (0–10) to quantify pain
  - Assess pain, character and location, and its relationship to food intake, empty stomach, or other factors and what relieves the pain
  - Administer medications to reduce acid secretion and monitor effectiveness
  - Teach the importance of following through with medication regimen as ordered
- Knowledge Deficit
  - Instruct patient regarding importance of avoiding risk factors
  - Clarify causative factors related to PUD
  - Provide information about the symptoms of complications of PUD and to have the patient call the health care provider immediately if any should occur

GLANDULAR AND HORMONAL DISORDERS

Disorders of the Adrenal Gland
Addison's Disease

Addison's disease is adrenocortical insufficiency due to the destruction of the adrenal cortex (primary adrenal insufficiency) or caused by impaired pituitary secretion of ACTH resulting in an inadequate secretion of cortisol (secondary adrenal insufficiency).

Causes

- Autoimmune disease (immune system makes antibodies that gradually destroy the cells of the adrenal cortex)
- Chronic infections (TB, histoplasmosis, or cytomegalovirus)
- Cancer (metastatic)
- Hemorrhage into the adrenal gland
- Tumors
- Bilateral adrenalectomy
- Sudden withdrawal of long-term corticosteroid therapy

Signs and Symptoms

- Severe and chronic fatigue
- Nausea, vomiting, and diarrhea
- ↓ appetite with weight loss
- Light-headedness due to ↓ BP

- Orthostatic hypotension
- Hyperpigmentation of skin
- Changes in menstruation cycles
- Addisonian crisis (adrenal crisis)
  - Symptoms of the disease become exacerbated due to stress
  - Severe pain in the lower back, abdomen, or legs
  - Vomiting or diarrhea
  - Severe dehydration
  - ↓ BP with loss of consciousness

Diagnostics
- Health History and Physical Examination
- Laboratory
  - Short ACTH stimulation test (serial serum samples obtained at intervals after injection of ACTH)
    - Patients with adrenal insufficiency are unable to respond to stimulation by producing more cortisol.
- Imaging
  - CT scan

Patient Care Management
- Medical
  - Hormones
    - Prednisone or cortisone
    - Aldosterone (Florinef)
    - Androgen replacement (Dehydroepiandros-terone)
- Multidisciplinary
  - Home health nursing to assess ability to administer medications and home safety
  - Physical therapist to help patient build strength and begin to be more independent

Nursing Management

- Fluid Volume, Deficient
  - Intravenous therapy (0.09% saline solution or 5% dextrose in saline)
  - Monitor for signs of dehydration ($\downarrow$ BP, $\uparrow$ HR, poor skin turgor, dry mucous membranes, low urine output)
  - Assess laboratory results (electrolytes, glucose)
  - Intravenous hydrocortisone (48–72 hours followed by oral agents long term)
  - Monitor nausea, treat to prevent dehydration
- Injury, Risk of
  - Monitor for signs of Addison's crisis ($\downarrow$ BP, $\uparrow$ HR, shock)
  - Assess ambulation and ability to perform self-care
  - Assist with ADLs as needed
  - Initiate fall precautions as needed
- Knowledge Deficit
  - Instruct patient and family regarding disease and importance of continuing with medication therapy long term, including the risks and benefits of corticosteroids
  - Encourage use of medical alert jewelry
  - Instruct family about signs of Addison's crisis and to seek medical attentions if they occur
  - Demonstrate to patient and family how to administer cortisol injections
  - Instruct patient and family to contact health care provider if experiencing stress, infection, or other illness so cortisol doses may be adjusted

Cushing's Syndrome

Cushing's syndrome is a hypermetabolic disorder of the adrenal cortex which involves an excess of cortisol and primary aldosteronism (excess of aldosterone). This disorder occurs with long-term secretion or exposure to excessive adrenocortical hormones, particularly cortisol and related corticosteroids, and to a lesser extent androgens and aldosterone.

Causes
- Prednisone therapy
- Tumors producing ACTH

Signs and Symptoms
- Fat deposits on faces and bodies
  - "Moon face" appearance
  - "Buffalo hump" on upper back
- Obese appearance with slender arms and legs
- Acne and purple striae on the face
- Thin skin
- Infections with poor wound healing
- Sudden weight gain
- Hypertension with left ventricular hypertrophy
- Hirsutism
- Pathologic fractures

Diagnostics
- Health History and Physical Examination
- Laboratory
  - Serum and urine cortisol (high)
  - Electrolytes
  - Glucose
  - 24-hour urine cortisol
- Imaging
  - CT scan & MRI

Patient Care Management
- Medical
  - Mitotane (Lysodren) an adrenal cytotoxic preparation, which suppresses adrenal gland function and helps to reduce blood glucose and blood pressure

- Aminoglutethimide (Cytadren) can be used to decrease production of adrenal hormones
- Gradual withdrawl or reduction of cortico-steroids (relief of symptoms caused by long-term corticosteroid use)
- Surgery
  - Transsphenoidal microsurgery (for pituitary tumors that are stimulating excessive ACTH production)
- Other
  - Radiation therapy

Nursing Management

Nursing responsibilities include understanding the care required for the patient who is postoperative and who has received radiation therapy (See Appendix #1: Nursing Process: Patient Care for the Postoperative Patient Following General Surgery.)

- Fluid Volume, Excess
  - Accurate I&O
  - Monitor lung sounds (crackles), $\downarrow$ O_2 sat, $\uparrow$ RR, and $\uparrow$ work of breathing
  - Assess for presence of edema
  - Daily weights
- Infection, Risk for
  - Monitor for signs of infection
    - $\uparrow$ WBC, $\uparrow$ Temperature
    - $\downarrow$ wound healing (exudate, inflammation, $\uparrow$ pain)
- Knowledge Deficit
  - Inform patient why serum electrolytes and glucose need to be monitored at regular intervals
  - Explain to patient the rationale related to body changes (hirsutism, acne, "moon face," "buffalo hump")
  - Allow patient to express fear and concern related to changes in appearance and feelings of depression

or suicide. Consider referral to social services or psychiatry for further follow up.

Pheochromocytoma

Pheochromocytoma is a rare, usually nonmalignant tumor of the adrenal medulla that causes hypertension by producing an excess of epinephrine (adrenalin) and norepinephrine. Triggers include emotional stress, trigger foods, abdominal pressure, tobacco, histamine, and glucagon.

Signs and Symptoms

- Hypertension
- Profuse sweating
- Nausea
- Headache
- Tachycardia and palpitations

Diagnostics

- Health History and Physical Examination
- Laboratory
  - Serum and urine 24-hour catecholamine metabolites (high)
  - Assays of free or unconjugated catecholamines
- Imaging
  - CT scans and MRI

Patient Care Management

- Medical
  - Management of hypertension
  - Alpha-adrenergic blockers (blocks excess hormone and lowers blood pressure after surgery)
- Surgery
  - Laparoscopic surgical removal of the tumor

Nursing Management

Routine postoperative care is required for a patient who has had the adrenal tumor removed. (See Appendix #1.)

- Injury, Risk for
  - Monitor BP
  - Assess for associated symptoms (headache, nausea, alteration in consciousness)
  - Notify health care provider if change in level of consciousness occurs
  - Avoid palpation of abdomen
- Knowledge Deficit
  - Explain purpose for surgical removal of tumor and expected postoperative care
  - Encourage patients to maintain a low-sodium, moderate-carbohydrate, low-fat diet to counteract the effects of excess hormone
  - Instruct patient and family of need for long-term hypertensive therapy despite removal of tumor

Disorders of the Parathyroid Gland

The parathyroid glands are four small, highly vascular glands located behind the thyroid gland, which regulate the blood calcium level by releasing parathyroid hormone (PTH). PTH is a small protein that acts directly on both the bone and kidneys where it stimulates release and reabsorption of calcium. It also acts indirectly on the intestines, causing them to reabsorb calcium.

Hyperparathyroidism

Primary hyperparathyroidism, the most common problem of the parathyroid glands, is a relatively common disorder that occurs when one or more of the parathyroid glands oversecrete parathyroid hormone. This occurs due to a benign tumor, an adenoma, or hyperplasia in one or more of the parathyroid glands.

Secondary hyperparathyroidism occurs when another medical condition causes the parathyroid glands to produce too much PTH in response to chronically low levels of circulating calcium. These include kidney failure, malabsorption problems, and rickets (severe vitamin D deficiency).

Signs and Symptoms

- Muscle weakness and lethargy
- Dyspepsia
- Nausea and constipation
- Bone tenderness, bone cysts
- Polyuria
- Osteopenia (mild loss of bone density) and osteoporosis (moderate to severe loss of bone density resulting in "brittle bones")
- Bone fractures

Diagnostics

- Health history and physical examination
- Laboratory
  - PTH (high)
  - Serum calcium (high)
  - Alkaline phosphatase (low)

Patient Care Management

- Medical
  - Treat underlying cause (renal failure)
    - Vitamin D
    - Cinacalcet (Sensipar)
    - Paricalcitol (Zemplar) for use during dialysis
- Surgery
  - Radioguided parathyroidectomy (removal of disease gland)
- Multidisciplinary
  - Pharmacist, the nutritionist, the endocrinologist, and the genetic counselor, as well as nursing

Nursing Management

Nursing management for the patient with hyperparathyroidism includes understanding routine postoperative care. (See Appendix #1.)

- Injury, Risk for
  - Monitor alertness and ability to ambulate safely
  - Carefully turn and lift patients to avoid fractures
  - Implement fall precautions
  - Accurate I&O
  - Monitor laboratory results (calcium and PTH)
- Knowledge Deficit
  - Instruct patient and family regarding disease and necessary treatment
  - Encourage patient to avoid calcium containing medications
  - Encourage patient to keep follow-up appoints for evaluation and laboratory tests
  - If removal of gland, instruct patient to modify diet with calcium-rich foods
  - Encourage patient to maintain daily exercise and brief exposure to sunlight

Hypoparathyroidism

Hypoparathyroidism is a rare condition that occurs when the parathyroid glands do not make enough parathyroid hormone.

Causes
- Injury to the parathyroid gland
- Surgery to thyroid gland
- Infections
- Unknown cause

Risk Factors
- Family history and heredity
- Neck surgery (especially thyroid)
- Presence of other disease

Signs and Symptoms
- ECG changes (prolonged QT interval)
- Weakness

- Muscle cramps, particularly of wrists and feet
- Abnormal paresthesias with tingling, numbness, and burning of hands
- Excessive nervousness
- Loss of memory
- Headaches
- Malformations of the teeth and fingernails
- Chvostek's sign (spasms of facial muscles)
- Trousseau's sign (contraction of carpal muscles with mild compression of the nerves)

Diagnostics

- Health history and physical examination (including nutritional history and calcium intake)
- Laboratory
  - Serum calcium (lowered) and phosphorus (high)
  - PTH immunoassay (lowered)
  - Vitamin D metabolites

Patient Care Management

- Medical
  - Oral calcium, calcitriol (an active form of an artificial vitamin D), and high doses of oral vitamin D daily
  - Intravenous calcium

Nursing Management

- Injury, Risk for
  - Monitor ECG changes
  - Monitor RR, O_2 sat, and work of breathing (due to weakness)
  - Keep emergency airway equipment at bedside
  - Monitor gait, strength, and ability to safely ambulate
- Knowledge Deficit
  - Instruct patient and family regarding disease and required treatment (e.g., lifelong calcium and vitamin D replacement)

- Emphasize to patient the importance of safety and fall prevention
- Encourage patients to obtain daily brief exposure to sunlight
- Encourage patients to verbalize concerns regarding chronic nature of disease and offer community resources as appropriate

Disorders of the Hypothalmus and Posterior Pituitary Gland
Diabetes Insipidus

Diabetes insipidus (DI) involves a permanent or transient deficiency in the synthesis or release of ADH or a decreased renal responsiveness. This deficiency is caused by the destruction of the back or "posterior" part of the pituitary gland (where ADH is normally released), an insensitivity of the kidneys to that hormone, or it can also be induced iatrogenically by various drugs.

Risk Factors
- Tumors
- Trauma
- Surgery
- Infection
- Pregnancy
- Congenital defects and genetic disorders

Signs and Symptoms
- Polyuria (excretion of large amounts of dilute urine)
- Polydipsia (excessive thirst)
- Signs of dehydration
  - Dry mucous membranes
  - Poor skin turgor
- Headache, lethargy
- Nausea
- Hypovolemic shock
  - $\uparrow$ HR $\downarrow$ BP

Diagnostics
- Health History and Physical Examination
  - Genetic evaluations
- Laboratory
  - Serum and urine levels of ADH
  - Serum electrolytes ($\uparrow$ sodium)
  - Serum ($\uparrow$) and urine ($\downarrow$) osmolality
  - $\downarrow$ urine specific gravity
  - Water deprivation (determines whether DI is neurogenic or nephrogenic in nature)
- Imaging
  - MRI (rule out pituitary tumor)

Patient Care Management
- Medical
  - DDAVP (vasopressin)
  - Intravenous hydration
  - Electrolyte replacement
  - Diet modification (low-sodium and low-protein diet)
- Surgery (for tumors)

Nursing Management
- Fluid Volume, Deficient
  - Accurate I&O
  - Assess for signs of dehydration ($\uparrow$ HR, $\downarrow$ BP, poor skin turgor, dry mucous membranes)
  - Intravenous fluid replacement
  - Oral fluids as tolerated (assess for risk of aspiration)
  - Monitor electrolytes
  - Hormone replacement
- Injury, Risk of
  - Initiate fall precautions
  - Assist with ambulation and activity as needed

- Knowledge Deficit
    - Instruct patient and family regarding nature of the disease and the importance of hydration and strategies to ensure the availability of fluid at all times
    - Encourage use of Medic Alert jewelry and a medical identification card

Syndrome of Inappropriate Antidiuretic Hormone (SIADH)

SIADH is an excess secretion of anti-diuretic hormone (ADH), which is a potentially life-threatening condition. In persons with this syndrome, ADH secretion continues even when serum osmolality is decreased, causing marked water retention and dilutional hyponatremia.

Risk Factors

- Central nervous system disorders
- Trauma, shock
- Stress
- Surgery
- Pulmonary malignancies, lymphoma, sarcoma
- Pulmonary infections (TB, bacterial pneumonia, lung abscess)
- Medications (barbiturates, general anesthetics, thiazide diuretics, antidepressants, and some chemotherapeutic agents)

Signs and Symptoms

- Headache
- Nausea and anorexia
- Thirst
- ↑ weight
- Oliguria
- Muscle cramps, weakness, and fatigue
- Mental confusion, irritability, and disorientation
- Seizures and coma

Diagnostics

- Health history and physical examination
- Laboratory
  - Electrolytes
  - Serum and urine osmolality
  - Urine specific gravity
  - Blood urea nitrogen (BUN)

Patient Care Management

- Medical
  - Fluid restriction
  - Intravenous electrolytes (3% normal saline)
  - Oral sodium replacement (food, salt)
  - Medications (demeclocycline or lithium, which blocks ADH)
- Multidisciplinary
  - Endocrinologist, neurosurgeon, primary care provider, nurses, diagnostic imaging staff, pharmacists, and dietitians comprise the team that will plan care for the patient with pituitary disorders.

Nursing Management

- Fluid Volume, Excess
  - Accurate I&O
  - Monitor urine specific gravity
  - Monitor lung sounds, presence of edema, and weight gain
  - Assess level of consciousness
- Injury, Risk for
  - Assess for gait disturbances and assist as needed
  - Implement fall precautions
  - Seizure precautions
- Knowledge Deficit
  - Patient and family education should include strategies to deal with SIADH as well as the underlying disease and related nursing care.

- Patients or their caregivers should be instructed on how to record the patient's daily weight and intake and output measurements and when to report changes to the health care provider.

Disorders of the Thyroid Gland
Hypothyroidism

Hypothyroidism is a hypometabolic condition in which the thyroid gland fails to produce adequate thyroid hormone, resulting in a slowdown of metabolism and cellular function.

- Primary hypothyroidism (thyroid gland fails to produce sufficient thyroid hormone to sustain normal metabolic function)
  - Causes
    - Hashimoto's disease (autoimmune disease)
    - Surgical removal of the organ
    - Therapeutic radiation as a result of treatment for hyperthyroidism
    - Cretinism (congenital hypothyroidism)
    - Aging
    - Iodine deficiency
    - Tumors of the thyroid gland
    - Discontinuation of thyroid hormone replacement therapy
- Secondary hypothyroidism (occurs when the cause is related to pituitary tumors and other pituitary disorders)
- Tertiary thyroid disease (originates at the level of the hypothalamus)

Risk Factors
- Familial history of thyroid disease
- History of autoimmune disease
- Pernicious anemia
- Aging

- Inadequate supply of dietary iodine
- Previous treatment for hyperthyroidism

Signs and Symptoms
- Fatigue
- Weight gain
- Cold intolerance
- Constipation
- Mental lethargy
- Dry skin
- Hair thinning or loss
- Enlargement of the thyroid gland (significant enlargement is called a goiter)
- ↑ TSH levels (pituitary will respond to an underproduction of thyroid hormone)
- ↓ free T_4 (FT_4) (thyroxine)
- Myxedema (severe hypothyroidism)
  - Profound lethargy
  - Muscle weakness
  - Facial edema
  - Thick tongue
  - Mental decline and personality change

Diagnostics
- Health history and physical examination
- Laboratory
  - TSH
  - Thyroxine level
    - Serum FT_4 (considered the best clinical measure of thyroxine levels)
  - Total T_3 and total T_4 (considered to be less reliable indicators of thyroid level)
- Imaging
  - Thyroid scanning
  - Ultrasonography

- Other
  - Fine-needle biopsy

Patient Care Management

- Medical
  - Oral synthetic thyroid hormone (levothyroxine)
  - Monitoring of serum TSH and FT_4 (6 to 8 weeks after therapy is initiated and regularly thereafter)

Nursing Management

- Fatigue and Activity Intolerance
  - Provide for periods of rest
  - Assist with care as needed
- Risk for Impaired Skin Integrity
  - Avoid use of soaps, astringents, or other agents such as alcohol
  - Liberally apply emollient skin lotion
  - Consider using an alternating air mattress if needed
- Constipation
  - Administer stool softeners as prescribed
  - Gradually increase fluid intake and fiber in diet
  - Increase activity level with short, frequent walks and mild exercise
- Hypothermia
  - Monitor the environment to provide a warm room for patient comfort
- Confusion, Acute
  - Reduce stimuli and mental demands while hormone deficiency is replaced
  - Instruct family about potential mood swings, depression, and irritability
- Knowledge Deficit
  - Provide instructions to patient and family in writing as well as orally
  - Instruct patient on administration of hormone replacement medication, signs and symptoms

of hypo- and hyperthyroidism, and self-care practices

- Instruct patient to take hormone replacement medication on an empty stomach for optimal absorption
- Advise patient to avoid use of sedatives, opioids, analgesic medications, or alcohol products, which would further depress metabolic functions and increase risk of myxedema crisis

---

Critical Alert

Patients should be advised they will be taking thyroid replacement therapy for the remainder of their lives and not to discontinue this medication without consulting with their health care provider. Immediately report signs of myxedema, a severe, life-threatening illness with symptoms including facial edema, thick tongue (macroglossia), mental confusion, irritability, severe mood swings, significant hypothermia (91°F to 95°F), severely slowed pulse and respirations, decreased blood pressure, profound neuromuscular weakness, anemia, and signs of psychosis, because the mortality rate is high.

Hyperthyroidism

Hyperthyroidism is a hypermetabolic condition in which the thyroid gland produces an excess of thyroid hormone and the body increases cellular function in response.

This condition may lead to thyrotoxicosis, a clinical syndrome that results when tissues are exposed to high levels of circulating thyroid hormone.

Causes

- Graves' disease (an autoimmune disorder)
- Toxic multinodular goiter
- Painful subacute thyroiditis caused by a viral infection
- Adenomas of the thyroid gland

Risk Factors

- Genetics
- Stress of pregnancy or viral illness

- Excessive iodine intake
  - A history of amiodarone therapy (contains 37% iodine)
- Excessive thyroid hormone replacement therapy

Signs and Symptoms
- ↑ appetite
- Unexplained weight loss
- Heat intolerance
- Exertional dyspnea
- ↑ HR, palpitations
- Fatigue
- Fine tremors of hand and tongue
- Nervousness, hyperactivity
- Goiter
- Thyroid storm (life-threatening condition in which the body decompensates in overwhelming thyrotoxicosis)
  - Sinus or supraventricular tachycardia
  - Hyperpyrexia (with temperature above 40°C [104°F])
  - Confusion, delirium, and coma

Diagnostics
- Health history and physical examination
- Laboratory
  - ↓ TSH
  - Thyroxine level
    - ↑ Serum FT_4, T_4, T_3
- Imaging
  - Thyroid scanning
  - Ultrasonography
- Other
  - Fine-needle biopsy

Patient Care Management

- Medical
  - Antithyroid drugs (propylthiouracil (PTU)) and methimazole (Tapazole, Carbimazole)
  - Radioactive iodine (destroys all or part of the thyroid gland and makes it unable to produce excessive thyroid hormone)
  - Beta-blockers or calcium channel blockers (to control cardiac arrhythmias such as tachycardia and/or atrial fibrillation)
- Surgical
  - Subtotal thyroidectomy

Nursing Management

- Anxiety
  - Decrease environmental stimuli and promote a restful environment
  - Eliminate chemical stimulants such as caffeine from diet
  - Administer antithyroid drugs as prescribed
- Imbalanced Nutrition
  - Monitor weight daily
  - Offer patient a well-balanced diet with nutritional supplements and nutritional consultation as needed
  - Teach patient about effects of hypo- and hyperthyroidism on weight
- Risk for Injury
  - Encourage patient to flush eyes with warm water at intervals while awake
  - Encourage patient to use artificial tears to keep eyes moist, and to cover eyes while sleeping
- Decreased Cardiac Output
  - Evaluate vital signs frequently
  - Maintain a restful, calm supportive environment

- Assess toleration of physical activity and work with patient to gradually increase activity as tolerated
- Monitor for signs of hemorrhage post thyroidectomy

Critical Alert

Following a thyroidectomy it is essential that during the immediate postoperative period, the patient be observed closely for signs of hemorrhage or swelling in the operative site, as well as damage to the vocal cords or parathyroid glands. Check behind the neck for signs of pooling blood.

The postoperative patient should be readily observable by the nurse and have a call bell in order to get immediate attention should symptoms of respiratory distress be noted. The location of the thyroid gland in proximity to the trachea and vocal cords also presents a threat to the airway, should swelling or hemorrhage cause obstruction. A tracheostomy set should be readily available in case of this emergency.

In the event of accidental removal of part or all of the parathyroid glands, intravenous calcium should also be readily available.

- Monitor for thyroid storm (if present, ICU care needed)
  - Severe fever
  - Restlessness, agitation
  - Atrial fibrillation, CHF, angina
  - HTN rapidly changing to hypotension
  - Diaphoresis
- Knowledge Deficit
  - Instruct patients (who receive radioactive iodine) to avoid close contact with other persons for a period of days
  - Instruct the patient that small children will need to have alternative care during this period
  - Instruct patient to use a private toilet and be instructed to flush two times after each use
  - Advise patients they should not be involved in handling food preparation for others and should

launder towels and linens they use separately from others

- Inform patients of signs and symptoms of hypothyroidism because radioactive iodine treatment is likely to result in hypothyroidism over a period of several weeks to months

- Inform patient about thyroid functioning, particularly symptoms of both hypothyroid disease and hyperthyroid disease since treatments for either condition may result in the opposite condition

- Patients need to understand that they should receive regular follow up laboratory work to assess thyroid function since treatments for hyperthyroidism, including antithyroid drugs, radioactive iodine, and surgery, may result in a significant decrease or cessation in thyroid hormone production over time

- Patients need careful instruction about the need for follow-up after treatment for thyroid disorders until there is evidence that hormone levels are normal and have stabilized

HEARING AND BALANCE DISORDERS

Hearing Loss

The most prevalent disorder associated with the structures of the ear is hearing loss. This disorder is estimated to affect approximately 30 million Americans. The degree of hearing loss can range from mild to complete.

General Causes of Hearing Loss

- Conductive: Sound waves cannot reach the inner ear for processing and interpretation.

- Sensorineural: The cause is damage to the auditory nerve or possibly damage to the small hair cells within the inner ear.

- Mixed: Both conductive and sensorineural hearing loss are caused by a dysfunction of both air and bone conduction processes.

Specific causes of hearing loss disorders include those that are mechanical, inflammatory, or obstructive in nature. The table on page 201 summarizes hearing loss and balance disorders.

Balance Disorders

The primary symptom of a balance disorder is the development of vertigo. Defined as an attack of dizziness, vertigo is often described as a "spinning" sensation. This sensation can last from 10 minutes up to several hours or days. Oftentimes, the most comfortable position for a patient experiencing vertigo is lying flat, immobilizing the head. Sudden head movements can precipitate nausea/vomiting. In addition to irritability, the patient might complain of tinnitus and reduced hearing on the involved side.

Causes of vertigo include benign paroxysmal positional vertigo (BPPV), labyrinthitis, Meniere's disease, and acoustic neuroma.

Patient Care Management

(The Signs and Symptoms and Patient Care Management are summarized in the table starting on page 201.)

Regardless of the nature of the disorder the patient with a hearing or balance disorder benefit from the multidisciplinary team. Team members include audiologists and therapists in occupational and physical medicine and speech and hearing.

Nursing Management

- Disturbed sensory perception: Auditory Communication: Verbal, Impaired

  - Assess degree of hearing loss

  - Speak clearly and slowly in a normal to deep voice; face the patient when speaking; use touch to gain the patient's attention

  - Respond to call light as soon as possible

  - Provide emotional support to the patient having difficulty coping with the new sensory deficit

  - Provide sensory stimulation; encourage expressing feelings of concern and loss for hearing deficit

- Risk for Falls, Risk for Injury

  - Assist the patient with ambulation and other activities of daily living

  - Utilize safety measures such as keeping bedside rails in elevated position and call light within reach

- Knowledge Deficit

  - Teach about disease process, medications, and treatments

  - Instruct or reinforce instruction on use of hearing aid

  - Teach to watch for visual cues if hearing impaired

  - Explain the cause for dizziness and vertigo

  - Teach family how to assist patient with ambulation and activities of daily living upon discharge

Common Disorders of the Ear

Disorder	Description	Signs & Symptoms	Patient Care Management
Benign paroxysmal positional vertigo (BPPV)	Formation of otoconia (small crystals of calcium carbonate) Causes: • Head injury • Infection (including adminis-tration of ototoxic medications such as Gentamicin) • Disorders of the inner ear • Degeneration due to advanced age • Viruses affecting the ear causing vestibular neuritis • Minor strokes involving ante-rior inferior cerebellar artery • Meniere's disease	• Onset caused by a change in the position of the head with respect to gravity • Dizziness or vertigo • Lightheadedness • Imbalance • Nausea	• Watch and wait since symptoms are intermittent • Modifications in daily activities: • Use two or more pillows at night • Avoid sleeping on the "bad" side • Get up slowly and sit on the edge of the bed when arising • Avoid bending down to pick up things and extending the head • Be careful when lying back such as in a dentist's chair or beauty parlor sink

(continued)

Common Disorders of the Ear (*continued*)

Disorder	Description	Signs & Symptoms	Patient Care Management

	Diagnosis:
	• Medical history
	  • Use of ototoxic medications and a review of what triggers the symptoms
	• Physical examination
	• Results of vestibular and auditory tests.
			Medications:
			  • Antiemetics
			• Surgery:
			  • Posterior canal plugging

Labyrinthitis	Infection of the labyrinth from a complication of otitis media	• Hearing loss on affected side • Tinnitus • Spontaneous nystagmus to the affected side • Vertigo with associated nausea and vomiting	• Systemic antibiotics • Stay in darkened room • Antiemetics • Antivertiginous medications

Disorder	Description	Signs & Symptoms	Patient Care Management
Meniere's disease	Either overproduction or decreased reabsorption of endolymphatic fluid causing a distortion in the inner canal system	• Tinnitus • Unilateral sensorineural hearing loss • Vertigo	• Dietary and Lifestyle Modifications: • Salt restrictions • Fluid restrictions • No smoking • Medications: • Antivertiginous medications • Antiemetics • Mild diuretics • Antihistamines • Antianxiety medications • Surgery: • Labyrinthectomy • Endolymphatic Decompression
Acoustic neuroma	Benign tumor of cranial nerve VIII	• Mild vertigo • Tinnitus • Gradual sensorineural hearing loss	• Surgical removal with resultant permanent hearing loss

HEART FAILURE (HF)

Heart failure is a common, chronic condition in which the heart is unable to pump enough blood to sustain the metabolic demands of the body. If untreated, the disease will progress resulting in increased symptoms, hospitalizations, and possibly death. The debilitating clinical syndrome of heart failure ultimately leads to common symptoms of poor activity tolerance, fluid retention, and fatigue, that limit quality of life.

A series of compensatory mechanisms are triggered when the heart's pumping action is compromised. The initial response to decreased cardiac output is the activation of the sympathetic nervous system (SNS) and the renin-angiotensin-aldosterone system (RAAS). Circulating levels play an important role in vasoconstriction, sodium retention, and toxic effects of the heart. In the early stages SNS and RAAS activation augments preload, ventricular contractility, and heart rate. But as cardiac function progressively worsens, these compensatory mechanisms are no longer able to maintain cardiac output and further compromise ventricular function. Increased cardiac wall stress, hypertrophy chamber dilation, increased myocardial oxygen consumption, and worsening myocardial ischemia occurs.

Heart failure (HF) is most commonly caused by hypertension, coronary artery disease, and dilated cardiomyopathies. HF may cause systolic and diastolic dysfunction, which may occur simultaneously and usually result in the same set of symptoms.

Systolic Dysfunction (Left Ventricular Systolic Dysfunction—LVSD)

Characterized by impaired ventricular function, which results in volume overload and decreased contractility. Diagnosed when the left ventricular ejection fraction (LVEF) (the proportion of blood ejected during each ventricular contraction compared with the total ventricular filling volume) is below 40% to 45%. Progressive adverse structural and neuro-hormonal changes occur within the heart, leading to deteriorating cardiac function and symptoms of low cardiac output and congestion.

Diastolic Dysfunction

Known as heart failure with preserved LVEF. Diastolic dysfunction seems to be related to a stiff, noncompliant heart with prolonged relaxation. Results in decreased filling, increased left ventricular end diastolic pressure, and reduced stroke volume at rest or during exercise. Common among elderly women, frequently associated with hypertension, diabetes, obesity, and atrial fibrillation.

Heart failure can occur as right, left, and/or biventricular depending on the extent and anatomy of the damage. Acute heart failure occurs suddenly, resulting in rapid congestion in the pulmonary vasculature and periphery, and decreased cardiac output leading to poor perfusion. Chronic heart failure can either occur insidiously or acutely and will lead to progressive cardiac dysfunction, progressive symptoms, and eventually death.

Left-Sided Heart Failure

Impaired pumping ability of the left side of the heart, which eventually backs the blood up into the pulmonary circulation. Elevated pressure and congestion in the pulmonary veins and capillaries result as the disease progresses. Symptoms result from pulmonary congestion.

Right-Sided Heart Failure

The inability of the heart to function on the right side, leading to a backup of blood, followed by congestion and elevated pressure in the systemic veins and capillaries. The most common cause of right-sided dysfunction is left-sided failure. Symptoms result from volume overload leading to ascites and lower extremity edema.

Biventricular Heart Failure

Global inability of both ventricles of the heart to pump blood effectively. Forward blood flow is compromised, leading to right- and left-heart failure symptoms.

Signs and Symptoms

- Dyspnea—key factor limiting their ADLs
  - Exertional dyspnea, orthopnea, paroxysmal nocturnal dyspnea, dyspnea at rest
- Cough, hemoptysis; pink frothy sputum due to pulmonary edema
- Crackles
- Jugular venous distention
- S_3—volume overload
- S_4—ventricular stiffness
- Tachycardia
- Chest pain
- Ascites/ positive hepatojugular reflux
- Nausea, anorexia, bloating, abdominal distention, right upper quadrant pain
- Decreased urine output, nocturia
- Weight gain; pitting edema
- Fatigue, restlessness, agitation, mental deterioration
- Poor energy, poor exercise tolerance

Critical Alert
The elderly may present with less common or overt symptoms, such as fatigue, poor concentration, disorientation, and failure to thrive.

Diagnostics

- Laboratory
  - CBC——Infection and anemia can exacerbate symptoms
  - Electrolytes, Creatinine—Baseline measurements for diuretic therapy
  - Liver Function Tests—Evaluate hepatic congestion
  - Thyroid Function Test —Hypo- and hyperthyroidism can exacerbate symptoms
  - B-type natriuretic peptide (BNP)—Correlates with severity of symptoms and prognosis
  - Lipid panel
- Chest x-ray—Pulmonary congestion, hypertrophy
- ECG—Dysrhythmia detection, ventricular hypertrophy, myocardial ischemia
- Echocardiogram—Evaluate size and function of chambers, wall motion, wall thickness, valvular structure and function
- Cardiac catheterization/PCI—Evaluate volume overload, pulmonary hypertension, CAD evaluation and treatment

Patient Care Management

- Treatment Goals for Acute Heart Failure
  - Rapid and thorough assessment of volume status, the extent of peripheral and organ perfusion
  - Identify precipitating conditions and prevent life-threatening conditions (cardiogenic shock, multiorgan failure, and death)
  - Relieve symptoms, stabilizing hemodynamic parameters, improving organ function
- Treatment Goals for Chronic Heart Failure
  - Alleviate symptoms of congestion
  - Improve perfusion

- Increase activity tolerance
- Improve quality of life
- Identify and treat precipitating conditions
- Decrease hospitalizations; reduce readmissions
- Slow or reverse progression of cardiac dysfunction
- Minimize risk factors
- Provide palliative care

Critical Alert

Factors that may precipitate or exacerbate heart failure are numerous and may be related to new or poorly controlled comorbid conditions, noncompliance, iatrogenic causes, or lack of adequate follow-up.

- Drug Therapy

Goal of medication therapy is to inhibit the neurohormonal response—SNS and RAAS, and relieve the symptoms of congestion.
  - ACE
  - ARB
  - Beta-adrenergic blockers
  - Diuretics
  - Digitalis
  - Aldosterone antagonists
  - Hydralazine and isosorbide dinitrate
  - Antiarrhythmics
    (See Appendix #22, Summary of Medications to Treat Heart Failure.)
- Procedural/Surgical Therapy
  - Cardiac catheterization to rule out CAD
  - Percutaneous coronary interventions
  - Implantable cardioverter defibrillator (ICD) to prevent sudden cardiac death

- Cardiac resynchronization therapy (CRT)—Biventricular pacemaker to help increase cardiac output if ejection fraction less than 35%
- Cardiac artery bypass surgery
- Cardiac valve replacement or repair
- Mechanical assist devices
- Heart transplantation

Critical Alert

Patients with heart failure need a multidisciplinary team approach to achieve optimal recovery and return to society. Close scrutiny is required by the team to provide optimal, evidence-based care. When heart failure reaches a terminal stage, palliative care is treatment done to reduce symptoms and suffering in end-of-life planning.

Nursing Management
Excess Fluid Volume

- Assess
  - Vital signs—Be alert for tachycardia and increased work of breathing
  - Lung sounds
  - Daily weight
  - Careful intake and output
  - Edema
- Limit sodium intake and fluids, as ordered
- Administer diuretics and evaluate electrolyte status

Alterations in Cardiac Output and Tissue Perfusion

- Assess
  - Vital signs
  - Skin color, temp
  - Heart Sounds
    - S_4—ventricular stiffness
    - S_3—volume overload
    - Presence of murmur

- Jugular venous distention
- Dysrhythmias
- Anxiety
- Administer oxygen as ordered

> **Critical Alert**
> Signs of abrupt decline in cardiac output include: resting tachycardia; narrow pulse pressure; cool extremities; altered mentation; hypotension; Cheyne–Stokes respiration; rise in BUN/creatinine; oliguria.

Activity Intolerance
- Monitor patient activity tolerance
- Encourage activities of daily living
- Space activities to allow for periods of rest

Knowledge Deficit
- Teaching plan includes
  - Dietary restrictions (fluids and sodium)
  - Importance of daily weight
  - Symptoms of increasing heart failure and when to notify health care provider
  - Review of medication regimens and side effects
  - Lifestyle changes to prevent a progression of the disease

    (See Appendix #23, Nursing Process: Patient Care Plan for Heart Failure.)

HEMATOLOGIC DISORDERS

Anemia

Anemia is defined as a decrease in the total body erythrocyte volume, usually measured by a decrease in hemoglobin protein, a decreased hematocrit, and/or a decreased red blood cell (RBC) count. The primary function of the erythrocytes is the transportation of oxygen on the hemoglobin molecules; thus, insufficiencies in the erythrocytes translate into an inability to maintain sufficient oxygen delivery to the tissues.

Causes

- Loss of blood volume
- Altered production of erythrocytes (hypoproliferative disorders)
- Altered (increased) destruction of red blood cells

Classifications

- Mild anemia (hemoglobin value of 10 to 12 g/dL)
- Moderate anemia (hemoglobin volume of 7 to 11 g/dL)
- Severe anemia (hemoglobin volume of < 7 g/dL and a hematocrit of < 25%)

Generalized Anemia

Despite the type of anemia, many clinical manifestations, diagnostics, and treatment goals will be the same and are discussed below. Specific disorders are presented in the following pages.

Signs and Symptoms

Signs and symptoms are related to anemic hypoxia (or decreased oxygen availability to the tissues specifically due to decreased concentration of functional hemoglobin or a reduced number of red blood cells).

- Abnormal paleness or lack of color of the skin
- ↑ HR (tachycardia)
  - Angina acute myocardial infarction
- ↑ RR(tachypnea)
- Breathlessness, or difficulty catching a breath (dyspnea)
- Lack of energy, or tiring easily (fatigue)
  - Exertional dyspnea or lack of endurance
  - Inability to engage in activities of daily living (ADLs)
- Dizziness, or vertigo, especially when standing
- Headache
- Irritability
- ↓ hemoglobin, ↓ hematocrit, ↓ RBCs

Diagnostics

- Laboratory
  - Complete blood count (CBC) (see chart)
  - Arterial blood gases (ABGs) (detects acid–base disturbances used in the evaluation of hypoxia)

Summary of Common Complete Blood Count Findings in Anemia

Lab Value	Normal Value	Expected Abnormality in Anemia	Rationale for Abnormality
Hemoglobin	*Women:* 12–16 g/dL *Men:* 13.5–18 g/dL	Decreased	Decreased hemoglobin production due to decreased erythrocyte production
Hematocrit	*Women:* 38–47% *Men:* 40–54%	Decreased	Decreased concentration of hemoglobin protein due to decreased erythrocyte production
Total RBC count	4.0–5.0 10^6/uL	Decreased	Reflects decreased total erythrocyte volume
Reticulocytes	0.5–1.5% of RBC count	Depends on etiology	Varies according to underlying etiology (acute or chronic, bone marrow involvement)

Patient Care Management

Comprehensive care of the patient with anemia requires the collaboration of an interdisciplinary team including registered dietitians, physical and occupational therapists, respiratory therapists, pharmacists, health care providers, and nurses. The overall treatment goal for anemia is to correct the tissue hypoxia by correcting the underlying abnormality.

Nursing Management

- Activity Intolerance
  - Assess for pallor, malaise, fatigue
  - Monitor laboratory values (e.g., hemoglobin, hematocrit, platelets)

> **Critical Alert**
>
> A significant drop in hemoglobin values (> 3 g/dL over a short period of time [< 24 hours]) should be reported immediately to the health care provider. This may indicate active blood loss. This finding is of particular concern if blood loss is not readily visible (e.g., from gums, emesis, or stool) suggesting internal bleeding. Patients should be immediately assessed for level of consciousness, lung sounds, and acute areas of pain.

- Assess normal activity pattern throughout day
- Provide assistance with activities
- Self-Care Deficit
  - Modify activities to coincide with patient's biologic energy cycles
- Impaired Gas Exchange
  - Monitor oxygen saturation levels and ABGs
  - Assess for dyspnea, ventilation depth, ↑ RR
  - Administer supplemental oxygen as needed
  - Assess for dizziness and cyanosis
  - Assess level of alertness and mental acuity
  - Administer blood transfusions (See Procedures and Therapies: Bleeding Precautions.)
  - Monitor for signs of transfusion reaction (See Appendix #33, Transfusion Reactions.)

- Risk of Injury, Falls
  - Monitor for unsteady gait, difficulty with transfers, orthopnea
  - Adjust environment to minimize risk of falls by placing necessary items within reach of patient, positioning bed in low and locked position, frequent observation
  - Reinforce patient instruction to call for assistance with ambulation
  - Assess vital signs (pulse, respirations, and BP) prior to ambulation
- Knowledge Deficit
  - Determine patient's previous knowledge of or skills related to his or her diagnosis and the influence on willingness to learn
  - Provide developmentally appropriate patient education that addresses underlying disease process, diet modification, medications, and activity modification

Anemia from Acute Blood Loss

Anemia from acute blood loss describes the loss of RBC volume due to RBCs leaving the circulating vascular space. It comprises a heterogeneous group of disorders ranging from "slow bleeds" to rapid trauma.

Causes

- Trauma
- Menorrhagia (excessive menstrual bleeding)
- Disorders of the gastrointestinal mucosa
- Slow cranial bleeding
- Internal hemorrhage

Signs and Symptoms

(See Generalized Anemia.)

- ↓ level of alertness
- ↓ urinary output

- Diaphoresis
- Bleeding into closed spaces (cranial vault)
  - Tenderness or severe pain
  - Swelling
  - Sudden changes in neurological status
  - Eventually death
- Gastrointestinal bleeding
  - Fecal occult blood in the stool
  - Melena (black tarry stools)

Diagnostics

- Health History and Physical Examination (determine cause of bleeding)
- Laboratory (See Generalized Anemia.)
- Imaging
  - CT scan, x-ray, MRI

Patient Care Management

- Medical
  - Treat underlying cause (e.g., gastric ulcer, cerebral hemorrhage, trauma)
  - Blood product administration
    - Given for: sudden decrease in hematocrit by more than 3%, significant observable hemorrhage, a hematocrit of < 25%, or severe impending hypovolemia

Nursing Management (See Generalized Anemia.)
- Cardiac Output, Decreased
  - Monitor for ↓ BP, ↑ HR, ↑ urine output
  - Assess quality of pulses
  - Monitor for presence of chest pain and ECG changes
  - Monitor accurate I&O
  - Maintain two large-bore IVs at all times

> **Critical Alert**
>
> Any patient reporting with sudden pain in the abdominal area, retroperitoneal area, or musculoskeletal fascial compartments or a change in level of consciousness should be immediately assessed for blood pressure, pulse, and respiratory rate changes. These may indicate bleeding into a closed space, which requires immediate medical intervention. Do not rely on changes in laboratory values because these may not accurately reflect blood loss.

Iron-Deficiency Anemia (IDA)

- Absolute iron deficiencies:
    - Excess iron loss (leading cause of IDA)
    - Iron absorption abnormalities
        - Surgical manipulation, Crohn's disease, celiac disease, liver disease
    - Insufficient dietary intake
- Functional iron deficiency:
    - Failure to supply enough iron to the bone marrow for erythropoiesis, despite adequate total body iron stores (e.g., chronic inflammatory condition)

        When any of the preceding situations occurs, demand for iron can exceed iron intake resulting in insufficient iron intake.

Signs and Symptoms (See Generalized Anemia.)

- Initially asymptomatic
- Pica (clay/dirt eating)
- Glossitis (tongue inflammation)
- Gastric atrophy
- Stomatitis
- Pagophagia (ice eating)
- Leg cramping

Diagnostics

- Health History and Physical Examination
- Laboratory
    - $\downarrow$ hemoglobin and hematocrit

- Microcytic erythrocytes ($\downarrow$ size of MCV, MCHC, and MCH)
- Bone marrow aspiration revealing absent marrow stores of iron
- $\downarrow$ serum iron, serum ferritin, and serum transferrin
- $\uparrow$ total iron binding capacity (TIBC)
- $\downarrow$ serum ferritin
- $\uparrow$ serum transferrin
- Positive fecal occult blood

Patient Care Management (See Generalized Anemia.)
- Medical
  - Dietary Modifications (red meats, fish)
  - Medication
    - Oral (ferrous sulfate)
    - Parenteral (for more rapid correction of depleted iron stores or patients with chronic kidney disease)

Nursing Management (See Generalized Anemia.)
- Knowledge Deficit
  - Instruct patient and family about signs and symptoms of GI blood loss and to report to health care provider
  - Explain administration techniques of oral and parenteral iron replacement

---

Critical Alert

During any administration of IV iron supplementation, if the patient reports any signs and symptoms of hypersensitivity or allergic reaction, stop the infusion, stay with the patient, monitor the airway, and call the health care provider immediately.

  - Encourage proper positioning (high Fowler's or sitting), mobilization, and fluid intake to minimize digestive problems with medications
  - Educate patient and family regarding importance of preventing constipation while taking supplements

- Encourage patient to take iron tablets with vitamin C (e.g., orange juice, strawberries) to help absorption
- Consult with clinical nutritionist for dietary recommendations and to prevent drug and food interactions that inhibit iron absorption.

Anemia of Chronic Disease (ACD)

Anemia is a common consequence of chronic diseases. The most common chronic diseases associated with anemia are cancer, chronic kidney failure, autoimmune disorders, and infectious diseases such as acquired immunodeficiency syndrome (AIDS). Chemical signals produced by invading bacteria or a virus, a tumor, or the body itself attack erythropoietic cells and organs to negatively impact erythrocyte production and iron metabolism. The result is a measurable decrease in erythrocytes, hemoglobin, and hematocrit, along with hypoxia, activity intolerance, and fatigue.

Signs and Symptoms (See Generalized Anemia.)

- Exacerbation of symptoms unique to the underlying disease process
  - ↑ myelosuppression
  - Infection
  - Left ventricular hypertrophy
  - Congestive heart failure
  - Headaches, loss of concentration, depression, and memory impairment

Diagnostics

- Health History and Physical Examination
- Laboratory
  - ↓ hemoglobin levels (8 and 9.5 g/dL)
  - ↓ total erythrocytes and reticulocytes (indicates diminished erythropoiesis)
  - ↓ ferritin and transferrin levels

Patient Care Management

The goal of therapy in ACD is maintenance of hemoglobin and hematocrit at sufficient levels to promote disease healing and prevent systemic complications. The target range for hemoglobin and hematocrit are Hgb 11 g/dL (Hct 33%) to Hgb 12 g/dL (Hct 36%).

- Medical
  - Blood transfusions
    - In severe anemia (Hgb < 8) or with obvious signs of bleeding (e.g., visible loss of blood or a significant drop in hemoglobin/hematocrit in a relatively short period of time)
  - Iron supplementation
    - Absolute iron deficiency
    - Patients being treated with erythropoietic agents
  - Erythropoietic agents
    - Exogenous forms of erythropoietin, the primary stimulating hormone of erythropoiesis produced in the kidneys
    - Chronic kidney disease and patients undergoing chemotherapy or immunosuppressive therapy

Nursing Management (See Generalized Anemia.)

Megaloblastic Anemias

Major Causes

- Folate deficiency (deficient dietary intake of folic acid)
- Vitamin B_{12} deficiency
- Pernicious anemia (malabsorption of vitamin B_{12})

Other Causes

- Intestinal malabsorption due to chronic GI inflammatory processes or surgical shortening
- General malnutrition
- Liver disease
- Chronic hemolytic anemias

- Anticonvulsant medications such as phenytoin that interfere with folate absorption
- Drugs that have antifolate activity including methotrexate and trimethoprim
- Chemotherapies with DNA suppression activity
- Alcohol abuse

Signs and Symptoms (See Generalized Anemia.)
- Gastrointestinal
    - Swollen and sore tongue (classically described as "smooth and beefy red")
    - Anorexia, nausea
- Integumentary
    - Hyperpigmentation over the hands and knuckles
- Neurological (vitamin B_{12} deficiency only)
    - Peripheral neuropathy
    - Unsteadiness, lack of coordination, ataxia
    - Confusion and memory loss
    - $\downarrow$ reflexes, positive Babinski's sign may be observed

Diagnostics
- Health history and physical examination
    - Determine dietary causes and problems with absorption
- Laboratory (See Generalized Anemia.)
    - Vitamin B_{12} ($<$100 pg/mL)
    - Folate level ($<$ 5 ng/mL)
    - Schilling test
        - Oral radioactively labeled vitamin B_{12} followed by 24 hour urine collection to determine vitamin B_{12} excretion
        - Parenteral dose may be indicated followed by 24 hour urine collection.
- Imaging
    - Various studies used to determine cause

Patient Care Management

- Medical
  - Medication review (for causative agents)
  - Dietary modifications
  - Vitamin supplementation
    - Oral or intravenous (for alcoholism)
  - Collaboration with clinical nutritionalist and pharmacists for dietary recommendations and monitoring of drug interactions

Nursing Management (See Generalized Anemia.)

- Risk for Injury, Falls
  - Assess sensation to extremities prior to ambulation
  - Implement fall precautions
- Knowledge Deficit
  - Instruct patient regarding risk factors and disease development, specifically during pregnancy and with advanced age
  - Patient education and reinforcement regarding dietary modifications and/or supplementation
  - Instruct patient in correct technique for IM injections of vitamin B_{12} and the importance of compliance with prescribed administration routine

Hemoglobinopathies

Hemoglobinopathy is a term used to describe a class of genetic red blood cell disorders characterized by abnormal hemoglobin, which can result in a variety of clinical problems, including hypoxia, accelerated RBC destruction, and decreased RBC production.

Sickle Cell Disease

Sickle cell anemia is the term given to a group of genetically based RBC diseases all characterized by misshapen "sickle-shaped" red blood cells. The source of the sickling is a malfunctioning hemoglobin molecule that twists the entire RBC from a soft, pliable, round donut shape into a long, hard, sticky elongated cell.

Sickle cells possess "sticky membranes" and unusual shapes that occlude small blood vessels that serve to further potentiate oxygen deprivation.

Signs and Symptoms

Onset of signs and symptoms is typically triggered by stressors such as infection, blood loss, or high altitudes.

- Pain
  - Bone and abdominal pain
  - Chest pain
  - Erections due to veno-occlusion
- Acute renal failure (due to arterial occlusion in the renal capillaries)
- Pulmonary tissue infarction (due to capillary occlusion and hypoventilation secondary to rib/sternal bone infarction)
- Splenomegaly (enlarged spleen) results from splenic sequestration
- Avascular necrosis (AVN), also known as aseptic necrosis of the large joints (due to interruption of the arterial supply of the femoral head)
  - Severe chronic joint pain
  - ↓ weight-bearing ability
  - Joint malformation
- Hemolytic anemia (due to the accelerated breakdown of red blood cells)
  - Splenomegaly
  - Jaundice
  - ↓ urine output
- Sickle cell crisis
  - Cells trapped by spleen lead to reduced circulating red blood cells
  - Widespread hypoxia
  - Severe pain
  - Possible organ failure

Diagnostics
- Health history and physical examination
- Laboratory
  - CBC
    - RBC morphology (to determine the prevalence of sickle cell hemoglobin)
    - Hemoglobin electrophoresis
    - $\downarrow$ RBCs
    - $\uparrow$ bilirubin

Patient Care Management
The cornerstone of sickle cell disease management is prevention of sickle cell crisis by ensuring adequate oxygenation via avoidance of triggering events at all times. Because patients are usually diagnosed as children, prevention of sickle cell crisis states should always involve collaboration with the parent. Interdisciplinary team members should include pharmacists, physical and occupational therapists, respiratory therapists, medical specialists such as hematologists, and the patient's primary health care provider.

- Medical
  - Oxygen therapy
  - Pain control
  - Hydration
  - Transfusions

Nursing Management (See Generalized Anemia.)
- Risk for Ineffective Tissue Perfusion: Cerebral, renal, cardiopulmonary, and abdominal organ
  - Frequently monitor neurological signs including level of consciousness, Glasgow Coma Scale, papillary changes, and cranial nerves
  - Assess for renal function (presence of edema, urine output, BUN, creatinine, urinalysis)
  - Report changes in assessment findings and laboratory data to health care provider

- Encourage oral fluid intake and administer intravenous fluid (dextrose 5% in water or in 0.45% normal saline)
- Assess peripheral pulses, heart tones, presence of jugular vein distention, and edema
- Encourage patient to avoid strenuous activity
- Assess for adventitious or diminished breath sounds
- Monitor respiratory rate and depth
- Administer high-flow oxygen therapy and assess oxygen saturation
- Obtain ABGs if O_2 sat falls below 80%
- Provide incentive spirometry every hour
- Assess for abdominal pain and tenderness
- Monitor for nausea, appetite, vomiting, and diarrhea
- Offer small, frequent meals

- Pain, Acute
  - Collaborate with patient to determine preferred pain control modalities
  - Assess pain, including rating and character frequently and reassess after any pain intervention
  - Administer pain medication on fixed schedule
  - Transfuse RBCs as needed
  - Monitor for transfusion reaction (See Appendix #33.)

- Knowledge Deficit
  - Explain cause of disease, including triggers and risks of sickle cell crisis
  - Describe activities/scenarios that can exacerbate hypoxic state emphasizing oxygenation and hydration
  - Teach family to recognize key physical symptoms of sickle cell crisis
  - Discuss appropriate use of oxygenation
  - Discuss appropriate use of pain medication to control pain

- Discuss role of balanced nutrition emphasizing need for key elements: vitamin B_{12}, folate, and iron
- Refer patient to dietitian for assistance in meal planning
- Discuss and explore appropriate physical exercise options that would maintain muscle/bone/ cardiovascular strength but limits risks of hypoxia

Thalassemia

Thalassemia refers to a group of hematologic genetic disorders characterized by a structural change (alpha or beta chains of the hemoglobin molecule are missing) in the hemoglobin molecule that subjects affected red blood cells to increased rates of hemolysis.

Signs and Symptoms (most common in beta-thalassemia major)

- Jaundice
- Splenomegaly
- Skeletal changes
- Pallor, tachycardia, and lethargy

Diagnostics

- Health history and physical examination
- Laboratory
  - ↓ hemoglobin and RBCs

Patient Care Management

- Blood transfusions
- Serum ferritin levels
- Intravenous or subcutaneous desferrioxamine (Desferal) to bind and neutralize excessive iron
- Intravenous and oral hydration
- Oxygen therapy

Nursing Management (See Generalized Anemia.)

Hemolytic Anemia

Hemolytic anemia is a term applied to wide range of diseases characterized by increased RBC destruction, or hemolysis. Infection, toxins, certain medications, injury, and other environmental stressors can all trigger minor increases in hemolysis, which then result in a decrease in circulating red blood cells, triggering hypoxia.

Causes

- Intrinsic causes
  - Deficiencies in metabolic protective enzymes (glucose-6-phosphate dehydrogenase deficiency)
  - Fragility and instability in the membrane structure (spherocytosis)
  - Increased hemolysis (hemoglobinopathies)
- Extrinsic causes
  - Infections, certain medications, autoimmune processes, toxins, and malignancies

Signs and Symptoms

- Hypoxia
  - Fatigue, activity intolerance
  - ↑ RR and HR
- Jaundice
- Hemoglobinuria (red-brown urine)
- Splenomegaly
- Hepatomegaly
- Acute renal failure (↓ and concentrated urine output)

Diagnostics

- Health history and physical examination
- Laboratory
  - CBC
    - ↑ reticulocytes (due to accelerated erythropoiesis)
    - ↓ reticulocytes (as bone marrow cannot replace RBCs)
    - ↓ RBC counts
  - ↑ serum erythropoietin

- ↓ Serum haptoglobin
- ↑ unconjugated bilirubin, ↑ increased lactate dehydrogenase (LDH), ↑ serum AST (SGOT)

Patient Care Management
- Medical
  - Oxygen therapy
  - Intravenous fluids
  - Removal of triggering agents (e.g., infection, toxins, medications)
- Surgical
  - Splenectomy (indicated if there are no identifiable triggering agents or in severe cases of acquired hemolytic anemia)

Nursing Management (See Generalized Anemia.)

Nursing care of the patient with hemolytic anemia has three main goals: avoidance of triggering factors in susceptible patients and prevention and treatment of complications.

- Injury, Risk for
  - Monitor I and O
  - Assess color and concentration of urine
  - Assess for left flank pain (suggests splenomegaly)
  - Monitor lung sounds, presence of edema, and skin turgor
  - Implement fall precautions as needed
  - Assess skin for breakdown and implement pressure ulcer prevention measures as appropriate

Aplastic Anemia

Aplastic anemia is a relatively rare disorder characterized by severe pancytopenia (low or absent red blood cells, white blood cells, and platelets) in both the periphery and bone marrow. Aplastic anemia is thought to be caused by damage to the hematopoietic stem cells (HSCs), resulting in their inability to reproduce and differentiate. Causes are either idiopathic (unknown), due to toxic exposure, infectious processes, or in relationship to another disease process.

Signs and Symptoms

- Pancytopenia
  - ↓ platelets
    - Mucocutaneous bleeding, easy bruising, and oozing from puncture sites
  - ↓ WBCs
    - Frequent infections
  - ↓ RBCs
    - Hypoxia
- Absent HSCs from the bone marrow

Diagnostics

- Health history and physical examination
- Laboratory
  - CBC
  - Bone marrow aspiration

Patient Care Management

- Medical
  - Immunosuppressive therapy
    - Antithymocyte globulin (ATG) and cyclosporine A (CsA)
  - Prophylactic antibiotics and antifungal medications
  - Iron chelation (to reduce excess iron stores)
- Surgical and procedural
  - Stem cell transplant

Nursing Management

(See Generalized Anemia, Thrombocytopenia, and Bleeding Disorders.)

Hemostasis, Disorders of

When the tight regulation of hemostasis is disrupted by disease, drugs, or environmental factors, the affected patient can present with abnormal bleeding, abnormal clotting, or in some cases both.

Disorders of Primary Hemostasis

Disorders of primary hemostasis include any problems affecting platelets or platelet interaction with the subendothelial vessel layer. All of these disorders result in prolonged bleeding times, resulting from slowed platelet plug formation.

Thrombocytopenia

Thrombocytopenia is defined as a decrease in the number of circulating platelets from the normal value of 150,000/iL.

Causes

- Impaired or suppressed production of platelets
  - Leukemia, lymphoma, multiple myeloma, metastatic cancers, and aplastic anemia
  - Chemotherapy, radiation therapy
  - Liver disease, exposure to viruses, drugs (e.g., thiazide diuretics)
- Accelerated destruction of platelets
  - Autoimmune (e.g., SLE, RA, HIV, multiple transfusions, drugs including depakote and heparin)
  - Non-autoimmune (e.g., prosthetic heart valves, thrombotic thrombocytopenic purpura [TTP], sepsis, and hemolytic uremic syndrome)

Signs and Symptoms

- Bleeding
  - Mucosal
    - Gums (following aggressive brushing or flossing)
    - Urinary tract
    - Nares

- Sputum after coughing
- Stool
- Cutaneous
  - Discoloration of the skin
  - Petechiae (small pinpoint lesions)
  - Purpura (larger group patches)
  - Ecchymosis
- Closed spaces
  - Cranium, pleural space, pericardial space, or abdomen

Diagnostics
- Health history and physical examination
- Laboratory
  - Platelet count
  - Bleeding time

Patient Care Management
- Medical
  - Treat the underlying cause
  - Platelet transfusion
  - Corticosteroids and IV immunoglobulin
- Surgical
  - Splenectomy

Nursing Management
Nurses in a variety of clinical settings must be familiar with the risks, early signs, and management of these diseases because they can occur as a side effect of a vast array of diseases and treatments.

Critical Alert

Patients who present with platelet counts of less than 20,000 μL are at imminent risk of internal bleeding. A drop in the platelet count below this level should be immediately reported to the health care provider as part of a comprehensive assessment including neurological, respiratory, cardiovascular, and abdominal symptoms. Prepare for possible platelet transfusion.

(See Appendix #35, Nursing Process: Patient Care Plan for Thrombocytopenia and Bleeding Disorders.) (See Procedures and Therapies: Bleeding Precautions.)

Immune Thrombocytopenia Purpura

Immune thrombocytopenic purpura (ITP) (previously referred to as idiopathic thrombocytopenic purpura) is an autoimmune disease marked by a decrease in the number of platelets due to destruction by antibodies produced against a patient's own platelets.

Signs and Symptoms (See Thrombocytopenia.)

Diagnostics (See Thrombocytopenia.)

Patient Care Management

- Medical
  - Remove the triggering event (if identifiable) and abatement of the immune response
  - Treat underlying disease process
  - Steroids (prednisone)
  - Intravenous immunoglobulin (IVIG)
- Surgical
  - Splenectomy

Nursing Management

(See Appendix #35.) (See Procedures and Therapies: Bleeding Precautions)

Heparin-Induced Thrombocytopenia (HIT)

Heparin-induced thrombocytopenia is an example of drug-induced, immune-mediated thrombocytopenia occurring in 3% of patients treated with unfractionated heparin for thrombosis. This disorder occurs most frequently in patients undergoing cardiovascular or orthopedic surgeries, because heparin is widely utilized to prevent thrombosis in these high-risk populations.

Signs and Symptoms

- ↓ Platelet count

Diagnostics

- Health history and physical examination
  - Clinical diagnosis of HIT is made on the basis of reduction of the platelet count, correlation with heparin administration, and when other causes (drugs, viruses, and bone marrow involvement) have been excluded.
- Laboratory
  - Platelet count
  - Anti-heparin platelet factor 4 (AHPF4) antibody

Patient Care Management

- Medical
  - Baseline platelet count prior to initiating heparin therapy
  - Frequent monitoring of platelet count
  - Cessation of all heparin therapy
  - Lepirudin (direct thrombin inhibitors)
    - Monitor PTT and INR
  - Warfarin (Coumadin)

Nursing Management

Nurses should carefully monitor the platelet counts of any patient receiving any form of heparin treatment. (See Appendix #35.) (See Procedures and Therapies: Bleeding Precautions.)

Von Willebrand's Disease (vWD)

Von Willebrand's disease is the most common inherited bleeding disorder and results from mutations in the essential clotting factor (von Willebrand's factor [Vwf]), which plays key roles in both primary and secondary hemostasis.

Signs and Symptoms

- Prolonged bleeding after minor cuts
- Bleeding from the gums
- Mucocutaneous bleeding (petechiae, ecchymosis)

- Prolonged bleeding times
- ↓ serum vWF (via ELISA test)
- Normal platelet count, PT, aPTT, and INR

Diagnostics
- Health history and physical examination
- Laboratory
  - Platelet count, PT, aPTT, and INR
  - ELISA test
  - Bleeding time

Patient Care Management
- Medical
  - Treat current symptoms
  - Desmopressin vasopressin analog (DDAVP), a synthetic hormone usually given by injection or nasal spray (prior to invasive procedures)
  - Transfusion of Factor VIII with fresh frozen plasma (FFP) or cryoprecipitate
    - Predisposes the patient to fluid overload and transfusion reactions

Nursing Management
(See Appendix #35.) (See Procedures and Therapies: Bleeding Precautions)

Disorders of Secondary Hemostasis

Disorders of secondary hemostasis refer to any disease process that disrupts the formation of the fibrin sheath via errors in the tissue factor (extrinsic) pathway or the contact activation (intrinsic) pathway. The most common cause of these disorders is deficiencies in quantity or quality of the clotting factors. Disorders of secondary hemostasis can occur days to weeks after an injury and in the deep subcutaneous layers, the muscles, and the joints.

Hemophilia

Hemophilia is a chronic condition that arises from the inheritance of mutated genes controlling Factor VIII or

Factor IX. Characteristic presenting symptoms are uncontrolled bleeding particularly into large muscle groups and joints.

Signs and Symptoms
- Prolonged bleeding and an inability to form clots
- Bleeding can have serious life-threatening consequences
  - Bleeding occurs deep in the tissues (joints and organs)
  - ↓ ICP
  - Hemiarthrosis (bleeding into the joints)
    - Leads to compartment syndrome
  - Oropharyngeal bleeding (into the esophagus)

Diagnostics
- Health history and physical examination
- Laboratory
  - CBC
  - Bleeding time
  - Platelet count, PT, aPTT, and INR
    - Only aPTT is prolonged or abnormal
  - Serum levels of Factor VIII and Factor IX

Patient Care Management
- Medical
  - Discontinue aspirin or other platelet interfering agents
  - DDAVP
  - Factor replacement therapy (via fresh frozen plasma)
  - Antifibrinolytics (most useful for mucosal and oral bleeding)

Nursing Management
(See Appendix #35.) (See Procedures and Therapies: Bleeding Precautions.)

Disseminated Intravascular Coagulation (DIC)

Disseminated intravascular coagulation is triggered by an injury or event leading to persistent activation of the clotting cascade. It manifests as widespread clot formation and thrombosis.

Triggers

- Sepsis
- Trauma (including surgery)
- Malignancy
- Toxin exposure
- Obstetric complications

Signs and Symptoms

- Bleeding from mucosa and catheter sites
- Petechiae, ecchymosis, and purpura
- Extremities with ↓ sensation and cool to the touch
- Altered level of consciousness
- Hemoptysis
- Pain described as swelling, sharp
- Shortness of breath/tachypnea
- Fatigue
- ↓ BP and ↑ HR

Diagnostics

- Health history and physical examination
- Laboratory
  - PT, aPTT (prolonged)
  - INR (increased)
  - Fibrinogen (decreased)
  - Clotting Factors V, VIII, X, XIII (decreased)
  - Fibrin degradation products and D-dimer (positive)
  - Clotting inhibitors: Antithrombin III and protein (decreased)

Patient Care Management

- Medical
  - Complete removal of the underlying injury
  - Anticoagulant therapy
  - Replacement therapy
    - Transfusion of platelets, FFP, or concentrations of coagulation factors
  - Restoration of anticoagulant (antithrombin) pathways
    - Activated protein C and antithrombin concentrations

Nursing Management

(See Appendix #35.) (See Procedures and Therapies: Bleeding Precautions.)

- Fluid Volume, Risk for Deficient
  - Accurate I and O
  - Monitor vital signs for ↓ BP, ↑ HR
  - Assess skin turgor and level of consciousness
  - Maintain intravenous access at all times
  - Prepare for intravenous hydration and blood product administration
- Tissue Perfusion, Ineffective
  - Administer oxygen therapy and evaluate O_2 sats
  - Assess color, temperature, and moisture of skin
  - Monitor mental status
  - Assess skin condition frequently (including mucous membranes)
  - Administer heparin therapy
    - Monitor laboratory studies for effectiveness

HYPERTENSION

Hypertension

Blood pressure is defined as the pressure created by the circulating blood through the arteries, veins, and the chambers of the heart. High blood pressure is an elevation of systemic blood pressure that is noted to be sustained. Sixty-five million adult Americans or one-third of the general adult population in the United States have hypertension. If high blood pressure remains undiagnosed and untreated, it has a high morbidity and mortality rate.

Classification of Blood Pressure for Adults

BP Classification	SBP (mmHg)	DBP (mmHg)	Lifestyle Modification Encouraged
Normal	<120	and <90	
Prehypertension	120–139	Or 80–89	Yes
Stage 1 hypertension	140–159	Or 90–99	Yes
Stage 2 hypertension	>160	Or >100	Yes

Risk Factors

- Cigarette smoking
- Obesity
- Physical inactivity
- Dyslipidemia
- Diabetes mellitus

- Microalbuminuria or estimated GFR < 60 mL/min
- Age (older than 55 years for men and 65 years for women)
- Family history of premature cardiovascular disease (men under age 55 and women under age 65)
- Gender
- Sodium intake
- Excessive alcohol consumption
- Atherosclerosis

Contributing Factors
- Modifiable Factors
  - High sodium dietary intake
  - Overweight
  - Excessive alcohol consumption
  - Low potassium intake
  - Smoking
- Nonmodifiable Factors
  - Family history
  - Age
  - Race

Causes
- Sleep apnea
- Drug-induced or -related causes
- Chronic kidney disease
- Primary aldosteronism
- Renovascular disease
- Chronic steroid therapy and Cushing's syndrome
- Pheochromocytoma
- Coarctation of the aorta
- Thyroid or parathyroid disease
- Unknown

Complications
- Cardiac
    - Left ventricular hypertrophy
    - Angina or prior myocardial infarction
    - Prior coronary revascularization
    - Heart failure
- Neurologic
    - Stroke or transient ischemic attack
- Renal
    - Chronic kidney disease
    - Renal failure
- Peripheral arterial disease
    - Peripheral ischemia
- Retinopathy
    - Vision changes leading to blindness
- Aortic artery aneurysm

Hypertensive Emergencies
- Hypertensive crisis (diastolic BP 120–130)
- Hypertensive encephalopathy (multifocal cerebral ischemia)
- Dissecting aortic aneurysm

Signs and Symptoms
- Asymptomatic (initially)
- Headache or dizziness
- Sleepiness
- Nausea & vomiting
- Irritability
- Visual disturbances

Diagnostics
- Health history and physical examination
    - Serial blood pressure checks

- Complete workup to determine target organ damage

Patient Care Management

A comprehensive plan includes addressing all factors that influence the occurrence of hypertension. This includes dietary restrictions, weight reduction where appropriate, medication regimen, exercise program, and finally stress reduction. Additionally, an evaluation needs to be made to determine if the patient is able to follow through with the lifestyle changes, monitoring of his blood pressure, and maintaining contact with the health care team.

- Medical
  - Dietary modifications
    - DASH (Dietary Approaches to Stop Hypertension)
    - $\downarrow$ Na, saturated fat, cholesterol, and total fat
    - Limit alcohol consumption
  - Exercise
  - Weight control
  - Stress reduction
  - Medications
    - Thiazide diuretics (Hydrochlorothiazide)
    - Potassium-sparing diuretics (Spironolactone)
    - Beta-adrenergic blocking agents (Propranolol, Atenolol)
    - Calcium channel blockers (Diltiazem hydrochloride, Nifedipine, Verapamil)
    - Angiotensin-converting enzyme (ACE) inhibitors (Captopril, Enalapril, Lisinopril)
    - Angiotensin II receptor blockers (Candesartan, Valsartan)
    - Central alpha agonists (Clonidine)
    - Vasodilators (Hydralazine, Fenoldopam, Nitroprusside)

Nursing Management

- Imbalanced Nutrition: More than Body Requirements
  - Discuss with the patient realistic goals for weight reduction and an exercise program that is age dependent
- Impaired Tissue Perfusion, Potential for
  - Monitor for changes in vital signs (e.g., ↑ BP, ↑ HR)
  - Monitor for worsening signs of HTN. (e.g., headache, visual changes, changes in renal function)
- Knowledge Deficit: Risk of Noncompliance
  - Teach the patient to report to the health care provider the use of herbal products and OTC medications prior to taking them because they frequently change the action of the hypertensive drugs
  - Teach the patient to monitor the amount of alcohol consumed per day/week because many hypertensive drug labels warn about the consumption of alcohol
  - Instruct the patient to read medicine bottle labels and to follow the directions for pulse and blood pressure assessment prior to taking the dose of medication
  - Instruct the patient/family about potential side effects of the prescribed therapeutic agents
  - Instruct patient/family regarding indications that necessitate contacting health care provider (e.g., headache, fainting, dizziness, follow-up appointment, renewal of prescription)
  - Demonstrate how menu planning is carried out using a prescribed diet plan such as the DASH diet. Frequently, a referral needs to be made to a therapeutic dietitian for assistance
  - Teach patient that health beliefs and practices influence lifestyle choices

IMMUNOLOGIC DISORDERS

Acquired Immunodeficiency Syndrome (AIDS)

Acquired immunodeficiency syndrome (AIDS) is the syndrome of opportunistic infections that occurs as the final stage of infection with the human immunodeficiency virus (HIV). This retrovirus is rapidly replicated and affects CD4 T cells (help cells) rendering the patient immune compromised and at risk for opportunistic infections (caused by organisms native to the environment).

Risk Factors

- Unprotected sex with an HIV-infected male or female
- Sharing of injection equipment
- Blood product recipient (especially prior to screening in 1985)
- Infants born to mothers with HIV infection (via exposure to blood during delivery or breast milk)
- Needlestick injuries

Signs and Symptoms

- General
    - ↑ Temperature, night sweats, fatigue, weight loss
    - Lymphadenopathy (swollen lymph nodes)
- Respiratory
    - ↑RR, dyspnea on exertion, adventitious breath sounds, hypoxemia
    - Cough (productive with blood-tinged sputum or nonproductive cough)

- Gastrointestinal
  - Inflamed oral mucosa
    - White patches in mouth, throat, tongue (bleed if scraped)
    - Redness in oral cavity
    - Pain and difficulty swallowing
    - Symptoms progress to esophagus
  - Abdominal pain and cramping
  - Nausea, vomiting, diarrhea (bloody), anorexia, weight loss
  - Chronic weakness
  - Wasting syndrome (10% or more body weight lost)
- Neurologic
  - Forgetfulness, decreased attention and concentration, progressive impaired motor function
  - Headaches, sensory and visual deficits, dizziness, aphasia, seizures, personality changes
  - Pain and numbness in extremities
  - AIDS dementia complex
- Integumentary
  - Non-blanching, flat or raised purple-brown lesions (Kaposi's sarcoma)
  - Ulcer lesions of oral, nasal, genital, and perianal mucosa
- Visual
  - "Seeing spots," unilateral visual loss progresses to bilateral loss and blindness
- Gynecological
  - Genital itching
  - Vaginal discharge (foul smelling, blood tinged, white or yellow cheese-like)
  - Bleeding between menses or after intercourse
- Opportunistic Infections and Malignancies
  - Pneumocystis carinii pneumonia (PCP)
  - Mycobacterium tuberculosis

- Mycobacterium avium complex (MAC)
- Hepatitis B and C
- Candidiasis
- Herpes zoster and herpes simplex
- Kaposi's sarcoma
- Non-Hodgkin's lymphoma
- Primary lymphoma of the brain
- Invasive cervical carcinoma

Diagnostics
- Health history and physical examination
- Laboratory
  - CBC (evaluates for anemia)
  - WBC (evaluates for leucopenia)
  - Enzyme-linked immunosorbent assay (ELISA)
  - Western blot
  - Rapid HIV antibody tests
  - CD-4 cell count (viral loading test)
  - HIV-RNA concentration (viral loading test)
  - Sputum culture and AFB stain
  - TB skin test
  - Blood cultures
- Imaging
  - CT scan and MRI

Patient Care Management
- Medical
  - Antiretroviral drug therapy
  - Management of opportunistic infections and malignancies

Nursing Management
The nursing care of the patient with AIDS involves multiple physical as well as psychological and social support issues. A diagnosis of HIV/AIDS is psychologically devastating to patients, the vast majority of who are

15 to 45 years of age and have not previously confronted issues of mortality. HIV/AIDS also carries a social stigma that may result in rejection by family and friends and social isolation at a time when the patient faces issues of grief and fear of dying. Nurses have a primary role in addressing these needs, and providing skilled, compassionate nursing care that is respectful to the individual's values, culture, and right to make individual choices.

- Risk for infection
  - Assess for symptoms of infection and notify health care provider
    - ↑ HR, ↑ RR, ↑ Temperature
    - Chills and diaphoresis
    - Change in mental status
    - Cough and adventitious breath sounds
    - Changes in mucous membranes or skin
    - ↑ WBC (may be severely ↓)
  - Administer antimicrobial medications as prescribed
  - Administer antiretroviral medications
  - Adhere to standard precautions
  - Maintain fluid and nutritional intake
  - Maintain skin and mucous membrane integrity with frequent turning and oral care every 2 hours

---

Critical Alert

Frequent and thorough oral assessment and care by the nurse is essential for the patient with oral candidiasis to maintain intact mucous membranes and prevent the spread of systemic infection by oral lesions. Frequent and persistent vaginal candidiasis may be the first sign of HIV infection in a woman.

  - Maintain sterile technique during all invasive procedures (urinary catheterization, IV line placement)
  - Perform meticulous care of any invasive lines or catheters; change out catheters according to agency policy
  - Discontinue catheters/invasive lines as soon as possible

- Assist with mobility, out of bed three or more times a day unless contraindicated or turning every 2 hours
  - Assist with incentive spirometry, coughing, and deep breathing every 1–2 hours when awake
- Ineffective Airway Clearance
  - Assess ↑ RR, abnormal breath sounds, and hypoxemia
  - Assess for cough
  - Assess sputum (color, consistency, amount)

> **Critical Alert**
> Individuals who present with a persistent cough, night sweats, and fever should be tested for TB. If they have a positive TB test and the individual engages in high-risk behaviors, HIV testing should be discussed and encouraged.

  - Assess level of consciousness (restless, confused, somnolence)
  - Assess color of skin (e.g., dusky, cyanotic)
  - Administer oxygen therapy and position for optimal ventilation
  - Maintain hydration
  - Administer mucolytics and bronchodilators as prescribed
  - Report abnormal findings to health care provider
- Imbalanced Nutrition: Less than Body Requirements
  - Assess for significant weight loss or weight below normal for patient's height, weight, and age
  - Assess diet history, food likes, dislikes, and intolerances
  - Assess and report abnormalities of oral cavity, mucous membranes, and swallowing
  - Monitor fluid and electrolytes, serum protein, albumin, transferrin levels, hemoglobin/hematocrit
  - Monitor daily intake with calorie count
  - Consult with dietitian to determine patient's nutritional needs

Cancer

Few words evoke an emotional response as dramatic as the word *cancer*. The impacts, both physiologically and psychologically, cause considerable changes in the lifestyles of both patients and families. Nurses must possess a broad base of knowledge about the pathophysiology and psychosocial aspects of the disease and its treatment. Patients rely on nurses for support and assistance throughout all phases of their illness, from diagnosis to end-of-life care.

Bladder Cancer

Bladder cancer is the fourth most common cancer in men (over 50 years of age) and the ninth leading cancer in women. Tumors may develop on the surface of the bladder wall or grow within the bladder wall. Those that grow within the wall are invasive and usually infiltrate the bladder wall invading the underlying muscles.

Risk Factors

- Environmental carcinogens:
    - 2-naphthylamine
    - Benzidine
    - Tobacco use
    - Nitrates
- Industrial exposure:
    - Rubber workers
    - Weavers
    - Leather finishers
    - Hairdressers
    - Aniline dye workers
    - Petroleum workers
    - Spray painters
- Female specific:
    - Tobacco use
    - Use of hair dye
    - Ingestion of tap water containing nitrates

Staging

- Stage 0: Cancer cells are found only on the inner surface of the bladder wall.

- Stage I: Cancer cells have invaded the layer of connective tissue under the bladder wall but have not penetrated muscle or spread to lymph nodes or distant sites.

- Stage II: Cancer cells have invaded the muscle layer but have not passed through the muscle to reach the tissue layer surrounding the bladder, nor have cancer cells spread to lymph nodes or distant sites.

- Stage III: Cancer cells have spread into the outer layer of tissue surrounding the bladder and may also invade surrounding structures, but lymph nodes and distant sites are not involved.

- Stage IV: Cancer cells have spread to the pelvic or abdominal wall or metastasized to a distant location such as the lungs, liver, or bones.

Grading

- Well differentiated:
  - Cells resemble normal cells more closely
  - Tend to be less aggressive
  - Grow slowly and are termed low-grade tumors
- Poorly differentiated:
  - Cells have lost their ability to resemble the normal cell.
  - Cells are termed higher grade and are more aggressive.

Signs and Symptoms
Initial Signs

- Hematuria:
  - Gross
  - Painless
  - Intermittent

Advanced Signs

- Suprapubic pain after voiding

Diagnostics
- Health history and physical examination
- Laboratory
  - Urinalysis (determine presence of RBCs and malignant cells)
- Imaging
  - Cystoscopy (with anesthesia) for biopsy of tumor
  - CT scan (identifies nodal involvement)
  - Ultrasound of bladder

Patient Care Management
- Medical
  - Intravesicular chemotherapy (bladder washed with antineoplastic agent)
  - Intravesical immunotherapy: instilled into bladder to stimulate immune system to destroy cancer cells
  - Systemic chemotherapy and radiation therapy may be required for advanced disease
- Surgery
  - Transurethral resection with electrical destruction
  - Segmental bladder resection (removal of portion of bladder)
  - Radical cystectomy (removal of entire bladder)
    - Urinary diversion is created using the intestinal tract (ileal conduit)

Nursing Management
Nursing management of the patient with bladder cancer requires an understanding of multiple aspects.

(See Appendix #36, Nursing Process: Patient Care Plan for Cancer.)

Specific nursing care for patient with bladder cancer is related to the care of the patient who has had an ileal conduit and bladder surgery.

(See Procedures and Therapies: Bladder Surgery and Ileal Conduit.)

Bone Cancer

The most common types of primary bone cancer include osteosarcoma, chondrosarcoma, and Ewing's sarcoma. Osteosarcoma has a greater incidence in males than females and the tumor most often develops in the arm, leg, or pelvis. Chondrosarcoma is a cancer of cartilage cells that may present anywhere in the body where there is cartilage, but the most common sites are the pelvis, leg, and arm bone. Ewing's sarcoma is a primary malignant bone tumor in the pediatric and adolescent population. Ewing tumors form in the cavity of the bone and most often present in the long bones of the leg and arm.

Signs and Symptoms

- Pain
  - Mild to severe
  - Pain and swelling, fever, fatigue, anemia, and leukocytosis (Ewing's sarcoma)
  - Intermittent and dull (chondrosarcomas due to being slow-growing tumors)
- Swelling
- Limited range of motion (ROM)
- Joint effusion
  - Tender to palpation and warm to touch with superficial blood vessels noticeable

Diagnostics

- Health history and physical examination
- Lab tests will include chemistry and CBC. Serum alkaline phosphatase is generally elevated. In some situations, the hematologic lab values will be altered
- Imaging
  - Bone scan (detects the extent of the malignancy)
  - CT and MRI (demonstrates soft tissue involvement and the exact location of the tumor)
  - Chest x-ray and lung scan (detects metastasis)

- Other
  - Bone biopsy
  - Arteriography

Patient Care Management

The treatment of bone cancer is best achieved by a multidisciplinary team. The objective or the goal is to slow the growth of the tumor by destroying and removing the lesion. Depending on the specific type of bone tumor, chemotherapy, surgery, radiation, or a combination of these treatments may be used.

Nursing Management

(See Appendix #1, Nursing Process: Patient Care Plan for the Postoperative Patient Following General Surgery; Appendix #36.)

Brain Cancer

Brain tumors may be primary or metastatic. Primary tumors are those that originate in the brain. These tumors rarely, if ever, travel to other areas of the body, remaining only in the brain. Metastatic tumors are those that originate in other areas of the body and travel to the brain. Examples of these are tumors that originate in the lung or breast tissue and metastasize to the brain.

Diagnostics

- Health history and physical examination
- Imaging
  - CT scan and MRI

The following table summarizes the classifications of the most common brain tumors.

Classification of Brain Tumors

Type	Average Age at Onset	Symptoms	Treatment	Prognosis
Meningioma	Age 40–60s	Dependent on location and size Seizures Headaches	Surgery Radiation for residual or recurrence (gamma knife, cyberknife)	Excellent with resection
Astrocytoma	Variable	Dependent on location and size	Surgery Radiation for residual recurrence	3–7 years with treatment, dependent on grade and extent of resection
Glioblastoma multi-forme (GBM)	Age 50–60s	Dependent on location and size	Surgery Radiation Chemotherapy	12–18 months with treatment

(continued)

Classification of Brain Tumors (*continued*)

Type	Average Age at Onset	Symptoms	Treatment	Prognosis
Oligodendroglioma	Age 40–50s	Dependent on location Seizures	Surgery Radiation Chemotherapy	5–10+ years with treatment
Ependymoma	All ages (60% are children)	Signs and symptoms Increased ICP Hydrocephalus	Surgery Radiation Chemotherapy for recurrence May need shunt	7–8+ years with surgery, less with recurrence

Pituitary adenomas	Variable	Hormone abnormalities dependent on area of pituitary affected. Visual disturbances. Headaches	Medical. Surgical possible. Radiation possible	Excellent
Acoustic neuromas	Age 40–50s	Hearing loss	Surgery. Radiation for residual (gamma knife)	Excellent
Metastatic tumors	Variable	Dependent on location, size, single or multiple	Surgery if single metastasis or symptomatic. Radiation (gamma knife). Chemotherapy	Usually poor, dependent on single or multiple and identification of primary disease

Nursing Management

(See Procedures and Therapies: Care of Craniotomy Patients for Brain Tumor.)

(See Appendix #36.)

Breast Cancer

Breast cancer is defined as the formation of a malignant glandular tumor as a result of an uncontrolled growth of abnormal cells in the breast tissue. The malignant cells over time destroy normal breast tissue. Cancer arises from the epithelial cells that line the ducts and the lobules.

In situ: Cancer confined to the ducts or lobules.

Invasive or infiltrative: Cancer starts in the lobules or ducts, but breaks through the walls to invade the surrounding fatty tissue of the breast. The most common type of breast cancer is invasive ductal carcinoma.

Paget's disease: Rare form of breast cancer that is characterized by infiltration of the nipple epithelium.

Inflammatory breast cancer: Highly malignant form of cancer because of its aggressive nature and fast-growing character. The skin of the breast, which looks red, feels warm and has a thickened appearance resembling an orange peel.

Risk Factors

- Age
- Family history
- Age at first pregnancy
- Age of menarche
- Age of menopause
- Obesity
- Hormone replacement therapy
- Alcohol consumption
- Sedentary lifestyle

Signs and Symptoms

- Painless mass
  - Located in the upper outer quadrant of the breast where the majority of glandular tissue is found
  - Described as a thickening in the breast tissue found during self-breast exam or showering
- Unusual lump in the axilla or above the clavicle
- A persistent skin rash, flaking or eruption near the nipple area (Paget's disease)
- Dimpling, pulling, or retraction in one breast, creating an asymmetrical appearance
- Burning, stinging, or prickling sensation in the breast
- Nipple abnormalities (spontaneous discharge, erosion, inversion, or tenderness)

Diagnostics

- Health history and physical examination
- Imaging
  - Mammography
  - Breast ultrasound
- Other
  - Breast biopsy

Patient Care Management

- Medical
  - Radiation therapy
  - Chemotherapy (oral and parenteral)
- Surgery
  - Lumpectomy
  - Mastectomy (removal of breast)
    - Modified radical (removal of breast and surrounding lymph nodes)
    - Radical (removal of breast, surrounding lymph nodes, and chest wall muscles)
  - Breast Reconstruction (done immediately after surgery or delayed)

Nursing Management

Nursing responsibilities focus on caring for patients with breast cancer who have had surgery, including issues surrounding body image disturbance. In addition, the nurse needs to understand the care associated with chemotherapy, radiation therapy, and end-of-life care.

(See Appendix #1; Appendix #36.)

Colon Cancer

Adenocarcinoma is the most common type of colon cancer and accounts for 95% of colon tumors. Adenocarcinomas grow irregularly and form hard, nodular areas. The cancer is spread first by local invasion and direct extension. Any tissue or organ in the neighboring area can be affected, such as the liver, duodenum, small intestine, pancreas, and the abdominal wall. The most common sites for metastasis of colon cancer are the liver, lungs, brain, and bones.

Risk Factors
- Race ($\uparrow$ incidence in African Americans)
- Gender ($\uparrow$ incidence in males)
- Dietary
    - $\uparrow$ intake of animal protein, fat, and calories
    - $\downarrow$ intake of folic acid, selenium, vitamin D, and calcium
- Chronic inflammation of irritable bowel syndrome (IBS)
    - Presence of C-reactive protein (CRP), which is marker of inflammation
- Daily alcohol consumption

Signs and Symptoms
- Usually asymptomatic until it is well advanced
- Depend on the location of the tumor and its stage of growth

- The most common symptoms:
  - Change in bowel habits
    - Constipation
    - Diarrhea
    - Change in the caliber of the stools
    - Bleeding in the stool
- Weight loss, fatigue, abdominal pain, and anorexia (with advanced disease)
- Anemia
- Bowel obstruction and bowel perforation

Diagnostics

- Health history and physical examination
- Laboratory
  - Fecal occult blood test (evaluated annually for those age 50 or greater)
  - Complete blood count (CBC)
    - Evaluates anemia and leukocyte response to inflammation
  - C-reactive protein
  - Carcinoembryonic antigen (CEA)
    - Too insensitive and nonspecific to be useful in screening or diagnosing but is useful in monitoring a patient's response to treatment.
- Imaging
  - Sigmoidoscopy every 5 years or colonoscopy every 5 to 10 years
  - CT scan
    - Detects possible metastasis in distant locations such as the liver or lungs
- Other
  - Tissue biopsy (done during colonoscopy and is almost 100% accurate in diagnosing this type of cancer)

Patient Care Management

Prevention of colon cancer is the primary goal of collaborative care, followed next by early detection and treatment. Prevention and early detection of colon cancer is done through educating the public about ways to decrease the risk, such as eliminating alcoholic beverages on a daily basis; increasing the amount of fruits, vegetables, and fiber; daily exercise and weight control; and possibly a daily low dose of aspirin.

- Medical
  - Chemotherapy (adjunctive therapy after colon resection)
  - Radiation therapy
    - Appears to prolong survival in patients with more advanced cancer, particularly rectal tumors
    - Used before surgery to shrink large tumors and make them easier to resect
- Surgery
  - Abdominoperineal resection with a colostomy
  - Laser photocoagulation (avoids colostomy)
  - Tumors of the rectum require removal of the rectum, sigmoid colon, and anus, necessitating a sigmoid colostomy for fecal elimination

Nursing Management

Nursing responsibilities focus on caring for patients who have undergone colon cancer surgery, including issues surrounding the placement of a colostomy. In addition, the nurse needs to understand the care associated with chemotherapy, and radiation therapy, and end-of-life care.

(See Appendix #1; Appendix #3, Nursing Process: Patient Care Plan for the Patient with Colon Cancer Having Surgery; Appendix #36.)

Esophageal Cancer

The development of esophageal cancer is facilitated by any process that allows food and drink to remain in the esophagus for prolonged periods, by ulceration and metaplasia usually caused from esophageal reflux, and by long-term exposure of the esophagus to irritants. Malnutrition causes mucosal changes that promote neoplastic changes.

Esophageal cancer can occur anywhere along the esophagus, but it is more common in the middle and distal portions.

Risk Factors

- Long-term alcohol use
- Tobacco use
  - Pipe and cigar smokers have a higher risk than cigarette smokers
- Deficiencies of trace elements and vitamins, particularly zinc and vitamin A
  - Seen in malnutrition from poor economic conditions, special diets, or alcoholism

Signs and Symptoms

- Dysphagia
  - Begins with difficulty swallowing solid food
  - Progressing to difficulty swallowing soft foods and liquids
  - Late in the disease, drooling may be noted because the patient can no longer swallow her saliva
  - Painful swallowing (odynophagia) is described as a steady, dull, substernal pain
- Heartburn
- Chest pain
- Regurgitation

Diagnostics

- Health history and physical examination
  - Assess patterns of dysphagia
- Laboratory
  - Complete blood count (CBC) to evaluate for anemia

- Serum albumin to evaluate nutritional status and liver function
- Aspartate aminotransferase (AST), alanine aminotransferase (ALT), bilirubin, alkaline phosphatase to evaluate liver metastasis
- Imaging
  - Barium swallow may be done initially to identify narrowing of the esophageal lumen or abnormal mucosa
  - Endoscopic visualization and biopsy
  - CT scan or MRI to assess for metastasis to other organs

Patient Care Management

The goal of therapy for the patient with esophageal cancer is to control dysphagia and maintain or improve nutritional status.

- Medical
  - Radiation and chemotherapy
    - If done preoperatively can shrink the size of the tumor, making removal easier
- Surgery
  - Removal of the affected area of the esophagus and re-anastomosis of the remaining esophagus to the stomach
  - Tumors in the upper esophagus usually require a tracheostomy and possibly a radical neck dissection with laryngectomy
  - Palliative surgery
    - If the cancer is extensive and has invaded the local tissue and metastasized to distant organs
    - Attempts to relieve pain and dysphagia
  - Complications
    - Hemorrhage
    - Shock
    - Infection

- Pneumonia
- Peritonitis due to leakage at the anastomosis sites or through the mediastinal space

Nursing Management

Nursing care for the patient with esophageal cancer will focus on assessing the severity of the symptoms, providing support once diagnosis is made, and educating the patient and family on lifestyle changes needed to facilitate palliative care. Understanding the nursing care of the patient who receives chemotherapy, radiation therapy, and surgery for esophageal cancer is essential when developing a plan of care.

(See Appendix #1; Appendix #2, Nursing Process: Patient Care Plan for Postoperative Esophageal Cancer; Appendix #36.)

Gastric Cancer

The majority of gastric cancer develops in the distal portions of the stomach and can be attributed to *H. pylori* infection. Because the stomach has a rich blood and lymphatic supply, the cancer spreads via the portal vein to the liver and through the systemic circulation to the lungs. Metastasis has also been found in bone, ovarian, and peritoneal tissue.

Risk Factors

- Gender (twice as prevalent in men)
- Race (highest incidences in Hispanics, African Americans, and Japanese Americans (who have retained the traditional diet)
- Genetics
- Chronic gastritis, gastric ulcer
- Atrophic gastritis
- Gastric polyps
- Pernicious anemia
- Dietary factors (use of nitrates used to preserve meats)
- Lack of hydrochloric acid (achlorhydria)
- History of gastric resection

Signs and Symptoms

There are rarely any symptoms associated with gastric cancer and patients seek medical attention when their health fails and the disease is in the advanced stage.

- Anorexia
- Indigestion and heartburn
- Weight loss with patient becoming cachectic

Diagnostics

- Health history and physical examination
- Laboratory
    - Complete blood count (CBC) usually indicates anemia
- Imaging
    - Upper endoscopy
    - Abdominal ultrasound (if mass felt on examination)
- Other
    - Biopsy

Patient Care Management

The medical management of gastric cancer involves identification of the cancer and in most cases is followed by surgical removal.

- Medical
    - Chemotherapy or radiation therapy
        - Helps prevent development of metastatic disease
        - Considered palliative in patients with advanced disease to help shrink the tumor and provide pain relief
- Surgery
    - Partial gastrectomy (removal of a portion of the stomach)

- Total gastrectomy (removal of the entire stomach where the esophagus is anastomosed to either the duodenum or the jejunum)
  - Complications
    - Dumping syndrome (the pylorus is bypassed and a food bolus rapidly enters the duodenum or jejunum)
    - Anemia due to changes in absorption of vitamins and minerals

Nursing Management

Nursing care of the patient with gastric cancer is mostly supportive. Understanding the care of the patient who receives chemotherapy, radiation therapy, and surgery for gastric cancer is essential. Additionally, the nurse must be aware of the interventions needed to care for a patient with a feeding tube as well as those required for a patient who undergoes an endoscopy.

(See Appendix #1; Appendix #4, Nursing Process: Patient Care Plan for Gastric Cancer and Gastric Resection; Appendix #36.) (See Procedures and Therapies: Endoscopy; Nasogastric Tube; and Tube Feedings.)

Head and Neck Cancer

Head and neck cancer is one of the more uncommon cancers; however, the challenges the patient, family, and health care team face during diagnosis, treatment, and recovery are intense and persistent. If detected early, head and neck cancer is treatable and curable. The predominant cell type in head and neck cancer is squamous cell cancer. Cells change from the normal fast growing dividing cells into altered cells that grow along tissue planes and into adjacent structures.

Risk Factors
- Alcohol
- Ultraviolet light

- Tobacco
  - Cigarettes, cigars, or pipes
  - Smokeless tobacco ("snuff" or chewing tobacco)
  - Exposure to secondhand smoke (called passive smoking)
- Irritation to the lining of the mouth caused by poorly fitting dentures
- Poor nutrition: a diet low in fruits and vegetables
- Human papillomavirus (HPV) infection
- Immune system suppression
- Gender: more common in men than in women

Signs and Symptoms
- Sore throat without fever
- Unilateral earache
- Change in voice or articulation
- Dental changes
- Weight loss
- Mass in the neck

Diagnostics
- Health history and physical examination
  - Length of time and sequence of each symptom
  - 12 cranial nerves are evaluated carefully as they give important clues to the invasion and location of the cancer
- Imaging
  - Panendoscopy includes tumor mapping and biopsy to confirm histologic diagnosis:
    - Bronchoscopy
    - Esophagoscopy
    - Nasal endoscopy
    - Examination of the oral cavity
    - Anatomical mapping of the cancer

Patient Care Management

A multidisciplinary team of experts including oto-laryngologists, medical oncologists, radiation oncologists, social service, clinical nurse specialists, speech pathologists, nurses, and dentists or maxillofacial prosthodontists provides a collaborative approach to providing care for patients with head and neck cancer.

- Medical
  - Chemotherapy
  - Radiation therapy
  - Combination therapy
- Surgery
  - Laryngectomy (partial or total)
  - Temporal bone resection
  - Maxillary (with or without orbital exoneration) or bimaxillary resection
  - Skull base resection
  - Neck dissection (remove tissues or structures that have cancerous cells or will likely develop cancerous growth)

Nursing Management

Effective management of the patient with head and neck cancer requires an understanding of postoperative care, cancer care, and specific issues related to this unique disease.

(See Appendix #1; Appendix #36.) (See Procedures and Therapies: Nasogastric Tube; Tube Feedings; and Tracheostomy.)

- Ineffective Airway Clearance
  - Monitor for $\uparrow$ RR, $\downarrow$ O_2 sat, and work of breathing
  - Assess lung sounds
  - Suction as needed, note amount and characteristics of sputum
  - Tracheostomy care per policy and as needed

    (See Procedures and Therapies: Tracheostomy.)

Patients who have reconstruction surgery with flaps require special nursing management. When assessing a reconstruction flap, it should be pink and warm with brisk capillary refill (<2 seconds). Signs of potential problems with a flap include:

- Blue or cyanotic is a sign of venous congestion.
- White indicates no arterial supply.
- Deep red is a sign of partial venous congestion with a vigorous arterial supply.

Leukemia

Leukemia is classified as either acute (aggressive with severe symptoms) or chronic (slowly progressing with fewer symptoms). The type of leukemia depends on the stem cell line affected: lymphoid or myeloid. (See table starting on page 269.)

Nursing Management

(See Appendix #36.)

Liver Cancer

Cancer of the liver develops from the liver's parenchymal cells (hepatocellular carcinoma) or from the cells in the bile ducts (cholangiocarcinoma). This type of cancer can be nodular, massive, or diffuse, and is most closely related to cirrhosis or hepatitis B and C. Hepatocellular carcinoma metastasizes to the heart, lungs, brain, kidneys, and spleen.

Risk Factors
- Hepatitis B and C
- Mycotoxins (mold on corn, peanuts, and grain)
- Excessive smoking and drinking
- Prolonged use of anabolic steroids
- Arsenic-contaminated water

Signs and Symptoms
- Weakness
- Anorexia with weight loss

Four Common Forms of Leukemia

Cancer		Signs and Symptoms	Diagnostic Technique	Prognosis	Treatment
Acute lymphocytic leukemia (ALL)	Most common in children *Etiology:* Radiation Chemicals Drugs Viruses	Anemia: Malaise Fatigue Neutropenia: Fever Bone pain Thrombocytopenia: Bleeding Bruising CNS involvement (10%) due to meningeal infiltrates	Peripheral blood smear: • CBC with differential • Bone marrow biopsy	Complete remission: 80–90% Cure: 30–40% Children achieve cure at rate of 60–85%	Chemotherapy: • Induction therapy to achieve remission • CNS treatment if needed • Postremission therapy Bone marrow or stem cell transplantation

(*continued*)

Four Common Forms of Leukemia (*continued*)

Cancer		Signs and Symptoms	Diagnostic Technique	Prognosis	Treatment
Acute myeloid leukemia (AML)	*Etiology:* Radiation Chemicals Drugs Viruses Certain genetic disorders increase incidence of acquiring AML	Anemia: Malaise Fatigue Neutropenia: Fever Bone pain Thrombocytopenia: Bleeding Bruising Anemia is usually present when health care provider sees patient for the first time. Recurrent infections not resolved with antibiotics.	Peripheral blood smear: • CBC with differential • Bone marrow biopsy	Patients over 70 years of age are intolerant of induction therapy. WBCs $>100,000/mm^3$ related to increased mortality during first week of therapy.	Chemotherapy: • Induction therapy to achieve remission • Postremission therapy Biotherapy: monoclonal antibodies Bone marrow or stem cell transplantation

| Chronic lymphocytic leukemia (CLL) | B-cell lymphocytes undergo a malignant transformation Few cases are of the T-cell line | 25% of patients are symptom free Evidence of disease found on routine examination and laboratory work Frequent respiratory and skin infections | Peripheral blood smear:
 • CBC with differential
 • Flow cytometry to evaluate immunopheno-type of cells
 • Bone marrow biopsy (for prognostic information) | Survival is often determined by the severity of disease when diagnosed. No pattern of predictability of disease course. | Often difficult to decide when to begin treatment. Treatment is aimed at alleviating symptoms, not cure. Treatment for complications:
 • Antibiotics
 • IV immunoglobulin
 Chemotherapy
 Splenectomy or radiotherapy (rarely done)
 Bone marrow or stem cell transplantation |

(continued)

Four Common Forms of Leukemia (*continued*)

Cancer		Signs and Symptoms	Diagnostic Technique	Prognosis	Treatment
Chronic myeloid leukemia (CML)	Myeloproliferative disorder Presence of Philadelphia chromosome Three stages: 1. Chronic 2. Accelerated 3. Blast crisis	Chronic Phase: Fatigue Pallor Dyspnea Anemia Night sweats Weight loss Sternum pain Accelerated: Chronic symptoms recur after treatment. Blast crisis: Aggressive and terminal phase that includes above symptoms with increased severity.	Peripheral blood smear: • CBC with differential • Bone marrow biopsy	Chronic phase lasts 3–4 years. Once blast crisis occurs, median survival is < 6 months. 85% of patients die during blast crisis due to complications such as bleeding and infections.	Chemotherapy Biotherapy: interferon bone marrow or stem cell transplantation

- Fatigue and malaise
- Abdominal pain
- Ascites
- Jaundice
- Palpable mass in the right upper quadrant
- Signs of liver failure

Diagnostics
- Health history and physical examination
  - Especially important since initial signs and symptoms are subtle
- Laboratory
  - AST and ALT (elevated)
  - Alpha-fetoprotein (AFP) (elevated in advancing disease)
- Imaging
  - Magnetic resonance imaging (MRI) and computed tomography (CT) scans
- Other
  - Liver biopsy is done to determine the tumor type

Patient Care Management
- Medical
  - Chemotherapy
    - Systemic
    - Directly into liver
- Surgery
  - Surgical Resection
    - Only if the tumor is localized and in a lobe of the liver that can be removed (e.g., if the tumor is in the posterior section of the right lobe, it cannot be removed because the right hepatic vein is located in this area).

Nursing Management

A goal of nursing care for patients with liver cancer is prevention whenever possible. In those patients who have a risk factor for liver cancer, such as chronic infection with HBV or HCV, the risk for developing liver cancer can be reduced if they abstain from alcohol. Most of the nursing interventions for a patient with liver cancer are similar to those for patients with cirrhosis and liver failure.

(See Appendix #1; Appendix #6, Nursing Process: Patient Care Plan for the Patient with Cirrhosis; Appendix #36.) (See Procedures and Therapies: Endoscopy; Nasogastric Tube; and Tube Feedings.)

Lung Cancer

Globally, lung cancer is the most common form of cancer; however, in the United States it is the second most common occurring malignancy. Common metastatic sites for all types of lung cancer include liver, bone, adrenal glands, and the brain. Efforts to combat the prevalence of lung cancer have been targeted at preventing exposure to known risk factors.

Risk Factors
- Tobacco smoke
- Radon
- Asbestos

Signs and Symptoms
- Respiratory
  - Cough and sputum production
  - Dyspnea
  - Wheezing
  - Hemoptysis
  - Chest pain
- Dysphagia
- Hoarseness

- Pain
- Fatigue and weakness
- Nausea and anorexia
- Disturbed sleep, memory impairments, and night sweats

Diagnostics
- Health history and physical examination
- Laboratory
  - CBC, liver enzymes, and chemistries (to detect comorbidities, possible metastatic disease, and complications commonly found with lung cancer)
  - Sputum cytology
- Imaging
  - Chest x-rays and chest CT scans
- Other
  - ECG
  - Pulmonary function tests
  - Lung biopsy (via bronchoscopy)
  - Transthoracic needle aspiration (TTNA)

Patient Care Management
- Medical
  - Chemotherapy, radiation therapy, or a combination of the two
- Surgical
  - Surgical resection of lung mass (lobectomy)

Nursing Management
Nursing management of patients with lung cancer is challenging and complex. The nurse must possess an appreciation of the care required for patients who have undergone surgical resection, those who receive

chemotherapeutic agents, and those who receive radiation therapy.

(See Appendix #1; Appendix #36.)

Lymphoma

Cancers of the lymphatic system (lymphomas) involve organs and tissues such as the lymph nodes, spleen, thymus, bone marrow, blood, and lymph. Malignant lymphomas are grouped according to the characteristics of the lymphocyte, such as Hodgkin's disease and non-Hodgkin's disease. (See following chart starting on page 277.)

Nursing Management

(See Appendix #36.)

Malignant Melanoma

Malignant melanoma is the most dangerous skin cancer because it is a rapidly growing invasive tumor that can metastasize to almost any organ in the body and result in death. It is a tumor involving melanocytes that is related to sun exposure.

Risk Factors
- Large number of typical moles
- ↑ Number of atypical moles
- Burns easily from exposure to the sun
- Freckles from sun exposure
- Difficulty tanning
- Family history of malignant melanoma
- Previous diagnosis of malignant melanoma

Signs and Symptoms
- Moles
  - Asymmetrical
  - Irregular borders

Cancers of the Lymphatic System

Cancer		Signs and Symptoms	Diagnostic Technique	Prognosis	Treatment
Non-Hodgkin's Lymphoma	Similar to Hodgkin's disease, but without the Reed-Sternberg cell *Etiology:* Infections Autoimmune disorders Environmental factors Typically female, Caucasian, and approximately 55 years of age	Painless lymphadenopathy (cervical or supraclavicular region) As disease worsens swelling and obstructive symptoms occur	Lymph node biopsy Chest x-ray Bone marrow biopsy Serum blood analysis: • Hepatitis B and C • CBC with differential • Chemistries	Indolent disease has most favorable prognosis. Highly aggressive disease requires high-dose therapy that increases risk of life-threatening complications.	Chemotherapy Biotherapy: monoclonal antibodies Bone marrow or stem cell transplantation

(continued)

Cancers of the Lymphatic System (*continued*)

Cancer		Signs and Symptoms	Diagnostic Technique	Prognosis	Treatment
Hodgkin's Lymphoma	Presence of Reed-Sternberg cells *Etiology:* Viral exposure Epstein-Barr virus most common Woodworking Most common in young adults, age 26–31 years Occasional peak in prevalence at age 60 years	Lymphadenopathy: Cervical Supraclavicular Mediastinal fever Night sweats Weight loss	Lymph node biopsy Staging laparotomy if receiving radiation Chest x-ray Bone marrow biopsy Serum blood analysis: • CBC with differential • Chemistries	If early stage, 20-year survival is near 80%. If receiving salvage therapy after relapse, survival is 80–95%.	Radiotherapy Chemotherapy Bone marrow or stem cell transplantation

- Variegated with shades of brown, tan, blue/black, or a combination of colors
- Larger than 6 millimeters in diameter
- Normal mole needs evaluation if:
  - Change in size
  - Change in shape
  - Change in color
  - Inflammation
  - Crusting or bleeding
  - Sensory changes

Diagnostics
- Health history and physical examination
- Laboratory
  - Skin biopsy
- Imaging
  - Chest x-ray, ultrasound, CT scan, and MRI (to detect metastasis)

Patient Care Management
- Medical
  - Chemotherapy
  - Radiation therapy
- Surgical
  - Removal with the intent to cure

Nursing Management
(See Appendix #1; Appendix #36.)

Multiple Myeloma
Multiple myeloma is one of the less common cancers of the hematopoietic system. The primary mechanism is a malignancy of the B-cell due to depressed antibody mediated immunity. (See following chart.)

Multiple Myeloma

Cancer	Signs and Symptoms	Diagnostic Technique	Prognosis	Treatment
Multiple myeloma	Most common in African Americans, age 70 Malignancy of B cell Immunodeficiency due to depressed antibody-mediated immunity	Findings are related to excess of Bence-Jones proteins. Infections: • Pneumonia • Urinary tract infection (UTI) • Systemic Skeletal: • Pain worse with movement • Hypercalcemia • Pathologic fractures	1. Serum electrophoresis to determine Bence-Jones proteins. 2. Serum immunoglobulin electrophoresis 3. Bone marrow biopsy: increase in abnormal, atypical, immature B cells. 4. Radiographic: osteolytic lesions bones	1. Incurable, sometimes treatable 2. 1/3 patients do not respond to therapy and die within weeks of diagnosis.	Chemotherapy Corticosteroids Immunotherapy Bone marrow transplant (autologous) Radiation therapy

Vertebral collapse

Renal failure:

- Proteinuria
- Obstructed distal and proximal tubules
- Hyperuricemia

Blood/bone marrow dysfunction:

- Anemia
- Hyperviscosity
- Coagulation disorders

Neurologic:

- Spinal cord compression
- Peripheral neuropathy

Nursing Management

(See Appendix #36.)

Pancreatic Cancer

Cancer of the pancreas is a rare cancer and holds a very high mortality rate. Most pancreatic cancer is ductal adenocarcinoma that develops from the exocrine cells in the ducts. Because of the vascular structure of the area, cancer cells infiltrate the portal vein, mesenteric artery, vena cava, and aorta, with metastasis to the liver.

Risk Factors

- Obesity
- Chronic pancreatitis
- Family history of pancreatic cancer
- History of abdominal radiation
- Cigarette smoking
- High-fat diet
- Diabetes mellitus

Signs and Symptoms

Most cases of pancreatic cancer are asymptomatic until the tumor invades surrounding tissue or obstructs the common bile duct.

- Jaundice
- Vague, diffuse epigastric pain that does not cause alarm
- Stools become light in color
- Urine becomes dark
- Pruritus results from the bilirubin in the skin
- Weight loss
- Steatorrhea
- Malnutrition

Diagnostics

- Health history and physical examination
- Imaging
  - Dual-phase spiral CT or an MRI

- Other
  - Percutaneous needle aspiration to get samples of the tissue for cytologic study
  - Laparotomy is performed to establish a definitive diagnosis and determine the extent of the disease

Patient Care Management

Treatment of pancreatic cancer is varied, ranging from surgical intervention to palliation.

- Medical
  - Radiation and chemotherapy
    - After surgery or for palliation (symptom relief)
- Surgical
  - Radical pancreaticoduodenal (Whipple) resection
    - Removal of the head of the pancreas, the duodenum, a distal portion of the stomach, a part of the jejunum, and the lower half of the common bile duct
    - Most pancreatic cancer is too advanced when first diagnosed for the Whipple procedure to be effective.

Nursing Management

Patients with pancreatic cancer require nursing care that focuses on palliation, comfort, and support. It is important to understand the routine care for postoperative patients in addition to the responsibilities associated with chemotherapy and radiation therapy.

(See Appendix #1; Appendix #36.)

Penile Cancer

Penile cancer is very rare in North America and Europe. Although the exact cause is not known, penile cancer is likely to be caused by two proteins produced by high-risk human papillomavirus that interfere with tumor suppressor genes.

Risk Factors

- Poor local hygiene
- Phimosis

- Human papillomavirus infection (risk for this infection is increased by sexual intercourse at an early age, many sexual partners, sex with a partner who has had many partners, or unprotected sex)
- Smoking
- Age (most cases occur in men over age 65)
- AIDS
- Not being circumcised

Signs and Symptoms
- Presence of lesion on penis

Diagnostics
- Health history and physical examination
- Imaging
  - Radiographic studies if metastatic disease is suspected

Patient Care Management
- Medical
  - Radiation therapy
  - Chemotherapy
- Surgical
  - Circumcision
  - Laser ablation for smaller lesions
  - Partial or total penectomy for larger lesions

Nursing Management
Nursing care depends on the extent of the cancer. Preoperative and postoperative education and emotional support are imperative.

(See Appendix #1; Appendix #36.)

Prostate Cancer
A man's lifetime risk for prostate cancer is 1 in 6, making this disease the most common cancer in men in the United States and the second leading cause of death.

The prostate has three zones that are surrounded by fibromuscular casing:

- Central zone
- Peripheral zone (70% of prostate and most common site for malignancy)
- Transitional zone

Prostate cancer occurs in two forms:

- Latent (slow growing)
- Aggressive (fast growing)

Signs and Symptoms

Asymptomatic if the cancer is of the slow growing type. Often signs and symptoms are not noticed until after metastasis has occurred. Common symptoms include:

- Frequent urination
- Urinary retention
- Trouble starting or holding back urine
- Weak or interrupted urine stream
- Dysuria
- Hematuria
- Painful ejaculation
- Nocturia
- Bone pain (lower back, hips, femur)

Diagnostics

- Health history and physical examination
  - DRE (digital rectal examination)
    - Used in combination with PSA to increase the likelihood of identifying a cancer
- Laboratory
  - PSA (prostate specific antigen)
    - Serum kinase that originates from the prostate epithelial cells
    - Not specific enough to diagnose prostate cancer as a single test

- Levels > 10 ng/mL have a 67% predictive value for prostate cancer.
  - Levels > 20 ng/mL suggest likely bone metastasis and a bone scan is recommended
- Imaging
  - Transrectal ultrasound guided biopsy is used to identify and help stage and grade the disease
    - Tumor Node Metastasis Staging System
    - Gleason Grading System
  - CT scans for Gleason scores > 6

Patient Care Management

The urologist is assisted by nurses, the oncologist, anesthesiologists, nutritionists, counselors, and community resources. The health care team should include the spouse or partner and the patient's family in all aspects of the plan of care.

- Medical
  - Consider the patient's age and any existing co-morbidities.
  - Slow growing tumor with co-morbidities:
    - No treatment or begin a program of "watchful waiting"
    - DRE and serum PSA would be done every 3–12 months.
    - Monitored for lower urinary tract symptoms and signs of metastasis
    - Transrectal ultrasound guided biopsy may be done every 3 years.
    - Lifestyle interventions to improve diet, exercise, and stress management can be instituted.
    - Support groups
  - Hormone therapy or orchiectomy (androgen suppression)
    - Decreases level of testosterone, thereby slowing disease progression

- Used in localized disease and for advanced, symptomatic metastatic disease
- Used to help relieve the pain and other symptoms of advanced disease
- Medications
  - Estrogen and the GnRH agonist

  (See Pharmacology Summary.)
    - Diethylstilbesterol (DES)
    - Leuprolide (Lupron)
- Vaccine: Provenge
  - Yet to be approved by FDA
  - Made of the patient's own cells and a protein that stimulates the immune system causing it to attack the cancer
  - Intended for those men with metastatic disease
- Chemotherapy is a last resort since it does not seem to alter survival.
- Radiation therapy
  - Brachytherapy (implant therapy)
    - Fewer side effects than radical surgery or external beam radiation, including less frequent occurrence of erectile dysfunction and urinary incontinence
    - Patient may experience swelling of the prostate that will alter urination patterns and can last up to 12 months
  - External beam radiation
    - Delivered over a period of 6 weeks
    - Side effects (occur near the end of treatment and last for up to 6 weeks after therapy is over)
    - Cystitis
    - Proctitis
    - Dermatitis

- Surgical
  - For more aggressive types and for the younger male
  - Radical prostatectomy or removal of the prostate, seminal vesicles, and adjacent tissues

Nursing Management

An understanding of the care of a patient who is postoperative is important as well as issues related to cancer.

(See Appendix #1; Appendix #36.)

- Ineffective Sexuality Pattern
  - Explain the effect of therapy on sexual function
  - Offer support and open communication with patient and his partner
  - Encourage patient to verbalize his concerns about sex and changes in his physical appearance
- Impaired Urinary Elimination
  - Indwelling catheter for urinary retention if needed
  - Catheter Care:
    - Maintain a closed sterile system
    - Keep drainage bag lower than bladder
    - Avoid kinks in drainage tubing
    - Secure to the patient's thigh with a stabilization device
    - Cleanse urinary meatus with soap and water twice daily
  - Encourage fluid intake to maintain urine output at 50 mL/hr
  - Accurate intake and output
  - Assess for excessive hematuria
  - Monitor laboratory data for infection and hemorrhage:
    - Hemoglobin/Hematocrit
    - WBC
    - Urinalysis

- Use incontinence pads and other equipment to keep patient dry
- Knowledge Deficit
  - Explain the purpose of equipment (e.g., urinary catheter, incentive spirometer, anti-embolic stockings) using return demonstration as appropriate
  - Explain that the urinary catheter is also a splint to help maintain the surgical reconnection of the urethra

Renal Carcinoma

Carcinoma of the kidney causes enlargement of the organ and eventually destroys it. Approximately 80 to 85% of all primary renal cell carcinomas originate within the renal cortex. Other locations include transitional cell carcinomas of the renal pelvis, parenchymal epithelial tumors, collecting duct tumors, and renal sarcoma.

Risk Factors

- Cigarette smoking
- Occupational exposure to toxic compounds
  - Cadmium
  - Asbestos
  - Petroleum by-products
- Obesity
- Acquired cystic disease of the kidney
- Genetic factors

Signs and Symptoms

Many patients are asymptomatic until the disease is advanced. When diagnosis is confirmed 25% either have metastases or advanced disease. Common presenting symptoms:

- Hematurea
- Pain
- Abdominal mass
- Weight loss

Common Metastasis

- Lungs
- Lymph nodes
- Liver
- Bones
- Brain

Diagnostics

Health history, physical examination, and radiographic imaging tests are the primary modes of diagnosing renal cancer.

Patient Care Management

- Medical
  - Chemotherapy:
    - Mostly ineffective
  - Radiation:
    - Only if disease has spread to distant organs or lymph nodes
  - Biotherapy:
    - More promising than chemotherapy but causes adverse reactions
- Surgical
  - Removal of kidney and surrounding cancerous tissue

Nursing Management

Specific nursing care for patient with renal cancer is related to the care of the patient who has had a nephrectomy with nephrostomy tube.

(See Appendix #1; Appendix #36.) (See Procedures and Therapies: Nephrostomy Tube.)

Reproductive System Cancers

(cervical, endometrial, ovarian, vulvar, vaginal)

(See Appendix #9, Comparison of Female Reproductive Cancers.)

Testicular Cancer

Cancer that forms in the tissue of the testis is the most common form of cancer in white men between the ages of 15 and 34. Besides age, other risk factors include familial history (especially siblings), prior personal history, cryptorchidism, Klinfelter Syndrome, natural exposure to gestational estrogen, and exposure to insecticides.

Signs and Symptoms
- Solid, painless, nontransluminating lump
- Dull discomfort or heaviness in the scrotum and lower abdomen
- Scrotum swelling
- Metastatic disease:
  - Cough
  - Hemoptysis
  - Weight loss

Diagnostics
- Health history and physical examination
  - First diagnosed as epididymitis or orchitis and treated with antibiotics
  - Testicular tumors have also been found coincident to sports injuries to the groin or genitals
  - A small number of men may first seek medical advice because of gynecomastia (enlargement of the male breast) caused by testicular tumors that secrete beta human chorionic gonadotropin (hCG).
- Laboratory
  - Serum markers (used to detect disease, monitor response to treatment and as a surveillance tool following treatment)
  - Beta human chorionic gonadotropin
  - Alpha fetoprotein
  - Lactic dehydrogenase

- Imaging
  - Ultrasonography of the scrotum to differentiate cancer from epididymitis or hydrocele
  - Chest x-ray
  - Computed tomographic (CT) scan of the abdomen

Patient Care Management

Treatment depends upon the type of tumor, the stage of the disease, and the presence of tumor markers. Combination therapy can result in 100% cure rates.

- Medical
  - Radiation therapy
  - Chemotherapy
- Surgical
  - Orchiectomy (total or affected side only)

Nursing Management

(See Appendix #1; Appendix #36.)

- Pain, Acute
  - Assess pain thoroughly using numeric scale and patient self-report
  - Instruct patient to inform the nurse when pain begins and if the pain is not relieved after interventions
  - Apply ice pack and scrotal support
- Risk for Impaired Tissue Perfusion
  - Assess surgical site for swelling, purulent drainage, redness, or ecchymosis
  - Monitor for ↑ HR, ↓ BP, and ↑ T
- Knowledge Deficit
  - Explain expected postoperative care (e.g., incentive spirometer, progressive ambulation, maintaining adequate nutritional intake)
  - Explain the purpose of preserving sperm in sperm bank

Cancer Emergencies

Oncologic emergencies occur as a result of the disease process or side effects of treatment. The following table presents the important emergencies along with a definition, clinical findings, and treatment options. The nursing management associated with cancer emergencies should focus on the specific condition and is presented throughout this text.

Oncologic Emergencies:
Signs and Symptoms, Treatment

Emergency	Signs and Symptoms	Treatment
Metabolic		
Disseminated intravascular coagulation (DIC)	Signs of bleeding and clotting	• Elimination of triggering event • Supportive measures (transfusion of blood products)
Hypercalcemia: serum calcium levels >9–11 mg/dL	Lethargy Altered mental status Nausea and vomiting Anorexia Polydipsia Constipation	• Hydration • Diuresis to enhance the excretion of calcium • Pharmacology: bisphosphonates (inhibit the action of osteoclasts) • Increased mobilization

(continued)

Oncologic Emergencies:
Signs and Symptoms, Treatment (*continued*)

Emergency	Signs and Symptoms	Treatment
Malignant pleural effusion; accumulation of fluid in the pleural cavity	Dyspnea at rest or activity Cough (non-productive) Chest pain Malaise Weight loss Fear of suffocation, anxiety	• Radiation or chemotherapy aimed at the primary tumor • Insertion of chest tube with drainage capability • Pleurodesis
Sepsis	Fever Chills Changes in blood pressure Rapid respiratory rate Mental cloudiness	• Recognition of impending shock is key • Infection control practices • Private rooms • Hemodynamic monitoring while in the intensive care unit (ICU) • Antibiotic therapy
Syndrome of inappropriate antidiuretic hormone (SIADH): endocrine paraneoplastic syndrome causing water imbalance	Hyponatremia Decreased serum osmolality Water retention Increased urine osmolality Normal skin turgor Normal blood pressure	• Treat underlying cause • Fluid restriction • Diuretic therapy

Emergency	Signs and Symptoms	Treatment
Hypersensitivity reaction (anaphylaxis): immunologic response to foreign substance or antigen; may be life threatening	Occurs within minutes of receiving certain chemotherapy agents Dyspnea Agitation Hypotension Laryngeal edema and spasm	• Prevention is the key • Careful monitoring of blood pressure, pulse, and oxygen saturation during infusion • Emergency equipment needs to be available
Tumor lysis syndrome: rapid lysis of malignant cells resulting in renal (e.g., acidosis), electrolyte (e.g., hyperuricemia, hyperkalemia), cardiac, and neurologic complications	Nausea and vomiting Edema Flank pain Hematuria Changes in blood pressure Lethargy Muscle twitching and weakness	• Prevention is the key • Pretreatment hydration • Pharmacologic therapy (diuretics, xanthine oxidase inhibitors, sodium bicarbonate) • Supportive measures for potential organ failure

(*continued*)

Oncologic Emergencies:
Signs and Symptoms, Treatment (*continued*)

Emergency	Signs and Symptoms	Treatment
Structural		
Increased intracranial pressure: volume of the brain, CSF, and cerebral blood volume increase	Signs and symptoms of increased intracranial pressure	• Pharmacologic therapy (osmotic diuretics, corticosteroids, anticonvulsants) • Surgery to relieve pressure and evacuate fluid • Radiation and chemotherapy to shrink tumor bulk
Spinal cord compression: malignancy that invades the epidural space and cauda equina	Signs and symptoms of cord compression are specific to the area of the cord being compressed	• Pharmacologic therapy (corticosteroids) • Radiation therapy to reduce tumor bulk • Surgery when bony instability occurs

Emergency	Signs and Symptoms	Treatment
Superior vena cava syndrome: obstruction of venous flow through the vena cava resulting in compression of intrathoracic structures, vascular congestion, and venous hypertension	Dyspnea Cough Feeling of fullness in the head Chest pain	• Pharmacologic therapy (fibrinolytic therapy) • Radiation therapy to reduce tumor bulk • Chemotherapy for specific cell types • Surgery (stents or bypass)
Cardiac tamponade: compression of the cardiac muscle by malignant fluid accumulation within the pericardial sac	Dyspnea Chest pain Tachycardia Cough	• Pharmacologic therapy (diuretics, corticosteroids, NSAIDS) • Removal of fluid via pericardio-centesis, pericar-diotomy, peri-cardiectomy

Latex Allergy

Latex allergies can occur as both a type I allergic reaction or as a type IV cell-mediated reaction in response to contact with products containing natural latex. Clinical manifestations occur either immediately or 4–48 hours after exposure.

Risk Factors

- Working in any industry using latex or rubber components (health care workers, housekeepers, hairdressers)
- History of hay fever or asthma
- History of allergy to bananas, avocado, kiwi, and strawberry
- Neural tube defects (e.g., myelomeningocele or spina bifida)
- Chronic bladder catheterization
- Multiple surgeries

Signs and Symptoms

- Redness of the exposed skin
- Urticaria and itching
- Asthma symptoms
- Conjunctivitis
- Progression to anaphylactic shock
- Delayed reaction symptoms
    - Dryness at the site of exposure, itching, and cracking of the skin
    - Redness, swelling, and scabbing of the fissures and cracks in the skin

Diagnostics

- Health history and physical examination
    - Recognition of previous exposure with associated symptoms
    - Recognition of risk factors

Patient Care Management

- Medical
    - Symptom relief with antihistamines and topical steroids
    - Treatment of anaphylactic shock

Nursing Management

Prevention of latex allergies is dependant upon the nurse to recognize those patients at risk and providing an environment that is latex free. Understanding the nursing responsibilities associated with anaphylactic shock is also necessary.

(See Appendix #10, Nursing Process, Patient Care Plan for SIRS, Sepsis, Shock.)

INFECTIOUS DISEASE

Infectious Disease

Infectious diseases remain a major cause of illness, disability, and death in this country and worldwide. Pneumonia, influenza, and septicemia were among the top 10 causes of death in the United States in 2003. Infections can range from mild to debilitating or death producing. The severity of the infection depends on the pathogenicity or disease-causing potential of the microorganism, the number of invading microorganisms, and the host defenses. Infectious diseases are constantly emerging and reemerging. Tuberculosis is an example of a reemerging disease.

Classifications
Community-Acquired Infection
An infection is acquired outside a health care setting.

Nosocomial Infection
An infection acquired during a hospitalization, which can lead to numerous complications in the hospitalized patient leading to a cost of many lives and billions of health care dollars. Patients who develop nosocomial infections are often critically ill with an increased susceptibility to infection. Many nosocomial infections are caused by multidrug-resistant organisms (MDROs).

Well-Known Resistant Organisms
- Methicillin-resistant *Staphylococcus aureus* (MRSA)
- Multidrug-resistant tuberculosis (MDR-TB)

- Penicillin-resistant *Streptococcus pneumoniae* (PRSP)
- Vancomycin-resistant enterococci (VRE)
- Vancomycin intermediate-resistant *S. aureus* (VISA)
- Vancomycin-resistant *S. aureus* (VRSA)

Nosocomial infections are related to the use of invasive devices such as urinary catheters, intravenous catheters, surgical drains, nasogastric tubes, and endotracheal tubes. Clean or sterile technique should be used when caring for anyone with invasive devices in order to avoid infection. Limit use of invasive devices and discontinue as quickly as possible.

Signs and Symptoms
Nonspecific Symptoms
- General malaise
- Fever
- Myalgia
- Fatigue

Localized
- Redness from increased blood flow to the area
- Heat due to increased blood flow to the area
- Swelling due to the fluid exudates that form in the interstitial tissue
- Pain caused by the pressure of the exudates and release of chemicals that irritate nerve endings
- Loss of function related to the pain and swelling

Systemic
- Fever
- Leukocytosis – Increase in the number of bands on a differential WBC count is known as a "shift to the left" and indicates an ongoing acute inflammation.

Infectious Disease, Diagnostics

Test and Normal Values	Expected Abnormality	Rationale for Abnormality
WBC count, $n = 5{,}000$–$10{,}000$ cells/mm^3	Elevated in acute infections, tissue injury, tissue necrosis. Decreased in viral infections, some bacterial infections, bone marrow depression.	WBC count increases in order to phagocytize or kill bacteria or cell debris.
• Neutrophils, $n = 50$–70% of the total WBC count; band, $n = 3$–6%	Neutrophils and bands are elevated in acute infections.	Neutrophils are the first WBCs to arrive at the site of infection. They have a short life span and must be continually produced when needed, so the immature neutrophil or band will be elevated.
• Basophils, $n = 0.5$–1.0% of total WBC count • Eosinophils, $n = 1$–4% of total WBC count	Elevated with allergic and parasitic responses. Do not respond to bacterial or viral infections.	Involved in phagocytosis of antigen-antibody complexes. Respond later in inflammation and help control the inflammatory process.

Test and Normal Values	Expected Abnormality	Rationale for Abnormality
• Monocytes, $n = 2$–8% of total WBC count • Lymphocytes, $n = 20$–40% of total WBC count	Elevated in allergic and parasitic reactions. Elevated with infection, tuberculosis, bacterial endocarditis. Elevated with some bacterial diseases, infectious mononucleosis, leukemia, some viral diseases.	Phagocytic cells that perform like neutrophils but start later and stay longer in the bloodstream. Function to fight chronic bacterial infection and acute viral infections. Responsible for immune reactions.
Erythrocyte sedimentation rate (ESR): *Males:* up to 15 mm/hr *Females:* up to 20 mm/hr	Elevated with acute and chronic infection, inflammation, cancer, tissue necrosis.	Nonspecific test that measures the rapidity at which red blood cells (RBCs) clump together. This process occurs more rapidly when there is an alteration in blood proteins due to inflammation. Therefore, an elevation indicates the presence of an inflammatory process.

(continued)

Test and Normal Values	Expected Abnormality	Rationale for Abnormality
Culture and sensitivity: Normally negative	Positive if pathogens are present in the specimen. The culture will identify the organism and the sensitivity will identify what antibiotic will work best.	If pathogens are present on the substance being tested, they will grow on a special culture medium and can be identified.
Gram stain: None with no organisms present	Differentiates between gram-negative and gram-positive organisms.	Useful for identifying the microorganisms so proper treatment can occur.
Febrile agglutinins: No agglutinins in titers < 1:80	Increased in infectious diseases such as rickettsial disease, salmonellosis, brucellosis, and tularemia.	A group of tests that helps identify the type of organism responsible for an infection based on antibodies.
Viral antibody tests: None with no organisms present	This is a group of tests for specific viruses. Will be elevated with viral infections.	Used to determine exposure to or existing viral infections that are difficult to culture. Includes several tests, each specific

Test and Normal Values	Expected Abnormality	Rationale for Abnormality
		to an organism and antibody reaction. They must be specifically ordered.
Fungal infection: Antibody tests negative	Elevated in the presence of a fungal-induced infection.	Looks for the presence of antibodies related to fungal infections or the presence of parasitic organisms.

Patient Care Management

- Evaluate for increased susceptibility to infection
  - All hospitalized patients, acute and long-term care
  - Very old or very young
  - Malnourished or poor hygiene
  - Chronic stress
  - Chronic illness (diabetes, COPD, etc.)
  - Immunosuppressed (cancer, HIV, etc.)
- Prevention
  - Limit use of invasive devices and discontinue as quickly as possible
  - Provide immunizations as appropriate
- Initiate special precautions
  - Resistant Organisms: Use appropriate measures
  - *Clostridium difficile*: Initiate contact precautions
  - Meningitis

- Neisseria meningitides:
    - Use droplet precautions for the first 24 hours of antimicrobial therapy; mask and face protection for intubation. (*Note:* This is the *only type of meningitis* that requires transmission-based precautions.)
- Enteroviruses: Use contact precautions for infants and children
- Mycobacterium tuberculosis: Use airborne precautions if pulmonary infiltrate; use airborne plus contact precautions if potentially infectious draining body fluid is present
- Respiratory Infections
    - In infants and young children, especially bronchiolitis and pneumonia (RSV, parainfluenza, adenovirus, influenza virus, human metapneumonia virus): Use contact plus droplet precautions; droplet may be discontinued when influenza and adenovirus have been ruled out.
    - Cough/fever/upper lobe pulmonary infiltrate (M. tuberculosis, respiratory viruses, Staphylococcus pneumoniae and/or S. aureus (MSSA or MRSA): Use airborne plus contact precautions, or resistant organism (RO) precautions for MRSA.
- For HIV-positive patients (or patients at high risk for HIV infection):
    - Use eye/face protection if aerosol-generating procedure performed or contact with respiratory secretions anticipated. Tuberculosis is more likely in an HIV-infected individual than in an HIV-negative individual. If tuberculosis is unlikely and there is no airborne infection isolation room or respirator available, use droplet instead of airborne precautions.
- For patients with history of recent travel (10 to 21 days) to countries with active outbreaks of SARS (avian influenza):
    - Use airborne plus contact precautions plus eye protection. If SARS and/or TB are unlikely, use droplet only instead of airborne.

National Guidelines for Standard and Transmission-Based Precautions

Category	Precaution
Standard Precautions	
Hand hygiene	Perform hand hygiene after touching blood, body fluids, secretions, excretions, and contaminated items whether or not gloves are worn.
Gloves	Wear clean, nonsterile gloves when touching blood, body fluids, secretions, excretions, and contaminated items. Put on clean gloves just before touching mucous membranes and nonintact skin.
Mask, eye protection, face shield	Worn to protect mucous membranes of the eyes, nose, and mouth during procedures and patient care activities that generate splashes or sprays of blood, body fluids, secretions, or excretions.
Gown	Wear a clean, nonsterile gown to protect skin and prevent soiling of clothing during procedures and patient care activities that may generate splashes or sprays of blood, body fluids, secretions, or excretions. Gowns should be impervious to fluids.
Patient care equipment	Handle used patient care equipment soiled with blood, body fluids, secretions, or excretions in a manner that prevents skin and mucous membrane exposure and contamination of clothing, and transfer of microorganisms to other patients and environments.

(continued)

Category	Precaution
Environmental control	Adequate procedures should be in place for routine care, cleaning, and disinfection of environmental surfaces.
Linen	Handle soiled linen in a manner that prevents skin and mucous membrane exposure and contamination of clothing.
Occupational health and bloodborne pathogens	Prevent injuries when using and disposing of needles, scalpels, and other sharp instruments or devices. Never recap needles or use any technique that involves pointing the sharp end toward part of the body. Use mouthpieces, resuscitation bags, or other ventilation devices as an alternative to mouth-to-mouth resuscitation.
Patient placement	Place a patient who contaminates the environment in a private room if possible. If not possible, place patients with the same diagnosis in the same room.
Transmission-Based Precautions	
Airborne precautions (TB, varicella, measles, and smallpox)	1. Place patient in private room with N95 respirator, monitored negative air pressure, 6 to 12 air changes per hour, and appropriate discharge of air outdoors. Keep room door closed and patient in room. 2. Wear respiratory protection when entering room. 3. If leaving the room, the patient should wear a mask. 4. Limit the movement and transport of the patient from the room.

Category	Precaution
Droplet precautions (meningitis or diphtheria)	1. Place patient in private room or in a room with cohort patients with the same disease. 2. Wear a mask when working within 3 feet of patient. 3. If leaving the room, the patient should wear a mask. 4. Limit movement and transport of patient from room.
Contact precautions (*Clostridium difficile* or wounds)	1. Place patient in private room or with a very low-risk roommate. 2. Wear gloves when entering room and remove gloves before leaving room. Then perform hand hygiene. 3. Wear a gown when entering the room and remove gown before leaving room. 4. Limit the movement and transport of the patient from the room. 5. Dedicate the use of noncritical patient care equipment to a single patient (blood pressure cuffs, stethoscopes, thermometer, etc.) 6. Any equipment removed from the room must be disinfected with hospital-grade disinfectant before being used with another patient. 7. *Clostridium difficile* is a frequent colonizer of the hospital environment. It is a spore former that can live in the environment for very long periods and is able to withstand many normal cleaning procedures.

(*continued*)

National Guidelines for Standard and Transmission-Based Precautions (*continued*)

Category	Precaution
Protective precautions – (immuno-compromised patients	Minimize exposures to pathogens. Limit time patient is outside the room for diagnostic procedures or other activities. When outside of room – patient wears mask. Strict enforcement of hand washing (visitors & hospital personnel). No one in room with any type of infection.

Nursing Management

> **Critical Alert**
> Hand washing done using the correct procedure and frequency has been shown to be the most important single action in preventing the spread of infection.

- Risk of infection
  - Initiate and follow isolation procedures as appropriate
  - Assess for signs and symptoms of infection
  - Obtain cultures appropriately, carefully following guidelines for proper handling
- Infection and risk of complications
  - Administer antibiotics and antipyretics
  - Manage fever and corresponding increase in metabolic demands (oxygen demand, tachycardia, increased caloric needs)
  - Encourage fluids to prevent dehydration
  - Provide high-calorie, high-protein diet
  - Space activities and allow for rest periods

- Knowledge deficit related to treatment of infection
  - Stress importance of taking all antibiotic as prescribed
  - Explain necessity of isolation procedures and risks of spreading infection
  - Provide emotional care for patients in precaution restricted rooms. Protective masks, gloves, and gowns may make the patient feel isolated and rejected
  - Teach proper wound care, signs and symptoms of infection include odor and exudate, fever, increased drainage, swelling, and lack of wound closure
- Knowledge deficit related to prevention and spread of infection
  - Teach about resistant organisms and the risks of transmission
  - Importance of frequent hand hygiene
  - Good hygiene, eating a well-balanced diet, exercising regularly, and getting an adequate amount of sleep will result in a stronger immune system and a greater resistance to infection
  - Avoid crowds and contact with susceptible persons
  - Use disposable tissues when coughing or sneezing
  - Use appropriate food-handling precautions
  - Clean equipment and eating utensils
  - Avoid contact with or sharing of body fluids through needles or razors
  - Use condoms during sexual activity

Inflammation, Sepsis, SIRS

Systemic Inflammatory Response Syndrome (SIRS)

SIRS is an organized immune response that can be triggered by infectious or noninfectious clinical insults including burns, pancreatitis, acute respiratory distress syndrome, surgery, and trauma.

Sepsis

Sepsis is a clinical syndrome defined as the presence of SIRS associated with a confirmed infectious process. Septic shock is a state of acute circulatory failure characterized by persistent hypotension. Severe sepsis is defined as sepsis with single or multiple organ failure.

Three principal actions occur within the body with sepsis: inflammation, coagulation, and fibrinolysis. The purpose of the inflammatory response is to protect the body from further injury and promote rapid healing. Vasodilation occurs near the injured area with vasoconstriction of arterioles resulting in increased microvascular permeability, allowing exudate to form at the site. Neutrophil activation and adhesion are initiated, which promote phagocytosis in order to clean the area and prepare for healing. Inflammation normally localizes an infection and kills the invading organism, but when inflammation is extreme it results in vascular congestion, endothelial injury and dysfunction, and overstimulation of the coagulation system.

Signs and Symptoms

- ↑ temperature with chilling
- Flushed skin that may be hot to the touch
- Bounding peripheral pulses
- Signs of shock

> **Critical Alert**
> ↓ Temperature indicates a worsening condition and grave prognosis.

Diagnostics

(See Shock section.)

Patient Care Management

(See Shock section.)

Shock

Shock is a condition where the body has lost its ability to perfuse tissues adequately. This results in both impaired oxygen and glucose use. Risk factors include significant injuries, catastrophic illness, age, and allergies.

Causes

- Alterations in the circulating volume of blood or plasma in the body
- Alterations in the heart's capability to pump
- Alterations in peripheral vascular resistance

Regardless of the cause of shock, the systemic response is detrimental and often leads to multiple organ dysfunction syndrome (MODS) and death.

Anaphylactic Shock

Anaphylactic shock results from an antigen–antibody reaction (hypersensitivity). The result is loss of vascular tone seen by vasodilatation of blood vessels. Because the blood has pooled in the periphery, perfusion to the tissues is markedly diminished or absent. In addition, other body systems will react to the toxin; specifically, the pulmonary system will respond with vasoconstriction, causing respiratory distress and potential respiratory collapse.

Cardiogenic Shock

Cardiogenic shock will develop when the heart has lost its ability to pump effectively, most commonly due to ischemia or cardiac arrhythmias.

Hypovolemic Shock

Hypovolemic shock results from significant fluid loss (severe dehydration or hemorrhage) that alters the amount of circulating volume in the body.

Neurogenic Shock

Neurogenic shock results from an imbalance between the sympathetic and parasympathetic stimulation of vascular smooth muscle, which results in vasodilation. The most common cause for neurogenic shock is spinal cord injuries.

Septic Shock

Septic shock is inadequate tissue perfusion due to an infectious process.

Signs and Symptoms

- Neurological
    - Altered mental status
    - Irritability
    - Seizures
    - Coma
- Pulmonary
    - ↑ RR, shallow respirations
    - Crackles from fluid shifts
    - ↓ O_2 sats despite an increase in oxygen administration
- Cardiovascular
    - ↑ HR, ↓ BP
    - Pulses
        - Thready, decreased, or absent

- • ↑ capillary refill time
  - • Cardiac dysrhythmia
- • Gastrointestinal
  - • Nausea, vomiting, absent bowel sounds
- • Genitourinary
  - • ↓ urinary output
  - • ↑ specific gravity
- • Integumentary
  - • Cool clammy skin
  - • Mottling, cyanosis
  - • Skin breakdown
- • Musculoskeletal
  - • Generalized weakness
  - • Wasting

Diagnostics

- • Health history and physical examination
- • Laboratory
  - • CBC (evaluates for presence of infection and inflammation)
  - • Electrolytes (evaluates for presence of organ dysfunction and glucose metabolism)
  - • Serum lactate (reflect tissue perfusion and presence of anaerobic metabolism)
  - • Coagulation studies (indicates cellular dysfunction and abnormal clotting cascade)
  - • Arterial blood gases (ABGs)
  - • Blood cultures and urinalysis (evaluates source of infection)
- • Imaging
  - • Chest x-ray, CT scan, MRI

Patient Care Management

To achieve optimal recovery and return to society, the patient in shock requires a multidisciplinary team that includes health care providers, nurses, pharmacists, social service personnel, physical therapists, and nutritionists. To prevent the complications related to shock and its sequelae, nurses and health care providers must be alert to all risk factors.

- Medical
  - Airway and ventilatory support
    - Oxygen therapy (100% nonrebreather mask, mechanical ventilation)
  - Circulatory support
    - Intravenous fluids
    - Vasoactive intravenous medications
    - Blood product administration
    - Continuous cardiac monitoring
    - Hemodynamic monitoring (PA catheter, CVP, Arterial line)
  - Antibiotic therapy
  - Intravenous stress dose corticosteroids (for patients with adequate volume replacement and who require vasopressors to maintain an adequate blood pressure)
  - Recombinant human activated protein C (rhAPC) (for patients who are at high risk of death with minimal risk of bleeding)
  - Glucose control
    - Maintain blood glucose < 150 mg/dL
  - Pain management
  - Stress ulcer prevention
    - H_2 receptors
  - DVT prophylaxis
  - Nutritional support
  - Laboratory (to evaluate response to therapy, see above laboratory tests)

Nursing Management

It is important to understand that some of the symptoms of these disorders are seen in other disorders, thus the nurse needs to be diligent in recognizing those patients who are at risk. Once the source or clinical insult has been identified, nursing care can be focused on the specific cause.

(See Appendix #10, Nursing Process: Patient Care Plan for SIRS, Sepsis, Shock.)

INTEGUMENTARY DISORDERS

Skin Infections
Cellulitis

This is a bacterial infection of the dermis and subcutaneous tissue layers due to a break in the skin. The causative organism is usually staphylococcus or streptococcus.

Risk Factors

- Loss of skin integrity (surgical wounds or trauma sites) compromised immune system

The most common sites of cellulitis are lower extremities, face, ears, and buttocks.

Signs and Symptoms

- Erythema with edema and indefinite border
- Edema
- Vesicles, blisters, or abscesses
- Regional lymphadenopathy
- Pain
- Fever, chills, headache, and vomiting

Diagnostics

- Health history and physical examination
- Laboratory
  - CBC ($\uparrow$ WBC and neutrophils)
  - Wound culture

Patient Care Management

- Medical
  - Rest and elevation of the affected site

- Antibiotics
- Pain medication
- Burrow's soaks

Nursing Management

- Impaired Skin Integrity
  - Monitor amount of inflamed surface area (measure daily)
  - Assist with repositioning and turning
  - Administer antibiotics and topical therapy as prescribed
  - Monitor nutritional status
- Pain, Acute
  - Assess pain level using 0–10 numeric scale
  - Offer pain medication and reassess accordingly
  - Offer nonpharmacological pain relief and reassess accordingly

Necrotizing Fasciitis

Necrotizing fasciitis (NF) is an infection of the superficial fascia or the connective tissue surrounding muscle and subcutaneous tissue, leading to fascial necrosis. It is commonly referred to as the "flesh-eating bacteria." Although relatively uncommon, it is significant because of the difficulty in recognizing it and the rapidity with which it spreads and can become fatal. This infection can occur at any age or in any location and is not specific to gender.

Risk Factors

- Simple minor injuries
- Complicated major surgeries or trauma
- Very young and very old
- Diabetes mellitus
- Atherosclerosis
- Chronic renal failure
- Obesity
- Immunosuppression

- Malnutrition
- Illicit drug injections
- Alcoholism
- Peripheral vascular disease

Once a break in the skin occurs and is contaminated, the organisms spread from the subcutaneous tissue along the superficial and deep fascia, facilitated by bacterial enzymes and toxins, which continue to break down tissue.

Signs and Symptoms for Necrotizing Fasciitis

Early Stage First 24–48 Hours	Advanced Stage 2nd–4th Day	Critical Stage 4th–5th Day
Flu-like symptoms such as fever, chills, myalgia, nausea, vomiting, and diarrhea. Abrupt localized pain beyond what would be expected. Patchy discoloration of skin that is violaceous to erythematosus without defined borders. Non-pitting edema outside the area of discoloration. Skin is essentially normal in appearance.	Skin swollen and tight and erythema is noted. Area becomes dusky blue in color. Blisters or bullae filled with purplish, foul-smelling, thin, watery fluid. Skin has paper-like appearance. There may be palpable crepitation due to the presence of gas. Spread of the infection—increasing wound size. Increased leukocytes. Decreased sodium.	Skin sloughs. Gangrene develops. Hypotension. Delirium. Loss of consciousness. Liver failure. Renal failure. Fever. Acute respiratory distress syndrome (ARDS). Coagulopathy. Fascia appears gray to grayish green. Elevated heart rate. Tissue necrosis.

Diagnostics

- Health history and physical examination
- Laboratory
  - CBC ($\uparrow$ WBC and neutrophils)
  - $\uparrow$ Creatinine phosphokinase (CPK)
  - $\uparrow$ BUN and Creatinine
  - Blood and wound cultures (positive for streptococcus)
- Imaging
  - CT scan and MRI (evaluates extent of fasciitis)
- Other
  - Tissue biopsy

Patient Care Management

- Medical
  - Admitted to ICU for close observation and hemodynamic monitoring
  - Antibiotic therapy
  - Intravenous immunoglobulin (IVIG)
  - Nutritional support
  - Wound care
    - Vacuum assisted closure device (wound VAC)
      - Negative pressure in the wound by applying suction
      - Suction drains interstitial edema fluid, thus decreasing pressure on capillaries and improving perfusion
      - Provides a mechanical stretch/distortion of the cells in the wound bed, which stimulates production of granulation tissue
      - Removes stagnant fluid in the wound, thus decreasing the bacterial burden in the healing wound bed

- Surgical
  - Surgical debridement (remove all necrotic tissue and prevent the spread of the infection)
    - As often as every 12 to 24 hours
  - Excision of organs or amputation may be necessary

Nursing Management

Nursing care for patients with necrotizing fasciitis requires excellent assessment, clinical decision making, and critical thinking skills.

- Impaired Skin Integrity
  - Assess skin for drainage, warmth, and redness
  - Assess skin lesions for changes
  - Implement an individualized treatment plan for the site of skin impairment. Use aseptic technique during treatments
  - Reposition every 2 hours, and assess for signs of further skin breakdown
  - Patient should be placed in a private room with contact isolation.
- Risk for Imbalanced Fluid Volume
  - Assess the patient's preoperative fluid status
  - Monitor vital signs ($\uparrow$ HR, $\uparrow$ RR, $\downarrow$ BP)
  - Monitor intake and output, daily weights
  - Assess for signs of edema in dependent areas or around lesions
  - Assess electrolyte levels
- Pain, Acute
  - Assess severity and quality of pain frequently using numeric scale 0–10
  - Provide pain relief as needed and reassess accordingly
  - Support the patient's use of nonpharmacologic interventions for pain relief
  - Plan care and activities around periods of pain

- Imbalanced Nutrition: Less than Body Requirements
  - Monitor food intake and consult with clinical nutritionist as needed
  - Assess the need for parenteral or enteral feedings
- Knowledge Deficit
  - Teach patient/family regarding ICU routines and expected treatment plan
  - Educate patient and family regarding wound care as appropriate
  - Consult with social services for support

Stevens–Johnson Syndrome

Stevens–Johnson syndrome (SJS) is a severe, acute, self-limiting skin reaction to infection or certain medications that occurs most commonly in children and young adults. It affects the epidermal layer of the skin and mucous membranes.

Causes

- Sulfonamides
- Betalactam antibiotics
- Penicillin
- Anticonvulsants
- Certain NSAIDs
- Allopurinol

Signs and Symptoms

- Flu-like symptoms (headache, rhinorrhea, cough, and body aches)
- Symptoms of an upper respiratory infection (fever, cough, headache, fatigue, sore throat, and malaise)
- Target skin lesions (bright-pink or red inner ring, a ring of lighter pink, and then a ring of dark pink)
  - Concentric macular exanthemas that focus on the face, neck, and extremities
  - Become blisters that grow together and break open

Diagnostics

- Health history and physical examination
  - Nikolsky's sign
    - Application of slight thumb pressure that leads to separation of the epidermis from the dermis when the thumb slides laterally on the skin
- Laboratory
  - Skin biopsy
  - Immunofluorescent studies (presence of immunoglobulin M [IgM] and C3 deposits in the vascular walls of the skin)

Patient Care Management

- Medical
  - Admission to burn unit if available
  - Withdrawal of the causative agent
  - Intravenous antibiotics
  - Intravenous glucocorticoids (controversial)
  - Intravenous immunoglobulin (IVIG)
  - Intravenous fluid replacement (similar to that initiated with the treatment of burns)

(See Burns section.)

  - Pain control
    - Topical anesthetics
    - Systemic medications
  - Dressings
    - Gauze with petrolatum or silver nitrate
    - Biologic skin covers (cadaveric allografts)
  - Nutritional support using TPN

(See Procedures and Therapies, Parenteral Nutrition.)

Nursing Management

Nursing care of the patient with Stevens–Johnson syndrome is very similar to that of a burn patient.

(See the Burns section for detailed nursing interventions.)

Wounds

Pressure Ulcers

According to the National Pressure Ulcer Advisory Panel (NPUAP), "A pressure ulcer is localized injury to the skin and/or underlying tissue usually over a bony prominence, as a result of pressure, or pressure in combination with shear and/or friction." The result is decreased circulation leading to vascular insufficiency, tissue anoxia, and cell death, resulting in tissue necrosis. Common sites of pressure ulcers are listed in following table.

Common Sites for Pressure Ulcers

Patient Position	Pressure Ulcer Sites
Supine	Scapula, occiput, sacrum, heels
Lateral	Ear, shoulder, trochanter, medial knee, malleolus, foot edge
Prone	Nose, forehead, chest, iliac crests, foot edge, toes

Risk Factors

- Restricted activity (e.g., quadriplegia, strokes, and fractured hips)
- Poor nutrition
- Moisture (e.g., incontinence, perspiration, wound drainage, or emesis)
- Comorbidities (e.g., diabetes mellitus, hypertension, respiratory disease, or vascular disease)

Signs and Symptoms

The signs and symptoms of pressure ulcers depend upon the stage (or depth) of the ulcer. See following table for pressure ulcer staging.

Pressure Ulcer Staging from the National Pressure Ulcer Advisory Panel

Stage of Wound	Guideline
Deep tissue injury (DTI)	Deep tissue injury is a new stage that is characterized by purple or maroon tissue over bony prominence areas from pressure or shear with intact skin. It often feels "boggy" (soft) or indurated (hard). It should be classified as a DTI, and close monitoring for further deterioration should be performed.
Stage I	Intact skin with nonblanchable area of redness. A keynote for other clues, especially for those with darker skin tones, is any change in color, warmth, edema, or pain over a bony prominence area of pressure.
Stage II	Classified most often as an open or fluid-filled blister. Partial thickness avulsion of skin into dermis layer and may present as a shallow open ulcer.
Stage III	Involves full-thickness loss in which the hypodermis or subcutaneous fat layer may be exposed. It may be shallow or deep, depending on the amount of hypodermis tissue.
Stage IV	Full-thickness wound with exposed tendon, muscle, and/or bone. Most often has slough (dead cells) or eschar (dead tissue).

Stage of Wound	Guideline
	Assessment for undermining and tunneling is prudent as they most often accompany this stage of wound. Again, one cannot use depth to determine the stage because certain anatomic locations may have less depth to tendon, muscle, and/or bone.
Unstageable	Eschar and/or slough that covers the wound area cannot be staged because the underlying tissue cannot be assessed. It is therefore classified as unstageable until the eschar is removed, and then the wound should be documented related to its defining characteristics.

Diagnostics

- Health history and physical examination
  - Identification of risk factors, including use of risk scale (Braden, Norton)
  - Determining stage (or depth)

Patient Care Management

A collaborative and comprehensive approach to wound care is essential. Many hospitals have wound care protocols, and others have wound care nurses or teams designed specifically to accomplish the task of leading the plan of care. Dietitians, case managers, social workers, consultative health care providers (cardiovascular, infectious diseases, surgeons, and plastic surgeons), nursing staff, and ancillary staff should be part of the plan of care, as all play a role in the prevention and treatment of pressure ulcers. The plan must focus on alleviating pressure, treatment of existing ulcer with sound wound care, education, nutrition, rehydration, mobility, and bed support surfaces (if applicable).

- Medical
  - Prevention by identification of risk factors
  - Wound care
- Surgical
  - Debridement

Nursing Management

Once a pressure ulcer develops, the nurse is responsible for assessing the wound at periodic intervals for improvement and response to treatment. The nursing process provides a framework for the management of patients with pressure ulcers. Risk assessment scores assist the nurse in determining appropriate interventions. (See following table with specific interventions.)

- Risk for Infection
  - Note the presence of exudates should be noted, paying particular attention to the amount, color, consistency, and odor
  - Monitor for ↑ temperature and WBC
- Impaired Tissue Integrity
  - Assess size of the wound with the patient in the same position each time. Document findings.
  - The wound's greatest length, greatest width, and depth at the deepest point should be noted
  - Identify any sinus tracts or undermining, and the presence of any foreign bodies in the wound
  - Note color of the wound which provides information about the vascular supply, presence of infection, nutritional status, and presence of healthy versus necrotic tissue.

Pressure Ulcers, Table of Interventions

Low Risk (15–18)

1. Keep skin clean and dry.
2. Use moisturizer on dry skin.
3. Do not massage bony prominences.
4. Protect skin from moisture; use underpads and briefs.
5. Use skin-protecting ointments (Aloe Vesta or equivalent) to protect skin exposed to urine, stool, or wound drainage.
6. Decrease friction and shear.
7. Increase mobility and activity as tolerated.
8. Assess skin daily.

Moderate Risk (13–14)

1. ALL OF THE ABOVE +
2. Wound care coordinator evaluation.
3. Use lift pads/trapeze (trapeze requires health care provider's order) to minimize friction and shear.
4. Consider a pressure reduction device on the bed and chair.
5. Consider utilizing a turning schedule.
6. Encourage proper dietary intake, and consider a dietitian consult.
7. If bed- or chair-bound, reposition the patient every 1 to 2 hours.
8. Protect heels and elbows; elevate heels off the bed surface, and use pillows between knees.
9. Increase mobility and activity in patients that are bed- or chair-bound.

(continued)

Pressure Ulcers, Table of Interventions
(*continued*)

High Risk (10–12)

1. ALL OF THE ABOVE +
2. Consult dietitian and wound care coordinator evaluation (must enter as consult evaluation in computer).
3. Elevate head of bed only as necessary for meals, treatments, and as medically necessary.
4. Obtain order from health care provider for pressure reduction/relief therapeutic bed.

Note: Low air loss beds do not substitute for turning.

Very High Risk (9 or below)

1. ALL OF THE ABOVE+
2. Obtain order from health care provider for pressure relief therapeutic bed.

LOWER RESPIRATORY DISORDERS

Asthma

Asthma is a chronic hyperreactive disorder of the airways (bronchioles) that is characterized by episodic reversible airflow obstruction and airway inflammation, persistent airway hyperreactivity, and airway remodeling (changes in wall structure). This inflammatory process causes recurrent episodes of wheezing, breathlessness, chest tightness, and coughing, particularly at night or in the early morning, in susceptible individuals. These episodes are usually associated with widespread but variable airflow obstruction that is often reversible either spontaneously or with treatment. The inflammation also causes an associated increase in the existing bronchial responsiveness to a variety of stimuli.

Intrinsic Asthma

(nonallergic asthma), is triggered by diverse nonimmune mechanisms, including respiratory tract infections, exercise, ingestion of aspirin, emotional upset, and exposure to bronchial irritants such as cigarette smoke, dust, chemicals, and fumes.

Extrinsic, or Atopic, Asthma

is initiated by a type 1 hypersensitivity response to an extrinsic antigen, such as pollens and allergens.

In many individuals the symptoms of asthma are reversible, but fibrosis of the lung may occur in some patients with asthma and these changes cause abnormalities of lung function. This decreases lung compliance and initiates a restrictive component to the lung disease.

Airflow obstruction can be caused by a variety of changes:

- Acute bronchoconstriction—Due to release of IgE-dependent mediator release upon exposure to aeroallergens and is the primary component of the early asthmatic response.

- Airway edema—Occurs 6 to 24 hours following an allergen

- Chronic mucous plug formation—Consists of an exudate of serum proteins and cell debris that may take weeks to resolve

- Airway remodeling—Due to long-standing inflammation and may profoundly affect the extent of reversibility of airway obstruction

Signs and Symptoms

Attacks vary from person to person, with many people being symptom free between attacks.

- Episodic wheezing, coughing, and feelings of chest tightness

- Acute immobilizing attacks, with use of accessory muscles for breathing, distant breath sounds caused by air trapping, and loud wheezing
  - Fatigue develops as the attack progresses
  - Skin becoming moist
  - Anxiety and apprehension becoming obvious
  - Dyspnea may be severe, and often the person is able to speak only one or two words at a time before taking a breath
  - Airflow is markedly decreased, breath sounds become inaudible with diminished wheezing, and the cough becomes ineffective despite being repetitive and hacking

Diagnostics

- Detailed history to rate severity and treatment options
- Sputum Gram stain and culture

- Pulmonary function tests (FEV1) (FVC)
- CBC
- ABG study

Patient Care Management
Goals of Therapy
- Achieve and maintain control of symptoms
- Prevent asthma exacerbations
- Maintain pulmonary function as close to normal levels as possible
- Maintain normal activity levels, including exercise
- Weight management: increased risk with an elevated body mass index (BMI)
- Avoid adverse effects from asthma medications
- Prevent the development of irreversible airflow limitations
- Prevent asthma mortality

(See Appendix #30, Summary of Medications to Treat Lower Airway Disorders.)

Nursing Management
During acute attack—Impaired gas exchange due to bronchospasm

- Monitor
  - Vital signs
  - Oxygen saturation and ABGs
  - Lung sounds
  - Air exchange and work of breathing
- Administer Medications:
  - Short-acting beta agonists—Quick relief medications are used to relieve acute asthma exacerbations and to prevent exercise-induced asthma symptoms.
  - Anticholinergics (used for severe exacerbations)
  - Systemic corticosteroids

- Long-term control inhaled medication
  - Corticosteroids
  - Cromolyn sodium
  - Nedocromil
- Long-acting beta agonists
  - Methylxanthines
  - Leukotriene antagonists
- Provide emotional support to patient and family

Knowledge Deficit Related to Disease Process, Prevention of Attacks

- Explain disease process and treatment plan
- Teach medication regime
- Teach about triggers, what drug to use when, proper inhaler technique, how to use a spacer with an MDI, and the importance of early use of corticosteroids in exacerbations
- Teach use of metered-dose inhalers, spacers, and importance of rinsing mouth after use
- Teach patient to monitor peak flow measurements with a diary for day-to-day management, which leads to better asthma control
- Discuss plans for possible emergencies at home or work
- Encourage a health maintenance routine that includes regular checkups, regular assessment of peak flow rates and use of a peak flow meter and awareness of individual triggers that cause bronchospasm or exacerbations

Chest Trauma and Thoracic Injuries

Chest trauma is the cause of nearly 16,000 deaths in the United States each year and the cause of death in 25% of all trauma patients. A fracture occurs because the pressure of an injury interrupts the bony integrity of the rib or the sternum. These injuries impair airway patency, breathing, and circulation. Rib fractures are the most common blunt thoracic injury in adults. These are frequently associated with other injuries such as flail chest, pulmonary contusion, and pneumothorax.

Flail Chest

A flail chest occurs when an injury causes a segment of the thoracic cage to be separated from the rest of the chest wall. This usually occurs when at least two fractures per rib occur (producing a free segment), in at least two ribs. In most cases, the severity and extent of the lung injury determine the clinical course and requirement for mechanical ventilation. Thus, the management of flail chest consists of standard management of the rib fractures and of the pulmonary contusions underneath. The patient with a sternal fracture is evaluated closely for underlying cardiac injuries.

Signs and Symptoms

- Severe localized pain, increased on movement of the ribs, deep breathing, coughing, or sneezing
- Shallow breathing, with splinting of the effected side
- Palpable defect and crepitation on movement or coughing with displaced fracture
- Tenderness along the sternum, ecchymosis, swelling, and the potential for a chest wall deformity
- Increased work of breathing and pulmonary shunting with hypoxia
- Severe respiratory distress

Diagnostics

- Chest x-ray
- ABGs
- Pulse oximetry
- CT scan

Patient Care Management

- Protecting the underlying lung
- Provide adequate oxygenation, ventilation, and pulmonary toilet
- Prevent pneumonia
- 100% oxygen via a nonrebreather face mask

- Oxygen saturation and ABGs are monitored
- Analgesia to insure adequate inspiration and clearance of secretions

Nursing Management

Potential for Respiratory Complication

- Monitor for dyspnea and hypoxia
- Pulse oximetry
- Lung sound assessment
- Provide pain medication

Knowledge Deficit

- Teach importance of deep breathing exercises
- Explain importance of pain medication and to notify nurse when needed
- Teach to call for assistance in case of increasing dyspnea and pain

Pulmonary Contusion

A trauma injury to the lung parenchyma, leading to edema and blood collecting in alveolar spaces and loss of normal lung structure and function. This blunt injury develops over 24 hours, leading to poor gas exchange, increased pulmonary vascular resistance, and decreased lung compliance. There also is a significant inflammatory reaction to blood components in the lung, and 50% to 60% of patients with significant contusions develop bilateral acute respiratory distress syndrome (ARDS).

Signs and Symptoms

- Clinical signs of contusion may be present—rib fractures, flail chest, or bruising
- Respiratory crackles
- Pain affecting the ability to ventilate and clear secretions

Diagnostics

- Rarely diagnosed on physical examination
- Chest x-ray—True extent may not be present for 24 to 48 hours

- CT scan—Most sensitive exam
- ABGs and/or pulse oximetry

Patient Care Management
- Close monitoring for hypoxemia
- Oxygen therapy
- Intubation and mechanical ventilation if necessary
- Fluid restriction to prevent pulmonary edema

Nursing Management
Potential for Ineffective Oxygenation
- Provide oxygenation
- Monitor lung sounds and notify health care provider for significant changes
- Oximetry
- Lung sounds
- Maintain fluid restriction—Careful intake and output
- Provide pain medication to encourage deep breathing

Knowledge Deficit
- Teach importance of deep breathing exercises
- Explain importance of pain medication and to notify nurse when needed
- Explain the reason for fluid restriction and careful intake and output

Pneumothorax
Pneumothorax results in a partial or complete collapse of the lung on the affected side. It is caused by a rupture in the visceral pleura or the parietal pleura and chest wall. As air separates the pleura, it destroys the negative pressure of the pleural space, disrupting the normal state of equilibrium. This may occur spontaneously or without obvious cause or as a result of trauma.

Spontaneous pneumothorax occurs unexpectedly in healthy individuals between the ages of 20 and 40. The cause of the pneumothorax is a ruptured, air-filled bleb or blister on the lung surface. Bleb rupture allows atmospheric air to enter the pleural cavity, resulting in a loss of negative pressure and collapse of the lung. Blebs on the visceral pleura rupture during sleep, rest, or exercise. Tension pneumothorax can develop with this rupture.

Tension pneumothorax is one of the rapidly developing complications of blunt chest trauma and occurs as a result of an air leak in the lung or chest wall. The air that enters the pleural space during expiration does not exit during inspiration due to the damaged tissue acting as a one-way valve. This increased pressure pushes the heart and mediastinal structures to the contralateral side. The mediastinal impinges on and compresses the contralateral lung. Hypoxia results as the collapsed lung on the affected side and the compressed lung on the contralateral side are compromised resulting in a diminished ability to effectively exchange gas. This hypoxia and decreased venous return caused by compression of the relatively thin walls of the atria impair cardiac function, thereby decreasing cardiac output and resulting in hypotension and, ultimately, hemodynamic collapse and death if untreated. In the hospital setting, tension pneumothorax can be caused by central venous catheterization and mechanical ventilation in which peak inspiratory pressure rises when the patient fights the ventilator. This more commonly occurs in patients with COPD receiving positive end-expiratory pressure (PEEP) during mechanical ventilation.

Traumatic pneumothorax occurs with penetrating chest injuries such as bullets or stab wounds, and fractured ribs that penetrate the pleura. Hemothorax is frequently associated with these injuries. A traumatic pneumothorax may also occur with fracture of the trachea, bronchus, or esophagus.

Hemothorax

Defined as blood in the thoracic cavity, it is one of the most common problems encountered following blunt chest trauma. Bleeding is caused by injuries to the lung parenchyma, such as pulmonary contusions and lacerations, which often are associated with rib and sternal fractures. Massive intrathoracic bleeding in blunt chest trauma usually stems from the heart, great vessels, or major systemic arteries. Chest surgery may cause what is classified as a traumatic pneumothorax as a result of air and fluid seeping into the pleural space. Hemothorax may emerge as a result of a malignancy that damages blood vessels. As air and blood separate the pleurae, it destroys the negative pressure of the pleural space disrupting the normal state of equilibrium. The lung recoils and collapses toward the hilus.

Signs and Symptoms
(Pneumothorax and Hemothorax)

Can be life threatening, depending on size of pneumothorax or hemothorax

- Pleuritic pain
- Breathlessness
- Breath sounds are unilaterally decreased or absent
- Respiratory distress, which can lead to respiratory arrest if untreated
- Increasing levels of agitation especially if this is a sudden event
- ↓ Cardiac output
- ↓ Blood pressure—Key sign occurring just prior to cardiovascular collapse
- ↑ Heart rate
- Late signs
  - Percussion note is hyperresonant, or very loud.
  - Tracheal deviation

Diagnostics
- Chest x-ray
  - Pneumothorax—Shows lung collapse and air in the pleural space
  - Hemothorax—Shows fluid accumulation in the pleural space or haziness if the quantity of blood is small

- CT scanning
- ABG—Evaluate hypoxia, hypercarbia, and respiratory acidosis

Patient Care Management
- Manage oxygenation to relieve hypoxia
- Lung reexpansion
  - Needle aspiration
  - Heimlich valve
  - Chest tube insertion and chest drainage device
- Mechanical ventilation if necessary

Nursing Management
Sudden Ineffective Tissue Oxygenation
- Respiratory assessment and rapid notification of health care team
- Pulse Oximetry/ABG's to evaluate hypoxia
- Observe for hypotension and tachycardia
- Provide maximal oxygen
- Prepare supplies for urgent lung reexpansion—Needle aspiration, Heimlich valve, chest tube with drainage device
- After insertion completed
  - Proper care of chest tube and drainage system per health care provider orders
  - Monitoring of lung sounds, vital signs, and pulse oximetry

> **Critical Alert**
> Never clamp a chest tube except under direct observation prior to removing the tube.

Anxiety due to dyspnea, pain, and sudden event
- Provide calming environment
- Explain rationale for all treatments
- Administer pain medication

Near Drowning

To be categorized as a near drowning the patient must survive for at least 24 hours after submersion. Immersion in water causes laryngospasm and pulmonary injury resulting in hypoxemia and its effects on the brain and other organs. Young adults typically drown in lakes, ponds, rivers, and oceans. Diving accidents are a common cause, and alcohol and recreational drugs have been implicated in many cases. After initial gasping, and possible aspiration, immersion stimulates hyperventilation, followed by involuntary apnea and laryngospasm leading to hypoxemia, cardiac arrest, and CNS ischemia. Inhalation of water causes pulmonary vasoconstriction, hypertension, destruction of surfactant, alveolar instability, and atelectasis.

Signs and Symptoms
- Hypothermia
- Tachycardia or bradycardia
- Hypotension
- Anxious appearance
- Tachypnea, dyspnea
- Hypoxia
- Metabolic acidosis
- Altered level of consciousness

Diagnostics
- History of situation, type of water, length of submersion
- ABG to assess level of hypoxia
- CBC
- Electrolytes
- Coagulation
- Chest x-ray to determine evidence of aspiration, pulmonary edema, or atelectasis

Patient Care Management

Alert and Oriented Patients

- Observed until the ABGs become normal and there is an absence of dysrhythmias

In Respiratory Failure Patients

- Intubate and mechanically ventilate
- Rewarm to 30°C (86°F)—Resuscitation efforts are not abandoned until rewarmed
- Decompress the stomach and prevent aspiration via nasogastric tube
- Treat for electrolyte imbalances, seizures, bronchospasm, atelectasis, dysrhythmias, and hypotension

Observe for Complications

- Acute renal failure
- Ischemic cerebral injury
- ARDS
- Pulmonary damage secondary to the drowning episode
- Cardiac arrest

Nursing Management

Risk of Tissue Hypoxia and Mental Deterioration

- Support oxygenation
- Assist with interventions
- Assess for signs and symptoms

Ineffective Family Coping

- Communicate the patient status to family members
- Explain rationale for oxygen therapy
- Explain the cause of symptoms—Hallucinations, ataxia, visual disturbances, headaches, and psychoses

Carbon Monoxide Poisoning

Carbon monoxide, or CO is an odorless, colorless gas that can cause sudden illness or death when fumes have built up in an enclosed space. It is found in combustion fumes such as those produced by cars and trucks, small gasoline engines, stoves, lanterns, burning charcoal and wood, and gas ranges and heating systems. Persons who attempt suicide or are victims of smoke inhalation are poisoned with carbon monoxide. Hypoxia rapidly occurs as the carbon monoxide easily binds to the hemoglobin, displacing the oxygen molecules.

Signs and Symptoms

- Headache
- Giddiness
- Tinnitus
- Weakness
- Nausea and vomiting
- Decreased level of consciousness

> **Critical Alert**
> Pulse oximetry *is not valid* because the hemoglobin is well saturated, but with carbon monoxide.

Diagnostics

- ABGs
- Chest x-ray
- Carboxyhemoglobin blood levels (greater than 40% are considered severe)

Patient Care Management

- Treat hypoxemia and induce release of carbon dioxide from hemoglobin
- 100% oxygen
- Hyperbaric oxygen therapy
- Intubation and mechanical ventilation may be required

Nursing Management
Risk of Tissue Hypoxia and Mental Deterioration

- Support oxygenation
- Assist with interventions
- Assess for signs and symptoms

Ineffective Family Coping

- Communicate the patient status to family members
- Explain rationale for oxygen therapy
- Explain the cause of symptoms—Hallucinations, ataxia, visual disturbances, headaches, and psychoses

Knowledge Deficit

- Educate regarding the dangers of smoking and advocate for the presence of smoke alarms
- Teach dangers of allowing exhaust fumes to be present in small enclosed places
- Upon discharge, instruct to seek assistance if they experience dyspnea, confusion, altered levels of consciousness, hallucinations, weakness, or nausea.

Chronic Obstructive Pulmonary Disease (COPD)

COPD is the fourth leading cause of death in America, most commonly caused by tobacco smoke exposure. COPD refers to a group of respiratory disorders characterized by chronic and recurrent obstruction of airflow in the pulmonary airways that is permanent and progressive (chronic bronchitis and emphysema). They coexist in many patients, although one disease may be predominant.

> **Critical Alert**
> Smoking cessation is the single most important factor in preventing COPD.

Chronic Bronchitis

This is hypersecretion of mucus and chronic productive cough that continues at least 3 months of the year for at least two consecutive years, most common in the winter months. Bronchial irritants contribute to increased secretions, edema, bronchospasm, and impaired mucociliary clearance. The mucous secretions are thicker and more tenacious than normal. Because of this, bacteria become embedded in the secretions where they reproduce rapidly. The bronchial walls become inflamed and thickened from edema and the accumulation of inflammatory cells. Airway enlargement and loss of elastic recoil in the alveoli cause air trapping and limiting airflow out of the lung.

Emphysema

This is identified by alteration of the lung architecture and destruction of alveolar walls. Lungs lose their elasticity and air spaces distal to the terminal bronchioles are abnormally enlarged or hyperinflated, causing limited airflow out of the lung and trapping of stagnant air. Portions of the pulmonary capillary bed necessary for gas exchange are eliminated. Airway resistance is increased because of compromised alveolar walls, or septa, especially during forced expiration. Hyperinflation of alveoli causes large air spaces (bullae) and air spaces adjacent to pleura (blebs) to develop. Additional airway narrowing can occur as a result of inflammatory hyperactivity of the bronchi with bronchoconstriction.

Signs and Symptoms
- Dyspnea
- Wheezing
- Increased work of breathing requiring accessory muscles use
- Ventilation/perfusion mismatching with decreased forced expiratory volume in 1 second (FEV_1)
- Productive cough

Diagnostics
- Chest x-ray
- CT scan
- Sputum Gram stain and culture

- Serum theophylline level
- CBC—Hemacrit levels to determine AAT levels
- Serum electrolytes, BUN, creatinine, liver function studies
- ABGs
- Pulmonary function tests
- FEV_1 (volume of air that the patient can forcibly exhale in 1 second) to FVC (forced vital capacity)

Patient Care Management

The goal is to improve daily living and the quality of life by preventing symptoms and the recurrence of exacerbations by preserving optimal lung function.

- Patient education and active involvement in therapy
- Smoking cessation
- Medication therapy
  - Bronchodilators
  - Theophylline to increase muscle function
  - Corticosteroids
  - Intravenous magnesium for bronchodilation by counteracting calcium-mediated constriction
  - Antibiotics
  - Beta-antagonists—Terbutaline (Brethaire, Bricanyl) and albuterol (Proventil)
  - Anticholinergics for bronchodilation ipratropium bromide (Atrovent) and ipratropium and albuterol (Combivent)
  - Glucocorticoid to decrease inflammatory response—Methylprednisolone (Solu-Medrol, Depo-Medrol) usually given intravenously to decrease the inflammatory response

(See Appendix #30.)

- Oxygen therapy maintain 90% saturation—Long-term and continuous therapy
- Physical therapy

346

> **Critical Alert**
>
> Occasionally, large increases in carbon dioxide can lead to deterioration of mental status, causing stupor and obtundation. In such cases, decreasing oxygen delivery is the wrong action. The CO_2 narcosis inhibits respiratory drive to the point that decreasing oxygen delivery leads to worsening of hypoxia. The correct action is immediate intubation and oxygenation.

Nursing Management

Ineffective Airway Clearance, Impaired Gas Exchange

- Assess breath sounds and work of breathing
- Monitor oxygen saturation and ABGs
- Encourage fluids to thin secretions
- Promote activities of daily living with rest periods
- Manage anxiety, encourage patient to verbalize

Risk of Infection

- Monitor for signs of infection
- Assess secretions for color, consistency, and quantity

Knowledge Deficit

- Teach and have patient demonstrate proper use of metered-dose inhalers
- Reinforce smoking cessation, provide referrals
- Teach to avoid triggers and exposure to infection
- Teach to use diaphragm more effectively and use pursed-lip breathing technique to keep the airways open longer
- Explain importance of oxygen therapy in the prevention of polycythemia vera, a condition that occurs when the hematocrit becomes elevated beyond the normal range as a compensatory mechanism of hypoxemia and the development of cor pulmonale that increases mortality in COPD.
- Review criteria for contacting the health care provider, and actions to be taken for increased symptoms

- Encourage involvement in pulmonary rehabilitation program for improved management of chronic disease

Cor Pulmonale

Cor pulmonale is defined as an alteration in the structure and function of the right ventricle caused by a primary disorder of the respiratory system. May occur acutely or as a chronic process. Disorders that lead to pulmonary hypertension are the common link between lung dysfunction and the heart dysfunction.

Causes

- Chronic lung disease (causes more than 50% of cases)
- Pulmonary embolism
- Interstitial lung disease
- Idiopathic primary pulmonary hypertension
- Blood disorders such as (polycythemia vera, sickle cell disease, and macrohemoglobinemia)

Diagnostics for Cor Pulmonale

Test	Expected Abnormality	Rationale
Chest x-ray	Enlargement of central pulmonary arteries; increased transverse diameter of the heart.	Changes in heart and pulmonary vessels are caused by pulmonary hypertension secondary to hypoxemia.
Echocardiography	Shows signs of chronic right ventricular pressure overload.	The right ventricle is strained by pulmonary hypertension.

Test	Expected Abnormality	Rationale
ECG	Incomplete right bundle branch block, low-voltage QRS, signs of right ventricular hypertrophy, and atrial and junctional dysrhythmias.	ECG changes are secondary to right atrial enlargement and hypoxemia.
Cardiac catheterization	Assesses degree of pulmonary hypertension and differentiates cor pulmonale from occult left ventricular dysfunction.	Chronic hypoxemia causes pulmonary hypertension.
Hematocrit	Abnormally elevated.	Polycythemia developed secondary to hypoxemia.
Serum Alpha 1-antitrypsin	Decreased.	Deficiency of AAT causes COPD symptomatology and leads to cor pulmonale.

Signs and Symptoms

Early Signs and Symptoms

- Asymptomatic until right ventricular pressures increase

- Significant signs and symptoms related to underlying lung disorder (e.g., dyspnea, exertional fatigue)
- Increased right ventricular pressure
- Left parasternal systolic lift
- Loud pulmonic component of the second heart sound (S_2)
- Murmurs of functional tri-cuspid and pulmonic insufficiency

Later Signs and Symptoms
- RV gallop rhythm (third [S_3] and fourth [S_4] heart sounds) augmented during inspiration
- Distended jugular veins
- Hepatomegaly
- Lower extremity edema
- Fatigue
- Dyspnea
- Chest pain on exertion
- Cough

Advanced Stages
- Hepatic congestion leading to anorexia, right upper quadrant abdominal discomfort, and jaundice

Physical Assessment Findings
- ↑ chest diameter
- Labored respirations with retractions of the chest wall and use of accessory muscles
- Hyperresonance to percussion
- Diminished breath sounds, wheezing
- Cyanosis (rarely)
- Split second heart sound, a systolic ejection murmur with a sharp ejection click over the pulmonary artery, along with a diastolic regurgitation murmur
- Third ventricular heart sound secondary to systemic venous congestion. This also may be reflected by distended neck veins

Patient Care Management

Treatment is directed at the underlying illness and optimizing oxygenation.

- Continuous oxygen therapy to relieve hypoxemic pulmonary vasoconstriction
- Diuretics to decrease right ventricular filling volume, caution with hypokalemia, metabolic acidosis, and a decline in cardiac output
- Vasodilator drugs including calcium channel blockers
- Theophylline for the weak inotropic effect to improve right ventricular ejection and decrease pulmonary vascular resistance
- Anticoagulation with warfarin in patients who are high risk for thromboembolism
- Phlebotomy is recommended for patients with severe polycythemia
- Cardiac medications

Nursing Management

Alteration in Oxygenation

- Provide continuous oxygenation—Careful to explain importance during exercise and sleep
- Administer medications to treat right ventricular hypertrophy, pulmonary hypertension, and underlying disease
- Monitor for deterioration
  - Labored respirations with retractions of the chest wall and use of accessory muscles
  - Diminished breath sounds, wheezing
  - Changes in heart sounds
  - Distended neck veins

Knowledge Deficit

- Teach management of oxygen equipment and medications
- Encourage involvement in pulmonary rehabilitation program for improved management of chronic disease

- Provide smoking cessation resources and importance of eliminating avoid exposure to secondhand smoke and respiratory pollutants
- Instruct when to call the health care provider

Cystic Fibrosis

Cystic fibrosis (CF) is the most common fatal recessive genetic disease among Caucasians. It affects mainly the exocrine (mucous) glands of the lungs, liver, pancreas, and intestines, causing progressive disability due to multiple-system failure. The typical features of CF lung disease are mucous plugging, chronic inflammation, and infection. CF is caused by a mutation in a single gene, the cystic fibrosis transmembrane conductive regulator (CFTR). This gene controls the production of a protein that regulates how salt is carried across the membranes that separate cells. The gene disturbance leads to production of unusually thick mucus that blocks bodily passages, particularly in the digestive and respiratory systems. About 12 million Americans are carriers of an abnormal CF gene; many of them do not know that they are CF carriers.

Signs and Symptoms
Pulmonary
- Persistent cough or wheeze
- *Pseudomonas aeruginosa* and/or *Staphylococcus aureus* in the sputum
- Hyperinflated lungs on chest x-ray
- Barrel chest and digital clubbing
- Chronic sinusitis
- Nasal polyps
- Recurrent episodes of pneumonia
- Chronic bronchitis

Gastrointestinal
- Frequent loose and oily stools
- Pancreatic abnormalities
- Cramps and abdominal pain

- Rectal prolapse
- Malnutrition and weight loss

Endocrine
- Glucose intolerance
- Polydipsia, polyuria, polyphasia

Reproductive
- Infertility in males
- High risk of complications with pregnancy
- Delayed sexual development

Diagnostics for Cystic Fibrosis

Test	Expected Abnormality	Rationale for Abnormality
Sweat test	Sodium chloride concentration in excess of 60 mEq/L.	Mucous plugging of the sweat duct causes malabsorption of sodium chloride. This is a diagnostic indicator of CF.
Chest x-ray	Shows densities or whiteout in areas of consolidation.	This is a diagnostic indicator of CF.
Fecal fat	Fecal fat concentration is elevated.	Pancreatic enzymes such as amylase, lipase, and trypsinogen do not reach the intestine to digest ingested nutrients. There is malabsorption of fat, protein, and fat-soluble vitamins. This results in steat-orrhea (fatty stool).

(continued)

Diagnostics for Cystic Fibrosis (*continued*)

Test	Expected Abnormality	Rationale for Abnormality
Pancreatic enzymes	Decreased.	Mucous plugging of the pancreatic duct results in fibrosis of the acinar glands of the pancreas. The exocrine function of the pancreas is altered and may be lost completely.
Pulmonary function studies	Show abnormal findings.	Tidal volume, vital capacity, and other functions are below normal related to the disease process.
Serum glucose	Elevated.	Diabetes mellitus may occur because the islets of Langerhans become fibrotic. CF-related diabetes affects 15% of patients with CF.
Semen analysis	Sperm count abnormally low.	Confirms infertility in males. CF causes maldevelopment of the vas deferens.
Genetic analysis	Positive for CF.	Confirms diagnosis.
Liver enzymes	Elevated.	Mucous plugging causes biliary cirrhosis late in the disease.

Patient Care Management

Early diagnosis and treatment are important in delaying the onset and severity. Careful history (CF in a sibling) and newborn screening is vital. Treatment measures are directed toward slowing the progression of secondary organ dysfunction and sequelae such as chronic lung infection and pancreatic insufficiency. Comprehensive multidisciplinary CF treatment programs have led to a dramatic increase in the median age of survival for those affected patients. Care is managed by a multidisciplinary team including the health care provider, nurse, respiratory therapist, physical therapist, and nutritionist. The patient and family members work closely with the team to develop a regimen that is successful. Involvement of the patient is critical.

- Chest physical therapy twice daily, more frequently with exacerbations (chest percussion and postural drainage)
- Nasal toilet
- Antibiotics to prevent and manage infections
- Mucolytic agents to prevent airway obstruction
- Pancreatic enzyme replacement and nutritional therapy

(See Appendix #30.)

- Screen patients for *Mycobacterium tuberculosis* infection with yearly PPD skin tests and treated prophylactically with the same regimen

Nursing Management
Risk for Ineffective Airway Clearance and Infection

- Monitor breath sounds, oximetry, and breathing effort
- Promote adequate airway clearance
- Administer medications as prescribed
- Encourage fluids
- Schedule chest physical therapy
- Encourage performance of ADLs

- Decrease exposure to infection
- Encouraged patients to wash hands frequently, especially after coughing

Knowledge Deficit
- Assist patients in gaining and maintaining independence by assuming responsibility for their own care
- Teach patient and family the disease process, methods of maintaining a clear airway, and the ADL regime
- Teach medication administration, proper use of inhalers
- Teach to prevent exhaustion and limit exposure to infection
- Home care instruction:
  - Postural drainage techniques
  - Aerosol-nebulation therapy
  - Breathing retraining
  - Controlled coughing techniques
  - Deep breathing exercises
  - Progressive exercise conditioning

Idiopathic Pulmonary Fibrosis

Idiopathic pulmonary fibrosis is a chronic, progressive, fibrosing interstitial lung disease of unknown etiology characterized by a poor prognosis and no proven effective treatment. Typically, when detected, IPF is already in an advanced stage. Patients who have IPF cannot develop normally with pulmonary gas exchange and have a much-reduced quality of life. Because of lack of an effective treatment, they rarely survive 5 years after being diagnosed.

Signs and Symptoms
- Progressive dyspnea upon exertion
- Cough
- Diminished stamina

- Weight loss and fatigue
- Interstitial infiltrates
- Abnormal pulmonary function test results indicating restrictive disease

Diagnostics

- Laboratory
  - Elevated hemoglobin value may reflect chronic hypoxemia secondary to IPF
  - Erythrocyte sedimentation rate elevation in 50% of patients
  - Serologic test results are nonspecific, but high titers may indicate connective-tissue disorders
- Imaging studies
- Pulmonary function tests demonstrate a restrictive ventilatory defect and decreased diffusing capacity bronchoalveolar lavage, echocardiography, and bronchoscopy to isolate or confirm diagnosis
- Lung biopsy

Patient Care Management

Management of IPF focuses preserving as much lung function as possible, and enabling the patient to engage in normal activities as long as possible.

- Preventing and treating complication (pneumothorax, infections)
- Oxygen therapy to improve exercise tolerance
- Corticosteroids
- Cytotoxics
- Antifibrotic agents
- Mechanical ventilation for acute respiratory failure
- Nutritional maintenance
- Immunizations
- Smoking cessation
- Pulmonary rehabilitation
- Lung transplant referral

Nursing Management

The main focus is on assisting the patient to remain functional and to maintain as much self-care and life management as possible. IPF does not have a positive prognosis, and the nurse must be aware of the psychosocial needs of the patient and family.

Ineffective Airway Clearance, Impaired Gas Exchange

- Assess breath sounds and work of breathing
- Monitor oxygen saturation and ABGs
- Promote activities of daily living with rest periods
- Manage anxiety, encourage patient to verbalize

Knowledge Deficit

- Teach to avoid triggers and exposure to infection
- Review criteria for contacting the health care provider, and actions to be taken for increased symptoms
- Encourage involvement in pulmonary rehabilitation program for improved management of chronic disease

Infections and Inflammatory Disorders

A variety of pathologies can affect the respiratory system. These respiratory alterations include infections, obstructive diseases, occupational diseases, chest trauma, restrictive disorders, and pleural, vascular, and malignant disruptions.

> **Critical Alert**
> Infections and inflammatory disorders of the respiratory tract are potentially life threatening and a significant cause of morbidly and mortality. The increasing number of resistant organisms enhances the complexity of treatments.

Acute Bronchitis

The sudden inflammation of the lower bronchial mucous membranes. Individuals who suffer from allergies, other respiratory illnesses such as chronic obstructive pulmonary disease (COPD), chronic sinusitis, chronic tonsillitis, or infected adenoids and smokers are at a higher risk.

- Most common viral triggers in adults
  - Adenovirus, influenza virus
  - Respiratory syncytial virus (RSV)
  - Parainfluenza virus
  - Enterovirus
  - Rhinovirus
  - Coronavirus
- Other causes
  - Pollutants such as ammonia and tobacco
- Common bacterial causes
  - *Streptococcus pneumoniae*
  - *Haemophilus influenzae*
  - *Bordetella pertussis*

Signs and Symptoms
- Viral bronchitis
  - Nonproductive cough, paroxysmal, aggravated by cold, dry, or dusty air
  - Wheezing and shortness of breath
- Bacterial bronchitis
  - Productive cough
  - Wheezing and shortness of breath
  - Fever
  - Pain behind the sternum that is aggravated by coughing

Diagnostics
- Health history and physical exam

Patient Care Management
- Treatment focuses on relieving symptoms
  - Antitussives to relieve cough
  - Analgesics

- Bronchodilators
- Increased fluid intake
- Incentive spirometer helps maintain oxygen and carbon dioxide exchange
- Additional treatment for acute exacerbations of chronic bronchitis and emphysema may include:
  - Beta-2 agonists
  - Anticholinergics
  - Antibiotic therapy (when indicated)
  - Corticosteroids
  - Aminophylline

(See Appendix #30.)

Nursing Management
Ineffective Airway Clearance, Impaired Gas Exchange

- Encourage fluids
- Administer medication
- Assess breath sounds and oxygen saturation
- Space activities to provide rest periods

Knowledge Deficit

- Teach importance of hydration to thin secretions
- Teach to avoid triggers, especially important in patients with chronic respiratory disorders

Influenza

A contagious disease caused by the influenza virus that may cause life-threatening complications such as pneumonia in high-risk populations. Influenza A and B epidemics typically occurs during winter months. Transmission of influenza occurs by small-particle aerosols, when an infected person coughs or sneezes and droplets are propelled through the air and deposited on the mouth or nose of people nearby. May also be spread when a person touches respiratory droplets on another person or an object and then touches his own mouth or nose before washing his hands.

Signs and Symptoms

- Abrupt onset, duration 2 weeks without complications
- Fever and chills—Persists for 3 to 4 days and occasionally 1 week
- Headache
- Fatigue
- Dry, nonproductive cough—May be associated with chest pain
- Sore throat
- Nasal congestion
- Myalgia
- Lung sounds are normal, unless complicated by pneumonia

Critical Alert
The elderly and patients with COPD are at an increased risk for pneumonia.

Diagnostics

- Health history and physical exam

Patient Care Management

- Relief of symptoms and prevention of secondary infection
  - Rest
  - Drink plenty of fluids
  - Avoid using alcohol and tobacco
  - Aspirin or acetaminophen for symptom relief
- Prevention
  - Vaccination of high risk population with antiviral injection

Nursing Management
Ineffective Airway Clearance, Impaired Gas Exchange

- Encourage fluids
- Aspirin or acetaminophen for symptom relief

- Assess breath sounds and oxygen saturation
- Space activities to provide rest periods

Knowledge Deficit
- Teach importance of hydration to thin secretions
- Teach importance of vaccination in high risk population

Lung Abscess

A lung abscess is a localized area of lung destruction caused by liquefaction necrosis usually related to pyogenic bacteria. Patients who present with this problem often have a history of pneumonia, possibly complicated by aspiration of oropharyngeal contents. Other causes include bacteremia seeding in the lungs, tricuspid endocarditis leading to septic pulmonary embolus, extension of hepatic abscess, associated with bronchial carcinoma, bronchial obstruction, TB, or fungal infections of the lung.

Signs and Symptoms

Often insidious, although more acute if a lung abscess follows pneumonia
- Spiking temperature with rigors and night sweats
- Cough with sputum that is often foul tasting, foul smelling, and blood stained
- Pleuritic chest pain
- Tachycardia
- Shortness of breath
- Lung sounds—diminished
- Decreased oxygen saturation if large/multiple

Diagnostics
- CT scan
- Pleural fluid and blood cultures
- Bronchoscopy may be used in the case of delayed drainage or suspected malignancy

Patient Care Management

- Health history and physical exam
- Evaluated for possible causes (severe periodontal disease infective endocarditis)
- Drainage of the lung abscess through postural drainage and chest physiotherapy
- Percutaneous chest catheter placement for drainage of the abscess
- Antibiotic therapy
- High in protein diet

Nursing Management
Impaired Gas Exchange Related to Lung Infection

- Assess
  - Work of breathing for worsening of condition
    - Inspect for accessory muscle retraction, cyanosis, grunting on expiration, and restricted chest movement
  - Lung sounds
- Maintain adequate oxygenation
  - Oxygen, as ordered
- Position patient for maximum lung expansion

Critical Alert
Restlessness or increased pulse may be the first signs of hypoxia. Breathlessness and cyanosis are later signs.

Pain Management

- Assess pain using numeric scale (0–10) to quantify pain
- Use pain control measures before the pain becomes severe to intervene early and with less medication

Knowledge Deficit

- Teach importance of spacing activities to optimize oxygenation

Pneumonia

Acute inflammation of lung tissue caused by inhalation of bacteria, viruses, fungi, protozoa, or parasites to the lung. May also be caused by lung insult from radiation therapy; aspiration of water, food, fluid, and vomitus; and inhalation of toxic gases, chemicals, and smoke. The inflammation causes exudate/fluid to fill the alveoli, thereby interfering with oxygen and carbon dioxide exchange causing hypoxemia. Pneumonia is the number one cause of death from an infectious disease, and frequently preceded by influenza. The increasing prevalence of drug-resistant organisms is of concern.

Hospital-acquired pneumonia (HAP) is an infection that occurs more than 48 hours after hospital admission. HAP has a mortality rate of 20% to 50%, most commonly caused by bacteria. *Community-acquired pneumonia* (CAP) is an infection that begins outside the hospital or is diagnosed within 48 hours after admission to a hospital in a person who has not resided in a long-term facility.

Risk Factors

- Advanced age
- Compromised immune system
- Chronic disease
- Underlying lung disease
- Alcoholism
- Decreased level of consciousness
- Smoking
- Malnutrition
- Immobility
- Crowded living conditions
- Exposure to day care
- Treatment in an ICU
- Endotracheal intubation
- Mechanical ventilation
- Contaminated respiratory therapy equipment

Signs and Symptoms

- Fever, chills, or hypothermia
- Respiratory rate greater than 20
- Heart rate greater than 100
- Crackles heard on auscultation
- Chest discomfort
- Dyspnea
- Rusty-colored sputum
- Cough
- Fatigue, muscle aches, headache, nausea

Diagnostics

- Chest x-ray
- Sputum Gram stain and culture (transtracheal aspiration; bronchoscopy with bronchoalveolar lavage; thoracentesis with pleural fluid sample)
- CBC
- ABGs
- Urine sample
- Serum electrolytes, BUN, creatinine, liver function studies

Patient Care Management

- Antibiotic therapy
    - Initiated while identifying the pathogen, later tailored to the specific pathogen
    - HAP—Methicillin-resistant *Staphylococcus aureus* (MRSA) is a consideration and vancomycin may be added to the combination antibiotic therapy
- Bronchodilators (aerosol route or with metered-dose inhalers)
- Oxygen and supportive therapies

(See Appendix #30.)

Nursing Management

Impaired Gas Exchange related to lung infection

- Assess
  - Vital signs
    - Temperature, assessment of fever
    - Tachycardia
  - Work of breathing for worsening of condition
    - Inspect for accessory muscle retraction, cyanosis, grunting on expiration, and restricted chest movement
  - Lung sounds—Auscultate for bronchial breath sounds, inspiratory crackles
- Maintain adequate oxygenation
  - Oxygen, as ordered
  - Evaluate pulse oximetry for trending
  - Check ABGs for hypoxia
- Position patient for maximum lung expansion
- Incentive spirometry
- Encourage fluids to thin secretions

Critical Alert
Restlessness or increased pulse may be the first signs of hypoxia. Breathlessness and cyanosis are later signs.

Knowledge Deficit

- Explain importance of oxygen, positioning, and incentive spirometry/coughing
- Teach importance of spacing activities to optimize oxygenation
- Importance of fluids and nutrient should be reinforced as appetite may be diminished
- Teach about all medications and importance of finishing antibiotic regime

Pulmonary Fungal Infections

Fungal infections of the lung caused by inhalation of contaminated soil resulting in pulmonary infections. Once in the lungs, the fungi elicit tissue responses ranging from acute exudative reactions to a prolonged chronic course, and disseminating to other organs and causing systemic infections. Additionally, individuals with fungal pneumonias may develop chronic pulmonary (e.g., cavitation, pleural effusions, bronchopleural fistulas) or extrapulmonary complications.

Risk Factors

- Travel to an area where fungal pneumonia pathogens are endemic
- Regular exposure to bird, bat, or rodent droppings in endemic areas
- Immunocompromised patients who have an increased risk for opportunistic infections, such as cancer and human immunodeficiency virus (HIV)
- Males

Signs and Symptoms

Acute Primary Disease—Mild self-limiting flu-like syndrome; dyspnea, nonproductive cough; pleuritic chest pain

Chronic (Cavitary) Pulmonary Disease—Immunocompromised: Productive cough; fever; night sweats; weight loss

Disseminated Infection—High fever; generalized lymph node enlargement; hepatosplenomegaly; muscle wasting; anemia, high white blood cell counts, and thrombocytopenia; ulcerations of the tongue and mouth and voice hoarseness; nausea, vomiting, diarrhea, and abdominal pain; meningitis becomes the most pronounced manifestation

Diagnostics

- Health history for exposure
- Culture or histology of fungal organism
- Chest x-ray—Nodular infiltrates that progress rapidly, cavitate, and cross lung fissures
- Lung scans—Perfusion defects consistent with fungal disease
- Skin tests similar to detect *Histoplasma* and *Coccidioides*

Patient Care Management

- Oxygen and supportive therapies
- Antifungal medication

(See Appendix #30.)

Nursing Management
Impaired Gas Exchange Related to Lung Infection

- Assess
  - Vital signs
    - Temperature, assessment of fever
    - Tachycardia
  - Work of breathing for worsening of condition
    - Tachypnea
    - Inspect for accessory muscle retraction, cyanosis, grunting on expiration, and restricted chest movement
  - Lung sounds—Auscultate for inspiratory crackles
- Maintain adequate oxygenation
  - Oxygen, as ordered
  - Evaluate pulse oximeter for trending
  - Check ABGs for hypoxia

Knowledge Deficit

- Explain importance of oxygen
- Teach importance of spacing activities to optimize oxygenation

Pulmonary Tuberculosis (TB)

Pulmonary tuberculosis (TB) is a highly communicable bacterial infection caused by *mycobacterium tuberculosis*. TB is transmitted via aerosolization when an infected person laughs, coughs, sneezes, spreading droplet nuclei that may be inhaled by others. The lungs are primarily involved but the disease can spread to other organs, characterized by the development of granulomas (granular tumors) and causing nonspecific pneumonitis. When the tubercle reaches a suitable site (bronchi or alveoli), it multiplies freely. A small percentage of those who are initially infected develop the disease (5% to 15%).

> **Critical Alert**
> Transmission of TB is rampant in crowded shelters and prisons where people weakened by poor nutrition, drug addiction, and alcoholism are exposed.

Signs and Symptoms
Frequently insidious, many patients do not become aware of symptoms until the disease is well advanced.

- Early symptoms: Lethargy, exhaustive fatigue, activity intolerance, nausea, irregular menses, and low-grade fever, symptoms may have occurred for weeks or months.
- Late symptoms: Dyspnea, Cough, sputum production, dull aching chest, weight loss, sleep disturbances, fever and night sweats

> **Critical Alert**
> Many elderly people whose general health has declined, develop active TB from TB infection that they had much earlier in life. Other elderly people, especially those with weak immune systems, become newly infected with *M. tuberculosis* and can develop active TB rapidly

Diagnostics
- Health history to evaluate exposure
- Physical exam
- Tuberculin skin test
- Chest x-ray
- Acid-fast bacillus smear, and sputum culture x 3

Patient Care Management
- Limit exposure to others—Negative pressure room/ Airborne isolation
- Anti TB medications

(See Appendix #30.)

Nursing Management

Risk for Spread of Disease

- Initiate and maintain airborne isolation—negative pressure room

Ineffective Airway Clearance

- Teach cough and deep breathing exercises
- Encourage fluids to thin secretions

Knowledge Deficit

- Explain to patient and family purpose and importance of airborne isolation
- Teach medication regime and importance of compliance

Occupational Lung Disorders

Exposure to toxic dust and particulate matter may cause a variety of respiratory disorders. Depending on the degree of intensity of exposure, smoking history, and underlying pulmonary disease, individuals may experience irreversible effects of chronic pulmonary disease after long-term exposures.

Occupational Asthma

Affects about 15% of the cases of adult asthma, it is difficult to recognize because the patient continues to experience symptoms when away from the source of exposure. Exposure to workplace chemicals irritants used in industry enzymes in food processing, detergents, pharmaceutical agents, gases, cereal grains.

(See Asthma for more information.)

Pneumoconiosis

The dusts of silica, asbestos, and coal are the most common causes of pneumoconiosis. Others include talc, fiberglass, clays, mica, cement, cadmium, beryllium tungsten, cobalt, aluminum, and iron. The dust deposits are permanent. Treatment is palliative and focuses on preventing further exposure and improving workplace safety.

Silicosis

Pneumoconiosis resulting from the inhalation of free silica and silica-containing compounds. It causes acute fibrosis of the lung tissue as well as fibrous nodules within the lung. Individuals are frequently asymptomatic. This occurs in coal mining and other industries involved in the extraction and processing of ore, preparation and use of sand, and manufacture of pipe building and roofing materials.

(See Pulmonary Fibrosis for more information.)

Coal Miner Pneumoconiosis (Black Lung or Coal Miner's Lung)

Pneumoconiosis caused by coal dust deposits in the lung. The disease affects about 4.5% of coal miners; about 2% have lung scarring causing restrictive disease. Its mild form is without symptoms except for chronic bronchitis. Its severe form consists of pulmonary fibrosis with dyspnea and wheezing often occurring. There is no specific treatment for the disease, and in complex cases patients may develop nodular lesions throughout the lungs. Patients experience a restrictive disease in which they cannot fully expand their lungs as well as an obstructive disease from secondary emphysema.

(See Restrictive Lung Disease.)

Asbestosis

Pneumoconiosis caused by exposure to microscopic fibers of asbestos. This progressive lung disease results in a diffuse interstitial fibrosis with diaphragmatic calcification. Fibrous tissue eventually obliterates the alveoli. Pulmonary function studies usually reveal a restrictive ventilatory defect and restricted lung volume as with silicosis. The patient experiences dyspnea and hypoxemia. The chances of arresting the disease are best in its early stages. Removal of the individual from the asbestos exposure is essential.

(See Restrictive Lung Disease.)

Signs and Symptoms

- Crackles of a dry quality can be auscultated in 70% to 90% of patients with diffuse interstitial fibrosis.
- Clubbing
- Chronic cough and sputum production, similar to acute bronchitis
- Shrinkage of the lung, which occurs with fibrotic changes, can cause a reduced vital capacity.
- Sputum is expectorated in large amounts and often contains varying amounts of black fluid, particularly with smokers.
- Respiratory failure
- Cor pulmonale

Patient Care Management

Identification and limitation to further exposure is key. There is no medical treatment for occupational lung diseases. Patient care management is related to the condition.

(See Asthma, Pulmonary Fibrosis, and Restrictive Lung Disease.)

Nursing Management

Activity Intolerance due to dyspnea and fatigue

- Teach proper use of oxygen therapy
- Provide smoking cessation resources
- Encourage involvement in pulmonary rehabilitation program for improved management of chronic disease

Pleural Effusion

The presence of fluid in the pleural space, which usually occurs secondary to other diseases. The source of the fluid usually is blood vessels or lymphatic vessels lying beneath either pleura, but may be an abscess or other lesion. A pleural effusion can cause compression atelectasis and displacement of mediastinal contents. An effusion may be a transudate or an exudate.

Transudate effusions are clear in color, have a low protein content, and are secondary to underlying diseases. Caused by heart failure, cirrhosis, nephrotic syndrome, and/or medical disorders leading to hypoalbuminemia.

Exudate effusions have a turbid appearance, are higher protein content and usually are caused by infection. Caused by malignancy, collagen vascular disease, pneumonia, pancreatitis, or pulmonary embolism.

Causes
- Heart failure
- TB
- Pneumonia
- Pulmonary infections
- Nephrotic syndrome
- Connective tissue disease
- Pulmonary embolism
- Fungal lung infections
- Neoplastic tumors

Signs and Symptoms
Depend on the underlying disease and the size of the effusion, symptoms varying from asymptomatic to severe breathlessness and pain.

- ↓ Breath sounds on affected side with dull percussion
- Pleural friction rub over the area of pleural inflammation that disappears with breath holding
- Asymmetric expansion of the thoracic cage, with lagging expansion on the affected side
- Anasarca
- Distended neck veins
- S_3 gallop rhythm
- Clubbing of the fingers
- Breast nodule or intra-abdominal mass

- Massive effusions (usually > 1,000 mL) findings:
  1. Mediastinal shift
  2. Displacement of the trachea and mediastinum to the contralateral side of the pleural effusion

Diagnostics

- Chest x-ray
  1. If more than 200 to 500 mL of fluid is present in the pleural space, blunting of the costophrenic angle
- CT scan
- Ultrasound
- Thoracentesis with pleural fluid obtained for biochemical, microbiologic, and cytologic analysis
  1. Protein and glucose concentration
  2. pH
  3. Bacteria, including acid-fast bacilli and cell content
  4. Cytologic testing reveals a malignant effusion about 80% of the time
- Closed-needle biopsy to identify tuberculosis and malignancies

Patient Care Management

As with any other life-threatening condition:

- Airway stabilization with adequate oxygenation and ventilation is the first priority.
- Thoracentesis is performed to remove fluid, if needed.
- Determine and treat the cause of the effusion
- Transudative effusions (most commonly caused by heart failure)
  - Treatment involves controlling the patient's heart failure before considering thoracentesis.
- Exudate effusions (most commonly have malignant cause) and fluid can accumulate rapidly and repeatedly.
  - Thoracentesis is done at frequent intervals to provide comfort and relieve dyspnea

Other Therapies for Management of Malignant Pleural Effusions

- Chemotherapy
- Radiation
- Intrapleural instillation of sclerosing agents
- Indwelling pleural catheters with intermittent drainage
- Chest tube drainage using the water seal system
- Pleuroperitoneal shunts
- Pleurectomy

Nursing Management

Potential for Impaired Gas Exchange

- Evaluate respiratory effort; assess chest expansion for symmetry
- Frequent lung sound evaluation, report pertinent changes
- Provide oxygen
- Monitor pulse oximetry

Pain Related to Chest Tube, or Pleural Drainage

- Provide pain prior to procedures and subsequently as needed
- Encourage positions of comfort

Chest Tube Management

- Monitors the system function and records the amount of drainage at frequent intervals
- Encouraged to turn frequently and ambulate to facilitate chest drainage.
- Monitors electrolytes for imbalances
- Monitor intake and output

Knowledge Deficit

- Teach purpose of chest tube drainage
- If applicable, teach home care of pleural catheter management and care of the catheter and drainage system

- Teach instructions on pain management
- Instruct when to call the health care provider

Pulmonary Embolism

Pulmonary embolism (PE) results when a thrombus breaks loose from an attachment and blocks a branch of the pulmonary artery, which impairs ventilation and perfusion, producing a life-threatening condition. The embolism can be a thrombus, air accidentally injected through an IV catheter, fat from bone marrow after a fracture, or amniotic fluid that has entered the mother's bloodstream after rupture of the membranes at birth.

Causes

Pulmonary embolism is a complication of a DVT, a common occurrence after surgery or trauma, childbirth, stroke, heart failure, myocardial infarction, atrial fibrillation, cancer, and prolonged immobilization. Other causes are oral contraceptive use, surgery especially involving the pelvic area, massive trauma, burns, cancer, stroke, myocardial infarction, and fractures of the hips or femur, and genetic mutations.

Signs and Symptoms

The clinical manifestations of PE depend on its size, location, and the amount of obstruction. Many patients with PE are completely asymptomatic.

- Pleuritic chest pain
- Pulmonary friction rub
- Fever
- Hemoptysis
- Dyspnea
- Diaphoresis
- S_3 or S_4 gallop
- Thrombophlebitis/lower extremity edema
- Atelectasis

Massive PE (May Be Fatal)

- Sudden crushing substernal chest pain
- Systemic hypotension

- Tachypnea
- Crackles
- Cyanosis
- Tachycardia
- Hypotension related to acute cor pulmonale
- Shock

Diagnostics for Pulmonary Embolism

Test	Expected Abnormality	Rationale for Abnormality
ABGs	Abnormal in some cases.	Altered gas exchange secondary to PE.
Pulse oximetry	Abnormal in some cases, normal in most cases.	Altered oxygen saturation secondary to PE.
CBC	White blood cell count may be normal or elevated.	Atelectasis and infiltrates occur, causing elevated white count.
ECG	Specific abnormalities with PE are tachycardia, tall, peaked P waves in lead 2, right axis deviation, and right bundle branch block. Most significant finding is tachycardia.	Hypoxemia secondary to PE causes cardiac abnormalities.

(continued)

Diagnostics for Pulmonary Embolism (*continued*)

Test	Expected Abnormality	Rationale for Abnormality
Chest x-rays	Usually normal initially. Within 24–72 hours atelectasis or infiltrates may be apparent as well as a small pleural effusion.	Altered perfusion pattern not visible via chest x-ray. In massive embolus dilation of the pulmonary vasculature near the embolus may be seen. Infiltrates and pleural effusions are visible later.
D-Dimer test	Positive.	The D-dimer test is a degradation product of cross-linked fibrin generated by plasmin cleavage. When levels are above 500 mg/L, the test is positive. This indicates activation of the fibrolytic pathway, meaning the body is trying to break down clots. Therefore the D-dimer test will be elevated in any condition such as disseminated intravascular coagulation (DIC), PE, DVT, and myocardial infarction where clots are formed. If the D-dimer is positive and the patient also has tachycardia, crackles, dyspnea, pleuritic chest pain, and cough, a PE diagnosis can be confirmed.

Test	Expected Abnormality	Rationale for Abnormality
V/Q scan	Diagnostic of abnormal perfusion pattern, or may be normal.	Perfusion pattern is altered by PE, but even if positive, this is not an acceptable end point in the diagnostic process.
Pulmonary angiogram	Positive.	Provides 100% certainty that an obstruction to pulmonary arterial blood flow does exist. A negative angiogram provides greater than 90% certainty in the exclusion of PE. This is still the most reliable diagnostic test for PE.
Ultrasonography and plethysmography	May detect presence of lower extremity DVT. Echocardiography reflects findings of right-sided heart failure.	Detection of lower extremity DVT helps confirm diagnosis of PE, but often cannot be visualized. Findings of right-sided heart failure consistent with PE.
Spiral CT scan	Positive.	This is a relatively new noninvasive diagnostic test that provides additional slices of the area visualized. In many patients a spiral or helical CT with intravenous contrast can visualize pulmonary vessels so well that an angiogram is not necessary.

Patient Care Management
Rapid Recognition and Therapy Based on Severity

- Oxygen (even with normal arterial PO_2)
- Pulmonary artery catheter insertion to evaluate cardiac output and fluid volume
- Fibrinolytic therapy
- Heparin therapy
- Long-term anticoagulation
- In the case of a cardiac arrest, CPR is not helpful.
- Emergency cardiopulmonary bypass, emergency thoracotomy

Preventive Therapy

- DVT risk assessment and prophylaxis therapy
- Long-term anticoagulation for patients who survive an initial DVT or PE
- Inferior vena cava (IVC) filters in patients with DVT who are unable to tolerate anticoagulants or have recurrent PE

Nursing Management
Risk for DVT and Pulmonary Embolism

- Assess all patients on admission and throughout the hospital stay for risks of PE and DVT
- Observe for signs and symptoms
- DVT prophylaxis and prevention
  - Early ambulation whenever possible
  - Active and passive range of motion exercises
  - Extremity elevation
  - Mechanical methods of prophylaxis (graduated compression stockings, intermittent pneumatic devices, and venous foot pumps)

Ineffective Tissue Perfusion and Impaired Gas Exchange

- Rapid assessment, recognition, and MD notification
- Oxygen

- Monitor vital signs and oximetry
- Administer anticoagulants

Knowledge Deficit
- Teach proper administration of medications
- Teach patient to monitor for bleeding and obtain blood tests as ordered
- Teach patient prevention while traveling
  - Avoiding constrictive clothing, and leg crossing
  - Changing positions frequently while seated
  - Smoking cessation
  - Stay well hydrated with water
  - Wearing compression stockings
- Teach reportable signs and symptoms
  - New onset shortness of breath, chest pain, anxiety, restlessness
  - New onset bleeding, headache, mental status changes

Pulmonary Hypertension

Pulmonary artery hypertension (PH) is a progressive disorder characterized by abnormally high blood pressure (hypertension) in the pulmonary artery increasing the resistance to blood flow through the lungs. There are two types of PH: primary (inherited), also referred to as idiopathic, and secondary, related to some other cause such as chronic heart or lung disease or blood clots in the lungs, or a disease such as scleroderma. Pulmonary artery hypertension is not curable, but it is treatable if diagnosed.

Risk Factors for Secondary Pulmonary Hypertension
- Chronic high-altitude exposure
- Obstructive sleep apnea
- Vasculitis
- Infectious diseases
- HIV

- Drugs and toxins
- Amphetamines
- Anorexigens
- Cocaine
- Toxic rapeseed oil ingestion

Signs and Symptoms

Symptoms of pulmonary hypertension may develop very gradually and often are nonspecific. Thus, patients may delay seeing a health care provider for years, and when seen their disorder may be misdiagnosed and treated for more common conditions:

- Exertional dyspnea
- Fatigue and lethargy
- Angina
- Syncope
- Raynaud's disease
- Edema
- Split second heart sound (S_2); right ventricular third heart sound (S_3)
- Jugular venous distention
- Liver congestion and peripheral edema

Diagnostics

- Chest x-ray
- Spirometry
- ECG
- Doppler ECG to assess right ventricular/pulmonary artery pressures and structural heart disease
- Ventilation/perfusion scanning to detect thromboembolic disease
- Pulmonary function tests
- CT
- Arteriography

Patient Care Management

Treatment is directed at the underlying disease instituted in the early stages

- Oxygen therapy
- Medications
    - Calcium (Ca) channel blockers to reduce pulmonary artery pressure or pulmonary vascular
    - Anticoagulants
    - Diuretics
    - Anticoagulants
    - Digoxin
- Lung transplantation (only cure for PPH)

Nursing Management

**Ineffective Airway Clearance,
Impaired Gas Exchange**

- Administer Oxygen
- Assess breath sounds
- Monitor closely work of breathing, report changes promptly
- Monitor oxygen saturation and ABGs
- Promote activities of daily living with rest periods
- Manage anxiety, encourage patient to verbalize

Knowledge Deficit

- Teach self-care regime to manage fatigue and weakness
- Instruct on medication administration
- Provide home oxygenation instructions, safety and administration
- Instruct on importance of medical follow-up
- Review criteria for contacting the health care provider, and actions to be taken for increased symptoms

Restrictive (Interstitial) Lung Diseases

Restrictive lung diseases (also known as interstitial lung diseases) result in reduced lung volumes, either because of an alteration in lung parenchyma or because of a disease of the pleura, chest wall, or neuromuscular apparatus.

Characteristics

- Reduced total lung capacity
- Vital capacity
- Resting lung volume
- Preserved airflow and normal airway resistance
- If caused by parenchymal lung disease, reduced gas transfer results in desaturation after exercise.

The mortality and morbidity from various causes of restrictive lung disease are dependent on the underlying etiology of the disease process. Factors that predict poor outcome include older age, male gender, severe dyspnea, history of cigarette smoking, severe loss of lung function, appearance and severity of fibrosis on radiologic studies, a lack of response to therapy, and prominent fibroblastic foci on histopathologic evaluation.

Intrinsic Lung Disease

A restrictive lung disease that effects the lung parenchyma. These diseases cause inflammation or scarring of the lung tissue (interstitial lung disease) or result in filling of the air spaces with exudate and debris (pneumonitis).

Causes

- Idiopathic fibrotic diseases
- Connective tissue diseases
- Drug-induced lung disease
- Primary diseases of the lungs (including sarcoidosis)

Signs and Symptoms

- Onset acute or insidious
- Progressive exertional dyspnea

- Dry cough (a productive cough is an unusual sign in most patients)
- Hemoptysis or grossly bloody sputum (diffuse alveolar hemorrhage syndromes and vasculitis)
- Wheezing (lymphangitic carcinomatosis, chronic eosinophilic pneumonia, and bronchiolitis)
- Chest pain (with rheumatoid arthritis, systemic lupus erythematosus, and some drug-induced disorders)
- Those with chest wall disorders:
  - Massive obesity and an abnormal configuration of the thoracic cage
  - Alveolar crackles
  - Inspiratory squeaks or scattered, late, inspiratory high-pitched rhonchi
  - Cyanosis at rest as a late manifestation of advanced disease
  - Digital clubbing

Diagnostics
Imaging Studies
- Chest x-ray
- CT scan
- Lung biopsy

Laboratory evaluations are completed to reveal positive findings in intrinsic lung diseases.

- Anemia can indicate vasculitis.
- Polycythemia can indicate hypoxemia in advanced diseases.
- Leukocytosis suggests acute hypersensitivity pneumonitis.

Patient Care Management
- Corticosteroids
- Immunosuppressive agents
- Cytotoxic agents

- Supplemental oxygen therapy, to alleviate exercise-induced hypoxemia and improves performance
- Antifibrotic therapies

(See Appendix #30.)

Nursing Management
Ineffective Airway Clearance, Impaired Gas Exchange

- Assess breath sounds
- Monitor oxygen saturation
- Promote activities of daily living with rest periods
- Manage anxiety, encourage patient to verbalize

Risk of Infection

- Monitor for signs of infection
- Assess secretions for color, consistency, and quantity
- Encourage fluids and diet

Knowledge Deficit

- Teach to avoid triggers and exposure to infection
- Reinforce smoking cessation, provide referrals
- Review criteria for contacting the health care provider, and actions to be taken for increase symptoms

Extrinsic Lung Disease

A restrictive lung disease that results in lung restriction, impaired ventilatory function, and respiratory failure. The cause of respiratory failure is multifactorial and is secondary to spinal deformity, muscle weakness, disordered ventilatory control, sleep-disordered breathing, and airway disease. As neuromuscular disorders occur and progress, the respiratory muscle weakness progresses.

Causes

- Diseases of the chest wall, pleura, and respiratory muscles

Signs and Symptoms

- Dyspnea
- Decreased exercise tolerance
- Recurrent lower respiratory tract infections
- Fatigue
- Dyspnea at rest
- Severe kyphoscoliosis
- Massive obesity
- Tacile fremitus, dullness upon percussion
- Decreased intensity of breath sounds
- Impaired control of secretions
- Pulmonary hypertension
- Cor pulmonale
- Acute and chronic respiratory failure
- In neuromuscular cases:
  - Accessory muscle usage
  - Rapid shallow breathing
  - Paradoxical breathing

Diagnostics

- Elevated creatinine kinase level that may indicate myositis
- Fluoroscopy procedures
- Pulmonary function testing
- Polysomnographic study for nocturnal hypoventilation or upper airway obstructions
- Bronchoalveolar lavage, lung biopsy, and surgical lung biopsy

Patient Care Management

- Maintain oxygenation
- Identify the cause of muscle weakness
- Minimize the impact of impaired secretion clearance
- Prevention and prompt treatment of respiratory infections

- Prevent severe gas exchange abnormalities during sleep
  - Noninvasive positive pressure ventilation via a nasal or oronasal mask during sleep
  - Permanent tracheotomy and ventilator assistance with a portable ventilator
- Treatment for massive obesity to improve in pulmonary function tests
- Mechanical ventilation for respiratory failure

Nursing Management

The main focus is on assisting the patient to remain functional and to maintain as much self-care and life management as possible.

Ineffective Airway Clearance, Impaired Gas Exchange

- Assess breath sounds
- Monitor closely work of breathing, report changes promptly
- Monitor oxygen saturation and ABGs
- Promote activities of daily living with rest periods
- Manage anxiety, encourage patient to verbalize

Risk of Infection

- Monitor for signs of infection
- Assess secretions for color, consistency, and quantity
- Encourage fluids and diet

Knowledge Deficit

- Teach to avoid triggers and exposure to infection
- Reinforce smoking cessation, provide referrals
- Review criteria for contacting the health care provider, and actions to be taken for increased symptoms

Sarcoidosis

Sarcoidosis is an inflammatory immune system disorder that affects multiple organ systems although 90% of patients present with pulmonary involvement. Exact cause is unknown; it is believed to occur when a person's immune system overreacts to an unknown toxin, drug, or pathogen that enters the body through the airways and triggers small areas of inflammation called granulomas (small inflammatory nodules).

Signs and Symptoms

- None (diagnosed by routine x-ray)
- Fever and night sweats
- Malaise
- Fatigue
- Weight loss
- Dry cough
- Wheezing
- Dyspnea

Diagnostics

- Chemistry and hematologic work-up including liver function tests
- TB skin test (to rule out TB)
- Chest x-ray
- CT scan
- Magnetic resonance imaging (MRI)
- Pulmonary function studies
- ABGs
- Oxygen saturation
- Fiber-optic bronchoscopy with transbronchial biopsies and culturing

Patient Care Management

Therapy is individualized based on the symptoms and organ systems involved. Many patients require no treatment; symptoms usually are not disabling and tend to disappear spontaneously. The decision to initiate drug therapy depends on the organ system involved and how far the inflammation has progressed. If the disease appears to be severe, corticosteroids are prescribed. Follow-up checkups are important to monitor the illness and side effects of medications.

Nursing Management

Impaired Gas Exchange Related to Lung Disease

- Maintain adequate oxygenation
    - Oxygen, as ordered
    - Evaluate pulse oximetry for trending
    - Check ABGs for hypoxia
    - Lung sounds—Auscultate for bronchial breath sounds, inspiratory crackles
- Position patient for maximum lung expansion

Knowledge Deficit

- Educate regarding administration of prednisone, the dangers associated with abrupt stoppage, and side effects such as weight gain, mood changes, hypokalemia, and muscle weakness.
- Instruct on disease and importance of follow-up appointments
- Review criteria for contacting the health care provider, and actions to be taken for increased symptoms

MALE REPRODUCTIVE DISORDERS

Prostate Disorders

- Common disorder of aging men, occurring in as many as 90% or men age 85 and older
- Nonmalignant, nodular growth of prostatic tissue that eventually compresses the urethra causing lower urinary tract symptoms (LUTS)
- As the urinary urethra constricts, it causes increased pressure to urinate, thereby causing bladder distention, eventual hypertrophy of the detrusor muscle, bladder diverticula, urinary stasis, infection, bladder stone formation
- If the obstruction is prolonged, hydronephrosis will occur and cause damage to the kidneys
- The exact cause unknown

Signs and Symptoms

- Urinary hesitancy and intermittency
- Weak urine stream
- Nocturia, frequency and urgency
- Sensation of incomplete bladder emptying
- Terminal dribbling of urine
- Overflow incontinence
- Complete urinary retention
- Hematuria if straining at urination is severe
- Enlarged rubbery prostate that has lost the median furrow

- Full urinary bladder palpable on abdominal examination
- Urinary tract infection
- Bladder stones and diverticuli
- Renal damage, insufficiency and failure after prolonged urinary retention

Diagnostics

- Patient self-report of symptoms using American Urology Association Symptom Index
- History and physical examination, including evaluation for neurological deficits and a digital rectal examination (DRE) of the prostate gland
- Serum blood urea nitrogen (BUN), creatinine, and urinalysis
- Post void residual urine measurement
- Uroflow rate studies that assess voiding patterns
- If hematuria, urinary tract infection, or signs of renal failure are discovered, then renal imaging, urine cytology studies, and cystoscopy
- Prostate specific antigen (PSA) is sometimes used to differentiate BPH from prostate cancer

Patient Care Management

Management depends upon the impact on the patient's quality of life, the presence of comorbidities (e.g., diabetes or heart disease), and the severity of the urinary problem.

Treatment modalities vary from watchful waiting (medication and treatments) to radical surgery.

- Nonpharmacology treatments:
  - Decreasing fluid intake at bedtime to decrease nocturia
  - Decreasing caffeine and alcohol intake because of the irritation to the urinary system
  - Urinary catheterization with standard or stiffer catheter for retention

- Dilation of the urethra may be necessary if catheterization unsuccessful
- Limiting prescription and over-the-counter drugs that may affect urination
- Pharmacology:
  - Alpha-adrenergic antagonists
    - Relaxing the bladder neck and prostatic muscle tone, thereby relieving obstruction
    - Does not affect the blood pressure
    - Specific agents:
      - doxazosin (Cardura)
      - terazosin (Hytrin)
      - tamsulosin (Flomax)
      - alfuzosin (Uroxatral)
  - 5 alpha-reductase inhibitors
    - Reduce the conversion of testosterone resulting in slower prostate growth
    - Specific agents:
      - finasteride (Proscar)
      - dutasteride (Avodart)
- Herbal remedies
  - Pygeum africanum (African star grass)
  - African plum tree bark
  - Rye grass pollens
  - Stinging nettle
  - Cactus flower
  - Saw palmetto
- Surgery
  - Transurethral resection of the prostate (TURP)
    - Via cystoscope, prostate tissue is cut.
    - Continuous bladder irrigation is needed to prevent blood clotting.
    - Postoperative side effects: erectile dysfunction, retrograde ejaculation, and incontinence.

- Thermoablation of the prostate: alternative operative therapies where microwave heat is used to coagulate prostate tissue

  - Transurethral microwave heat treatment (TUMT)

  - Transurethral needle ablation (TUNA)

- Transurethral vaporization of the prostate (TUVP)

  - Laser or electrical vaporization to destroy or remove prostate tissue

- Transurethral incision of the prostate (TUIP)

  - Surgical incisions are made in the prostate to enlarge the urethral opening

  - Less destructive than TURP and TUVP, making it a better choice for younger men

  - It is less likely to cause retrograde ejaculation or erectile dysfunction

Nursing Management

Routine postoperative nursing care can be found in Appendix #1, Nursing Process: Patient Care Plan for the Postoperative Patient Following General Surgery.

- Impaired Urinary Elimination

  - Catheter care:

    - Maintain a closed sterile system

    - Keep drainage bag lower than bladder

    - Avoid kinks in drainage tubing

    - Secure to the patient's thigh with a stabilization device

    - Cleanse urinary meatus with soap and water twice daily

  - Continuous bladder irrigation:

    - Use 0.9% normal saline 5 liter bags

    - Observe for excessive bleeding and clots

    - Notify health care provider for bright red irrigation returns

- Encourage fluid intake to maintain urine output at 50 mL/hr.
- Accurate intake and output; assess for excessive hematuria
- Monitor laboratory data for infection and hemorrhage:
  - Hemoglobin/Hematocrit
  - WBC
  - Urinalysis
- Pain, Acute
  - Assess pain thoroughly using numeric scale and patient self-report
  - Instruct patient to inform the nurse when pain begins and if the pain is not relieved after interventions
  - Instruct patient not to strain against the indwelling urinary catheter in an attempt to void
  - Stool softeners to prevent pain from straining
- Knowledge Deficit
  - Instruct patient and family regarding disease process and expected treatment
  - Instruct patient and family regarding purpose of indwelling catheter and bladder irrigation
  - Explain importance of notifying nurse if pain worsens or patient experiences urinary retention

Inguinal Hernia

Abdominal hernias are protrusions of abdominal contents through a weakness in the abdominal wall and are very common and usually congenital.

Reducible Hernias

- Mass appears on standing
- Reduces when supine

Incarcerated Hernias

- Contents cannot be replaced into the abdomen

Strangulated Hernias

- Irreducible hernia
- Blood supply to trapped bowel has been cut off
- Bowel obstruction occurs

Signs and Symptoms

Symptoms typically occur following an episode of trauma or coughing. The symptoms depend upon the severity of the hernia.

General Symptoms

- Visible bulge
- Discomfort or pain
- Tenderness
- Bowel obstruction and infarction

Diagnostics

Physical examination is considered the primary diagnostic tool. Abdominal x-ray and WBC may be done to determine the presence of a bowel obstruction.

Patient Care Management

Occasionally, when the hernia is small and asymptomatic, a watchful waiting approach will be taken. Otherwise medical management includes surgery to repair the hernia with placement of mesh to reinforce the repair. Surgery for hernia repair may be conventional or laparoscopic. Hernia repair surgery is considered elective unless incarceration occurs.

Nursing Management

Nursing care depends on the severity of the hernia. For patients who will be having surgery the nurse needs to provide general preoperative and post-operative care. (See Appendix #1.)

Sexually Transmitted Infections

(See separate section.)

Testicular Disorders

Annually, 1 in 4,000 males under the age of 25 experience testicular torsion. The process for the development of this problem begins with the congenital absence of attachment of the testicle to the tunica vaginalis. Without this attachment, the testicle hangs freely and can easily twist on the cord. The left testicle is more at risk because of the longer spermatic cord. This twisting causes the blood supply to the testicle to be closed off. Poor vascular supply will cause ischemia, necrosis, and loss of the testicle if it is not relieved within 6–12 hours.

Signs and Symptoms

- Sudden, severe pain in one testicle
- Nausea and vomiting
- Light-headedness

Diagnostics

Physical Examination

- Testicle will be high in the scrotum due to the shortening of the spermatic cord.
- The affected testicle may also feel larger than normal.
- Cremasteric reflex (the testicle will rise in the scrotum when the thigh near the scrotum is stroked) will be absent.

Doppler Ultrasound

- Confirms diagnosis

Patient Care Management

Pain Management
Immediate Surgery

- Orchiopexy:
  - Testicle and cord are untwisted.
  - If the testicle is viable it is anchored to the scrotum to prevent recurrence.
- Orchiectomy:
  - Removal of testicle if it is unviable

Nursing Management

Routine postoperative care is found in Appendix #1.

- Pain, Acute

> **Critical Alert**
> Sudden onset of testicular pain should be reported to health care provider immediately. Surgical intervention required within 6–12 hours to preserve testicle. Assess pain thoroughly using numeric scale and patient self-report.

  - Instruct patient to inform the nurse when pain begins and if the pain is not relieved after interventions
  - Apply ice pack and scrotal support
- Risk for Impaired Tissue Perfusion
  - Assess surgical site for swelling, purulent drainage, redness, or ecchymosis
  - Monitor for signs of bleeding and infection. ($\uparrow$ HR, $\downarrow$ BP, and $\uparrow$ T)
- Knowledge Deficit
  - Explain expected postoperative care (e.g., incentive spirometer, progressive ambulation, maintaining adequate nutritional intake)

MUSCULOSKELETAL DISORDERS

Muscular Dystrophy

Muscular dystrophies are a group of genetic myopathies caused by a protein deficiency in muscle membranes. This protein named dystrophin is required by muscles and muscle membranes to function properly. Therefore, a person with a muscular dystrophy has progressive muscle weakness leading to an inability to control any voluntary movement.

Myotonic Muscular Dystrophy

Myotonic dystrophy, or Steinert's disease, is the most common adult form of muscular dystrophy. It is caused by a defective gene that is transferred from one generation to another.

Sign and Symptoms

- Muscle wasting of the distal extremities, including hands, forearms, and feet and also the face and neck
- Cataracts
- Dysphagia
- Weakness of the diaphragm and an adverse reaction to anesthesia
- Decreased peristalsis
- Alteration or inappropriate insulin secretion, increased carbohydrate metabolism, and excessive sleeping

Diagnostics

- Health history and physical examination
  - Initial complaint may be a change in vision or difficulty swallowing
  - Weakness and myotonia
- Laboratory
  - Muscle biopsy
  - DNA testing (abnormal chromosome 19)

Patient Care Management

- Medical
  - Support of the wasting muscles
  - Avoid complications such as constipation from decreased gastric peristalsis, aspiration from difficulty swallowing, and decreased visual acuity from resulting cataracts
  - Medications to treat delayed muscle relaxation
    - Phenytoin (Dilantin)
    - Mexiletine (Mexil)
    - Carbamazepine (Tegretol)
    - Quinine
    - Procainamide (Pronestyl)

Nursing Management

Nursing care for patients with muscular dystrophy is aimed at supporting the patient's independence level, preventing complications, and preventing injury. Many aspects of care are required, including care by a nurse, nutritionist, physical therapist, occupational therapist, and orthotics technician, which will assist the patient to maintain mobility for as long as possible. For the caregiver, assistance from a financial counselor, psychologist, home health nurse, and access to respite care will decrease the chance of severe caregiver role strain.

- Aspiration, Risk for
  - Assess the patient's gag reflex prior to administering food or fluids

- Assess respiratory status before and after meals/drinking
- Provide thickened liquids
- Teach the patient and family the importance of eating small bites of food
- Cardiac Output, Decreased
  - Monitor heart sounds, skin color and temperature, capillary refill
  - Accurate I and O
  - Restrict fluids as needed
  - Schedule rest periods between activities
- Breathing, Ineffective
  - Observe for dyspnea (difficulty breathing), pallor or cyanosis, rate and depth of respirations, use of accessory muscles
  - Monitor O_2 sat levels
  - Encourage rest periods as needed
- Activity Intolerance Impaired Physical Mobility
  - Teach family to perform PROM exercises three times per day
  - Teach patient and family the need to maintain appropriate weight
  - Teach patient/family the importance of maintaining safety in the home by keeping it uncluttered
- Knowledge Deficit
  - Encourage patient and family to maintain a safe environment by not having clutter on the floor, removing throw rugs, electrical wires, toys, etc.
  - Explain the importance of eating a well-balanced diet to include protein, carbohydrates, minerals, vitamins; Eat a diet high in fiber and drink at least 2,500 mL fluid/day
  - Encourage patient to provide as much of own care as possible to maintain independence, but rest when needed
  - Explain the importance of moving joints as much as possible

Osteomyelitis

Osteomyelitis is an infection of the bone that requires aggressive early treatment to decrease the amount of bone or joint damage. Is a complex bone disorder with the potential for chronic and long-term effects.

Risk Factors

- Patients with compromised immune system
- Diabetes
- Peripheral vascular disease
- Malignancies
- Presence of prosthetic hardware within the bone
- Trauma or surgical procedures

Signs and Symptoms

- Fever
- Site has edema, warmth to touch, tenderness, and movement or joint limitations
- Generalized complaints of fatigue and malaise
- Subperiosteal abscess causing pressure and eventual fracturing of small pieces of bone

Diagnostics

- Health history and physical examination
- Laboratory
  - CBC ($\uparrow$ white blood cells and leukocytes, $\downarrow$ hemoglobin)
  - Blood cultures
  - Needle aspiration of bone with culture of material taken is essential to identifying the causative organism.
- Imaging
  - X-rays (demonstrate a swelling of overlying tissues and about 40% to 50% focal bone loss)
  - MRI, bone scan, ultrasound

Patient Care Management

- Medical
  - Treat the underlying cause
  - Immobilization of the affected bone
  - Pain medication
  - Antibiotics (parenteral for 4–6 weeks followed by oral)
  - Physical therapy
  - Nutritionalist consult
- Surgery
  - Incise the site and drain the abscess
  - Removal of dead bone

Nursing Management

Nursing care focuses on rest, immobilization of the affected part, and administration of analgesics, antipyretics, and antibiotics.

- Pain, Acute
  - Reduce lighting and noise, and provide room for the patient's significant others
  - Cultural and spiritual factors such as prayer, ritual, and music can also increase the patient's comfort
  - Medicate the patient with narcotics and NSAIDs
  - Elevate and support the affected extremity
  - Teach the patient to report increasing or uncontrolled pain
- Nutrition, Imbalanced: Less than Body Requirements
  - Facilitate education with a dietary consultant
  - Encourage frequent oral hygiene
  - Provide the patient with printed material outlining the dietary needs and restrictions
  - Promote the intake of protein foods with high biologic value: eggs, meats, diary products and foods high in protein and vitamins A, B, and C

- Knowledge Deficit
  - Teach the patient and family the importance of adhering to the therapeutic regimen
  - Stress importance of taking prescribed antibiotics as scheduled even if patient is feeling better
  - Teach the patient the signs and symptoms of any side effects that may occur
  - Stress importance of a safe environment to prevent falls and possible fractures
  - Teach the proper use of any assistive devices that may be required
  - Stress the importance of reporting signs of infection
  - Education for maintenance of long-term PICC catheter (for IV antibiotics) and the importance of aseptic technique should be emphasized

Osteoporosis

Osteoporosis is a skeletal disease that is characterized by low bone mass and deterioration of the bone tissue. This continued deterioration results in bone fragility and susceptibility to fractures.

Risk Factors
- Rheumatoid arthritis
- Glucocorticoids
- Chronic renal failure
- Sedentary lifestyle
- Increased life expectancy
- History of fractures
- Body weight
- Smoking and alcohol
- Physical inactivity and poor calcium intake

Signs and Symptoms
- Fracture after minor trauma or fall (hip, vertebrae, and wrist)
- Kyphosis
- Loss of height

- Pain aggravated by movement or jarring
- Pathologic fractures of the spine and femur
- Spontaneous wedge fractures
- Vertebral collapse producing pain that radiates around the trunk
- Sites of osteoporosis
  - Hand, wrist, spine, hip, knees, and feet

Diagnostics
- Health history and physical examination
  - Assessment of bone mass
- Laboratory
  - Biochemical markers (evaluates the process of bone modeling and remodeling)
  - CBC, serum calcium and phosphorus, urine calcium, and alkaline phosphatase
- Imaging
  - Bone mineral density tests
  - CT scan (evaluates the spine), ultrasound, regular x-rays, and, in rare cases, bone biopsy

Patient Care Management
- Medical
  - Prevent further bone loss and maintain function
    - Calcium and vitamin D
    - Pain medication
    - Anti-inflammatory medication (steroidal and NSAIDs)
    - Bisphosphonates
    - PTH
    - Estrogen and progestin
    - Exercise and diet

Nursing Management
Nursing care of the patient with osteoporosis is focused on the primary goals of maintaining independence and function, preserving bone mass, and preventing fractures.

The majority of the strategies focus on education and behavioral changes.

Nursing diagnoses for the patient with osteoporosis will be based on objective and subjective data collected during the assessment phase. Potential nursing diagnoses for osteoporosis include:

- Pain, Chronic
  - Assess pain on a numeric scale 0–10
  - Administer medications and reassess accordingly
- Injury, Risk
  - Implement fall precautions as needed
  - Encourage weight-bearing exercises
- Knowledge Deficit
  - Educate patient and family regarding prevention strategies, side effects of medications, and safety measures.

Paget's Disease (Osteitis Deformans)

Paget's disease is a chronic disorder that causes irregular bone breakdown and formation, which in turn causes the bones to weaken. This results in pain, bone deformities, fractures, and arthritis. The most common sites are the pelvis and tibia. Other less affected areas include the femur, clavicle, skull, and spine.

Signs and Symptoms
- Bone pain at the site
  - Constant and worse at night
  - Edema or deformity at the affected site
  - Hearing loss or deafness (if the ossicles of the ear are involved)
- Complications
  - Pathologic fractures
  - Hypercalcemia
  - Renal calculi
  - Spinal cord injury
  - Bone sarcoma

Diagnostics

- Health history and physical examination
- Laboratory
  - Alkaline phosphatase
  - Urinalysis ($\uparrow$ hydroxyproline concentration)
  - Bone marrow biopsy
- Imaging
  - X-rays
  - Bone scan
- Medical
  - Calcitonin injections
  - Diet high in protein, calcium, and vitamin D

Nursing Management

- Pain, Acute
  - Assess pain using numeric scale 0–10
  - Medicate for pain and reassess accordingly
  - Offer alternative pain relief strategies
- Knowledge Deficit
  - Educate the patient and family regarding prevention, importance of exercise, diet, and medication side effects

Rhabdomyolysis

Rhabdomyolysis is defined as a syndrome involving muscle necrosis or breakdown. The injured muscle fibers release myoglobin into the bloodstream, which alters the filtration in the kidneys, causing damage and failure.

Causes

- Trauma with muscle compression
- Surgical procedures in which there is a long period of muscle compression
- Immobilization (due to a coma or postictal state)
- Extreme physical exertion
- Snakebite
- Toxins

Signs and Symptoms

- Muscle pain (myalgia)
- Fatigue
- Fever
- Nausea and vomiting
- Dark-colored urine
- Complications
  - Acute renal failure due to tubular obstruction secondary to the myoglobulin pigments
  - Electrolyte imbalance:
    - Hyperkalemia and hyperphosphatemia due to the release of potassium and phosphate from the damaged muscles
    - Hypocalcemia due to deposited calcium salts in the muscle tissue. This electrolyte imbalance can be severe and patients often show other symptoms associated with hypocalcemia, such as disturbances in cardiac conduction or blood coagulation.
    - Hyperuricemia
    - Metabolic acidosis
    - Compartment syndrome (increased pressure in muscle compartment), may lead to permanent disability of the associated joint) due to edema of a limb and muscle.

Diagnostics

- Health history and physical examination
- Laboratory
  - ↑ CK levels (100 times normal or higher)
  - Urinalysis (presence of myoglobin)
  - Serum myoglobin

Patient Care Management

- Medical
  - Identification of underlying cause and prompt management

408

- Observation in ICU
- Management of acute renal failure
- Increased parenteral fluids

Nursing Management
- Fluid volume imbalance (See Renal Failure section)
  - Accurate I and O
  - Monitor for signs of fluid overload and deficit
  - Monitor for electrolyte imbalances
    (See Fluid and Electrolyte section.)
- Tissue perfusion, ineffective
  - Monitor skin color and temperature
  - Monitor mental status changes
- Knowledge Deficit
  - Explain to patient and family rationale for treatment plan including ICU routines
  - Encourage patient and family to ensure home environment is free of obstacles

MUSCULOSKELETAL TRAUMA

Amputation

Amputation is the surgical removal or traumatic loss of a body part. In the upper extremities amputation is rare and often associated with trauma, meningococcemia, and osteosarcoma. In the lower extremities, peripheral vascular disease, diabetes, and gangrene are the frequent causes for elective amputation.

(See Diabetes and Vascular sections for signs and symptoms, diagnostics, and patient care management.)

Types

- Below knee amputation (BKA)
  - Preferred because balance and coordination are more stable, gait is more natural, and there is a better potential for revisions if needed
- Above knee amputation (AKA)
  - Requires more energy to ambulate necessitating that the patient raise the hip and swing the prosthesis/leg forward for clearance because the leg plus prosthesis must remain straight.
  - In the elderly this may be a safety risk, and wheelchair mobility is a safer practice.
- Traumatic amputation
  - Sudden loss of the part and may require more extensive removal of tissue, bone, and muscle than amputation due to vascular insufficiency

Nursing Management

(See Appendix #38, Nursing Process: Patient Care Plan for the Orthopedic Surgical Patient.)

- Injury, Risk for
  - Monitor closely for skin integrity
  - Float remaining heel off of the mattress with pillows or a heel protection device
  - Stump care
    - Elevation of the stump and compression wrapping of the extremity to prevent edema

> **Critical Alert**
> The stump should be elevated for the first 24 hours to prevent postoperative edema. After 24 hours, keep the stump flat while in bed or extended while out of bed in a chair to prevent contracture of the nearest joint.

- Pain, Acute
  - Provide relief of phantom limb pain and reassess accordingly
    - Narcotics
    - Antiseizure medication
    - Antidepressants
    - Nerve block, spinal stimulation, use of transcutaneous electrical nerve stimulation (TENS) units, and biofeedback

Fractures

Fractures (breaks in the bone) are a discontinuity of the bone that may be complete or incomplete. A healing cascade begins with the blood that leaks out at the fracture site causing a hematoma rich in osteoblasts (cells that make bone). Healing time is dependent on the site and type of the fracture and on the underlying health of the patient. Typically healing will occur within 2 weeks up to 6 months.

Classification of Fractures
- Open
  - A tear in the soft tissue, exposing the bone to the outside environment

- All open fractures have the potential to be contaminated, and this increases the morbidity and mortality of the injury
- Closed
  - The soft tissue envelope, which may be damaged, does not communicate with the outside; in effect, there is no skin opening
- Non-displaced
  - Bone ends are touching each other, keeping anatomic alignment
- Displaced
  - Bone ends are not touching each other, compromising anatomic alignment
- Pathological
  - Weakened bone due to underlying disease process (e.g., malignancy) resulting in fracture
- Stress
  - Due to repetitive use most commonly seen with sports activities (e.g., track and field)

Signs and Symptoms (General)
- Pain at site of injury
- Deformity
- Numbness
- Compromised neurovascular status
  - Changes in pulse, color, and temperature of extremity

Diagnostics (General)
- Health history and physical examination
  - Assess for comorbidities and mechanism of injury
- Imaging
  - X-ray
  - CT scan

Patient Care Management (General)

- Medical
  - Immobilization
  - Casting
  - Splint
    - Traction
  - Pain control (narcotics)
- Surgery
  - External fixation
  - Open reduction internal fixation
  - Intramedullary rod (for long bone fractures)

Nursing Management

Nursing management of the patient with a fracture involves relief of pain and frequent reassessment of function related to the specific anatomical location involved.

(See specific fracture types for nursing interventions.)

Hip Fracture

A hip fracture is due to a break in the femoral head, neck, intratrochanteric, subtrochanteric, or acetabular region.

Cause

- Trauma (falls)
- Pathologic due to malignancy

Signs and Symptoms

- Pain
- Affected leg is shortened and externally rotated

Diagnostics

- Health history and physical examination
- Imaging
  - X-ray
  - MRI and CT scan (to evaluate for other injuries)

Patient Care Management

- Medical
  - Immobilization (maintain alignment of extremity)
  - Pain control
- Surgery
  - Total hip arthroplasty

Nursing Management

(See Appendix #38.)

- Injury, Risk for
  - Implement hip precautions

Hip Precautions

Posterior Hip Precautions	Anterior Hip Precautions
Hip abductor pillow while in bed.	Hip abductor pillow while in bed.
Do not bend hip greater than 90 degrees.	Take mini steps when walking.
Use an elevated toilet seat.	Do not assume a straddle position—like mounting a horse.
Do not sit in low chairs.	Do not twist or turn the body away from the operative side.
Do not twist or turn the body toward the operative side.	Do not turn leg and foot outward.
Do not turn leg and foot inward.	Do not lift operative leg up and out.
Keep operative leg straight when getting up and use one's arms to push up.	

- Knowledge Deficit
    - Educate the patient and family regarding safety within the home
        - Securely fastened safety bars or handrails for the bath and shower
        - A stable armchair with a firm seat cushion allowing the knees to remain lower than the hips
        - A raised toilet seat
        - A shower bench or chair
        - A sock aid and a long-handled shoe horn for putting on and taking off shoes and socks without excessively bending at the hip
        - A "reacher" to access items without bending at the hip
        - Removal of all loose carpets and electrical cords from walkways
        - Food and household items up to waist level to prevent bending

Pelvic Fractures

A fractured pelvis requires a large amount of force, which requires the provider to anticipate other serious injuries. Organs that can be injured during pelvic trauma include the bladder and urethra, vagina, prostate, and gastrointestinal system.

Signs and Symptoms
- Pain
- Rotation of the iliac crest
- Difference in leg length
- Blood from meatus (indicates urethral damage)
- Changes in rectal tone and bleeding
- Vaginal tearing

Diagnostics
- Health history and physical examination
- Imaging

- X-rays
- CT scan

Patient Care Management
- Medical
  - Determine hemodynamic stability of patient
  - External stabilization (pelvic binder)
  - Pain control
- Surgery
  - Pelvic angiography for embolization of arterial bleed
  - Reduction with surgical ring stabilization
    - External fixation or internal fixation

Nursing Management

Specific nursing interventions for a patient who has sustained a pelvic fracture are listed below.

(See Appendix #38.)

- Infection, Risk for
  - If open fractures, apply a sterile dressing immediately to help protect the open wound from further contamination
  - Postoperatively monitor for signs of infection such as warmth and redness, drainage with a foul odor, purulent drainage, increased pain, and fever
  - Notify health care provider immediately if signs of infection are noted
- Fluid Volume, Deficient, Risk for
  - Ensure type and crossmatch for blood products
  - Assess signs of fluid loss
    - ↑ HR, ↓ BP, ↑ RR
    - ↓ urine output
    - Change in mental status

- Saturated dressings
- ↓ hemoglobin/hematocrit (may initially be ↑ due to dilutional effect seen with dehydration)

Critical Alert

If there is blood at the meatus, do not attempt to insert a Foley catheter as the patient may be experiencing damage to the urethra.

- Injury, Risk for
  - If using a pelvic binder
    - Assess position of the binder and ensure smooth, direct contact between the patient and binder to avoid skin breakdown

---

Critical Alert

It is critically important to be careful when maneuvering the pelvis so as not to cause damage to the vasculature or neural bundles.

Complications of Fractures
Compartment Syndrome

Compartment syndrome is a condition where increasing pressure within the muscle compartments compromises circulation and the function of soft tissues, nerves, and vessels. This leads to anoxia and necrosis of the tissue, which in turn leads to more edema in the compartment and a subsequent increase in pressure. The progression will continue until a surgical release of the fascial envelope is performed. If pressure is not reduced, irreversible muscle damage and nerve damage can occur within hours and can also lead to life-threatening complications such as rhabdomyolysis and renal failure. The most commonly affected compartments are those of the tibia (lower leg), forearm, upper arm, hand, foot, and thigh.

Causes

- Bleeding into the compartment by fractured bone or torn muscle tissue
- Over hydration
- External pressure applied by the trauma itself, casts, dressing, burns (tight eschar), or even clothing

Signs and Symptoms

- "Five P's"
  - Pain out of proportion to the injury or pain with passive stretch of the muscle within that compartment
  - Pallor
  - Poor capillary refill
  - Paresthesia
  - Pulselessness in the affected extremity

Diagnostics

- Health history and physical examination
  - Neurovascular assessment
  - Intracompartmental pressure can be measured with a transducer

Patient Care Management

- Surgical
  - Emergency fasciotomy
  - Skin grafts or amputations may be required for severe cases

Nursing Management

(See Appendixes #1, Nursing Process: Patient Care Plan for the Postoperative Patient Following General Surgery and #38.)

Fat Embolism Syndrome

Fat embolism syndrome (FES) occurs when fat globules released from long-bone fractures enter the circulatory system. In the most severe cases, the emboli can produce multiple-organ failure from both a direct embolic effect and from activation of the inflammatory cascade.

Signs and Symptoms of Fat Embolus

Early Findings	Later Findings	Last Component
Hypoxemia Dyspnea Tachypnea	Neurologic abnormalities: Confusion altered LOC focal deficits Possible seizures	Petechial rash found most often on the head, neck, anterior thorax, subconjunctiva, and axillae

Diagnostics

(See section on Pulmonary Embolism.)

Patient Care Management

(See section on Pulmonary Embolism.)

Nursing Management

(See section on Pulmonary Embolism.)

Rhabdomyolysis

Rhabdomyolysis occurs when the injured skeletal muscle fibers break down and leak inflammatory mediators, such as myoglobin and creatinine kinase, into the circulation. It is most commonly seen with crush injuries but can occur with any massive soft tissue injury. Complications associated with rhabdomyolysis include acute renal failure and respiratory distress due to muscle weakness and fluid and electrolyte imbalances.

Signs and Symptoms

- Pain, tenderness, swelling, bruising, and weakness within the affected muscles
- Muscles feel soft and flabby
- Dark colored urine (due to myoglobin)
- General malaise
- Fever
- Nausea and vomiting

- Confusion and agitation
- Anuria

Diagnostics
- Health history and physical examination
- Laboratory
  - Serum creatinine kinase ($\uparrow$ at least 5 times normal)

Patient Care Management
- Medical
  - Parenteral fluids (maintain circulating blood volume and perfuse the kidneys while flushing the myoglobin)
  - Creatinine kinase levels should be obtained
  - IV Sodium bicarbonate infusion to alkalinize the urine
  - Dialysis as needed

Nursing Management
(See Renal section for nursing interventions associated with renal failure.)

NEUROLOGICAL DISORDERS

Acute Brain Disorders
Brain Tumors
(See Brain Cancer in Immunologic Disorders.)

Hydrocephalus
Hydrocephalus is an excessive accumulation of CSF in the intracerebral ventricles. It may be caused by over-production or inadequate drainage.

Types
1. Communicating hydrocephalus refers to large ventri-cles in a system with communication between all of the ventricles and the pathway for CSF. The cause of communicating hydrocephalus usually is due to blockage or malabsorption of CSF by the arachnoid granulations. Hydrocephalus is a common occurrence in brain trauma, some brain tumors, subarachnoid hemorrhage, and some encephalopathic conditions, including meningitis, encephalitis, and brain abscess.

2. Noncommunicating (also referred to as obstructive) hydrocephalus refers to a blockage somewhere within the CSF pathway. One or more of the ventricles may be larger than the other ventricles, depending on the level of the obstruction. The most common cause is space-occupying lesions, such as tumors.

Sign and Symptoms
Increased Intracranial Pressure
- Papilledema
- Headache

- Nausea and vomiting
- Incontinence
- Gait changes
- Difficulty with extraocular movements, particularly up-gaze
- Alterations in LOC

Diagnostics
- Patient's history and presenting symptoms
- CT scan of the head, without contrast
- MRI

Patient Care Management

Hydrocephalus Is a Surgically Treated Condition
- In emergency situations, an external ventricular drain is placed.
- Non-emergently—placement of a shunting device to remove extra spinal fluid
- Monitor for complicatons:
  - Obstruction of the proximal or distal
  - Infection
  - Disconnection
  - Overshunting resulting in slit ventricles and headaches
  - Subdural hematoma (SDH), in extreme cases
  - Undershunting

Nursing Management

Risk of Neurological Deterioration
- Ongoing accurate neurological assessment
- Report any changes in neurological status

(See Appendix #41, Nursing Process: Patient Care Plan for Acute Brain Disorders, and Appendix #42, Patient Teaching & Discharge Priorities for Acute Brain Disorders.)

Infectious Diseases of the Central Nervous System

Many infectious diseases may affect the nervous system. Meningitis, encephalitis, and cerebral abscesses are examples of infections of the central nervous system (CNS) that can be caused by a number of pathogens including common bacteria, fungi, and viruses. Infectious diseases may be acquired or nosocomial.

Meningitis

Defined as an inflammation of the meninges. *Bacterial meningitis* is an inflammation of the meninges caused by a bacterial pathogen. *Viral meningitis* is an inflammation of the meninges caused by viral pathogens, such as herpes simplex virus, mumps, measles, or any other virus. Bacteria can enter the meninges by various methods and structures. Bloodborne pathogens are the most common, entering via the bloodstream. Other bacteria enter the body via other structures, such as the sinuses or the inner ear, by dental procedures, or endocarditis. Cerebrospinal fluid is a common route for infection. A dural tear caused by trauma or surgery can create a route for the introduction of pathogens. Patients with skull fractures, for example, may experience rhinorrhea or otorrhea. If a route is available for CSF to leave the body, organisms have a route to enter the body. Unsterile technique during surgical procedures, including lumbar puncture, placement of an EVD, or collection of CSF from an EVD, is a method of introducing organisms into the CSF.

Signs and Symptoms

Meningeal Irritation, or Meningismus

- Headache is a common and early symptom
- Photophobia
- Nuchal rigidity, or stiff neck (Kernig's sign, and Brudzinski sign)

High Fever

Altered level of consciousness, such as lethargy, irritability, confusion, and seizures

Diagnostics
- Accurate history, focusing on recent illnesses:
  - "Flu-like"illness, systemic virus
  - Recent dental procedures, head trauma, and/or brain surgery
- CT scan of the head to rule out mass
- Lumbar puncture
- CSF Gram stain and culture

Patient Care Management
Bacterial Meningitis
- Antibiotics
- Dexamethasone

Viral Meningitis
- Supportive measures
- Relief of symptoms, such as fever or pain
- Respiratory and/or circulatory support

Encephalitis
An inflammation of the brain tissue by bacterial, viral, fungal, or parasites. The most common form of encephalitis in the United States is herpes simplex virus (HSV). Other types of viruses include arthropod-borne, such as those carried by mosquitoes. Another cause of viral encephalitis is postviral disease, from measles, mumps, or chickenpox. Prognosis is dependent on early diagnosis and treatment. Neurological deficits such as cognitive impairment, motor weakness, seizure disorder, swallowing difficulties, and personality changes are common.

Signs and Symptoms
Symptoms are usually more pronounced than those with meningitis.
- Severe headache
- Fever
- Nausea and vomiting

- Confusion
- Alterations in LOC, such as lethargy
- Focal deficits, such as motor weakness
- Seizures and bizarre behavior
- Increased ICP
- Death or severe neurological damage if untreated

Diagnostics
- Accurate history, focusing on recent illnesses
- Lumbar puncture
- CSF Gram stain and culture
- CT scan may show signs of hemorrhagic lesions
- Brain biopsy to diagnose HSV

Patient Care Management
Supportive Management of Symptoms
- Respiratory support
- Management of increased ICP
- Nutritional support
- Close evaluation of intake and output
- Monitor for systemic response to disease

Medication Therapy
- Antiviral agents (acyclovir or famciclovir)—started early in the disease
- Dexamethasone to reduce cerebral edema
- Phenytoin for seizure management
- Pain medications
- Antipyretics

Brain Abscess
A localized infection carried from other sites of the body extending into the cerebral tissue. An abscess can be introduced into the brain, such as infection, congenital abnormalities, or by penetrating wounds. An abscess may be caused by various agents, including bacteria, fungus, virus, and parasites. Almost half of all

abscesses are carried through the blood from other infected sources, as with pneumonia or endocarditis. The invading bacteria cause inflammation, cerebral edema, increased ICP, and necrosis. Prognosis is excellent if treated early and aggressively.

Signs and Symptoms
- Headache
- Generalized malaise
- Fever and chills
- Nausea and vomiting
- Neurological deficits correspond to the location of the lesion
  - Motor weakness
  - Sensory deficits
  - Cranial nerve weakness
  - Speech disturbances
- Alterations in LOC, such as confusion and lethargy
- Seizures

Secondary Symptoms Occur Due to the Expansion of the Space-Occupying Lesion
- Cerebellar lesions may result in ataxia, nystagmus, or postoccipital headache.
- Frontal lesions may result in contralateral hemiplegia, aphasia, or personality changes.
- Severe headaches indicating increased ICP
- Herniation syndromes may occur if left untreated.

Diagnostics
- Accurate history, focusing on recent illnesses and injury
- CT scan or MRI studies showing the encapsulated abscess
- Lumbar puncture usually *is not performed* because of risk of herniation.

Patient Care Management

Surgical Drainage of the Abscess

Supportive Management of Symptoms

- Respiratory and cardiovascular support
- Management of increased ICP

Medication Therapy

- Anitibiotics
- Steroids
- Pain medications
- Antipyretics

Nursing Management (General Infectious Diseases)

Decrease Risk of Infection

- Hand washing and universal precautions
- Identify patients at increased risk (immunosuppressed, elderly, critically ill, intubated patients)
- Initiate isolation procedures, if indicated
- Monitor for early signs of infection

Risk of Neurological Complications

- Assist with procedures using proper techniques
- Obtain cultures and initiate antibiotics promptly
- Monitor neurological status, report changes promptly

Knowledge Deficit

- Teach importance of hand washing to prevent spread of infection
- Explain procedures and treatment modalities

Seizures

Seizures are described as a single, temporary event that consists of uncontrolled, electrical neuronal discharge of the brain that interrupts normal brain function. Seizures may occur as a result of most acute brain disorders: a brain tumor; brain trauma such as a hematoma or concussion; or in conjunction with an infectious process such as meningitis, encephalitis, and abscesses. They also may be seen with other, nonneurological disorders, such as metabolic disorders including severe dehydration, electrolyte imbalances, or withdrawal from alcohol or drugs. Idiopathic seizures also may occur in the absence of underlying abnormalities. Epilepsy is a condition in which seizures occur spontaneously, and they can recur due to an underlying condition or without a known cause.

Signs and Symptoms

Generalized Seizures: Affect the whole brain, with bilateral, symmetric electrical discharges

- Alterations in mentation, behavior, sensation, or motor tonic-clonic
- Loss of consciousness
- Stiffening of the body, with jerking of all extremities
- Cyanosis
- Excessive drooling, biting of mouth and/or tongue
- Urinary incontinence
- Pupillary changes, with a gaze deviation (away from the side of a structural abnormality)
- Postictal stage characterized by extreme lethargy and no memory of the event

Partial Seizures: Can be simple or complex, with the differentiating factor being consciousness

Simple Partial Seizures

- Specific motor or sensory abnormalities
- Focal motor seizures or those with somatosensory components, such as the visualization of flashing lights or hearing of noises
- No loss of consciousness

Complex Partial Seizures

- May begin as a simple partial seizure
- Consciousness is impaired.
- Progression to a generalized seizure may occur.

> **Critical Alert**
> Status epilepticus has been described as "either continuous seizures lasting at least five minutes, or two or more discrete seizures between which there is incomplete recovery of consciousness." Status epilepticus is a medical emergency, because continued seizure activity could result in severe neurological injury due to cerebral hypoxia. It may result in respiratory and/or cardiovascular failure.

Diagnostics

- Detailed account of the event must be available
- Clinical presentation, medications, and past medical history
- Physical examination and neurological assessment
- MRI or CT scan, to rule out structural abnormality
- EEGs
- Wada tests
- Functional MRIs

Patient Care Management
Management of Status Epilepticus

- Termination of the seizure is of primary importance
- Short-acting benzodiazepines
- ABCs of life support

Immediate Treatment of an Underlying Condition

- Antiepileptic medications
- Surgical resection of an identifiable source

Nursing Management
Risk of Seizure Activity

- Observe and document event:
  - Were there precipitating events?
  - Where did the seizure start and did it progress to other areas?
  - What type of movement of the extremities?
  - Were there pupillary changes?

- Was there gaze deviation? If so, which direction?
- Was there incontinence of bowel or bladder?
- What was the patient's mental status (unconscious or awake and talking)?
- How long did the event last?
- After the seizure, what was the patient's mental status?
- Was there any motor weakness after the seizure?
- Safely administer medications
- Provide safe environment
- Be prepared to support ABCs with emergency equipment at bedside

Traumatic Brain Injury (TBI)

Traumatic brain injury is and has always been a major health problem, the largest number of TBI appears to be secondary to motor vehicle crashes, falls, and acts of violence, such as gunshot wounds and assault.

Skull Fractures

Categorized According to Type of Break and Severity

Linear skull fractures are simple breaks in the continuity of bone, with no displacement, and most commonly are seen in low-velocity impact situations. Linear fractures of the temporal bone may result in a tear of the middle meningeal artery, resulting in more serious brain injury, such as an epidural hematoma.

Comminuted skull fractures are fragmented interruptions of the skull resulting from multiple linear fractures with an area of bone depression at the point of impact. *Basal skull fractures* usually are an extension of a linear fracture into the skull base. The mechanism of injury is the same as linear skull fractures with a more serious result. The skull base is rough and uneven, and its texture may cause tears to the delicate dura. CSF may leak through the tear in the dura leaking from the nose or the ear. It is distinguishable by its characteristic halo sign, which appears as blood with a yellow ring around it.

Other Signs and Symptoms of Basal Skull Fractures

- Battle sign, which is ecchymosis, or bruising, over the mastoid bone
- Bulging tympanic membranes
- Presence of raccoon eyes, or periorbital ecchymosis
- Cranial nerve deficits, due to damage to various cranial nerves
- Damage to the olfactory nerve (CN I) results in decreased sense of smell
- Visual deficits, due to damage to the optic nerve (CN II)
- Facial weakness, due to damage to the facial nerve (CN VII)
- Decreased hearing, due to damage to the acoustic nerve (CN VIII)

Critical Alert
The presence of CSF leaking from the nose (rhinorrhea) or ears (otorrhea) is a serious complication. The patient with CSF leak is at risk for meningitis. Place head of bed at 30 to 45 degrees (unless contraindicated) and call MD.

Depressed skull fractures are the displacement of a comminuted skull fracture, frequently seen with other injuries to the brain. The degree of neurological symptoms depends on the degree and location of brain involvement. Hair, dirt, and other debris found within the wound present a risk for infection.

Diagnostics

- Physical assessment and knowledge of the mechanism of injury
- Skull x-rays
- CT scan

Patient Care Management

- Close observation for neurological deterioration
- Linear fractures usually do not require treatment.

- Open or comminuted fractures are considered contaminated, and careful wound debridement with surgical closure is required.

- Depressed skull fractures may require elevation of the depressed bone, debridement, and antibiotics.

Hematomas

Collections of blood. Intracranial hematomas are defined by their location, either epidural or subdural.

Epidural hematoma (EDH) refers to bleeding into the space between the skull and the dura, caused by the laceration of an artery or a vein. As bleeding occurs, an enlarging hematoma develops as the dura is stripped away from the inner table of the skull. Pressure is exerted on the brain tissue by the expanding lesion, with resulting neurological compromise. Immediate posttraumatic period of unconsciousness, followed by a lucid interval that can last from minutes to hours, is textbook presentation of EDH. A rapid deterioration in LOC may follow, characterized by sleepiness, confusion, obtundation, coma, and possibly death caused by the enlarging hematoma. Other possible signs and symptoms are an enlarging pupil on the same side of the injury (ipsilateral), increasing headache, seizures, motor weakness, and/or pathological positioning.

Subdural hematoma (SDH) is defined as bleeding between the dura and the arachnoid layers of the meninges. Usually are caused by the tearing of bridging veins located over the surface of the brain. SDHs are divided into three categories based on the amount of time between the initial injury and the presentation of signs and symptoms.

Acute subdural hematoma (SDH), neurological signs and symptoms up to 48 hours after injury. On CT of the head, the acute SDH appears as a hyperdense lesion. The most common signs are severe headache with possible gradual deterioration of LOC, starting with drowsiness and progressing through confusion, obtundation, and coma. Pupillary signs also may be present, most commonly an ipsilateral dilation, and sluggish reactivity. Hemiparesis of the contralateral arm and leg also may be present.

Subacute subdural, hematoma neurological signs and symptoms develop from 48 hours postinjury up to about 3 weeks. They are associated with less serious lesions, perhaps due to bleeding at a much slower rate. The blood in a subacute SDH appears isodense with hyperdense areas and a clear blood–fluid level on a CT scan.

Chronic subdural hematoma, neurological signs and symptoms develop over 3 weeks to several months. These are associated with minor head injuries, possibly occurring weeks to months prior to the presentation of neurological signs and with elderly, who may have atrophic brains. The SDH increases slowly in size, possibly from repeated small venous bleeds, until a significant mass effect develops and symptoms occur. The most common symptom is increasing headache, slowing mentation, confusion, and drowsiness. Seizures are a common presenting symptom.

Critical Alert

Patients with a diagnosis of SDH are at risk for expanding hematoma. Therefore, frequent neurological assessments are required (i.e., hourly until stable, then q2h). A decrease in neurological function, such as increasing confusion or lethargy, increasing motor weakness, or an enlarging pupil is a medical emergency. The doctor should be notified immediately.

Diagnostics

CT Scan of the Head

- Showing high-density elliptical-shaped mass adjacent to the skull

- Mass effect also is seen with a shift of the brain from the side with the EDH to the opposite side.

Patient Care Management

- Immediate surgical evacuation of large hematomas

- Small hematoma that may absorb

  - ICU monitoring with frequent neurological assessment

  - Serial CT scans to monitor the size of the hematoma

- Postoperative care in the ICU with close monitoring of neurological status
- Antiepileptic drugs (AEDs) may be warranted due to risk of seizures.

Cerebral Contusions

Contusions of the brain are defined as bruising of the brain tissue, often associated with other neurological injuries, such as skull fractures or hematomas. They may occur from blunt trauma, penetrating wounds, or acceleration/deceleration injuries. The injuries are referred to as coup, in which bruising occurs directly below the point of impact on the skull, or contrecoup, which occurs directly on the opposite point of impact. Contrecoup contusions usually have a coup component, in which case they are referred to as coup-contrecoup contusions. Contrecoup contusions occur as a result of the brain moving with the skull, and bruising itself during acceleration/deceleration movement. Signs and symptoms are highly dependent on the location, size, and the amount of cerebral edema associated with the lesion.

Diagnostics

- Physical assessment and knowledge of the mechanism of injury
- Skull x-rays
- CT scan

Patient Care Management

- Treatment dependent on the neurological condition
- Close monitoring of neurological assessment
- Monitoring of ICP due to cerebral edema
- Serial CT scans ("Blossoming" or expansion of the contusion may occur at approximately 3 days.)
- Seizure treatment if necessary

Concussion

Refers to a recognized collection of symptoms as a result of mild head injury. It is described as a temporary, neurological dysfunction caused by an external force to the head. It is also described as a "shaking of the brain."

Signs and Symptoms

- Confusion
- Possible brief loss of consciousness
- Headache
- Intellectual impairment
- Memory loss

Diagnostics

An accurate history of the event is essential, including questions such as length of period of loss of consciousness, if any; presence of confusion; and length of time until symptoms subside. No radiographic findings are associated with concussions. However, if the patient has a focal neurological exam, or an extended period of unconsciousness, the patient should be admitted to the hospital, and a CT of the head should be obtained to rule out other, more serious brain trauma.

Second-Impact Syndrome

Characterized by a second concussion, in an indeterminate time frame, that occurs before the brain can completely recover from the first concussion. It is caused by a loss of disordered autoregulation of the brain's blood supply as a result of the first injury. Because of poor brain compliance, persistent vascular congestion and increased ICP persist, the result can be massive cerebral edema and possibly death. It is for this reason that consideration must be made of the advisability of continuing risk-taking activities after receiving an initial concussion.

Postconcussion Syndrome

A condition that follows mild head injury and is characterized by one or more of the following symptoms: headaches, dizziness, vertigo, tinnitus, hearing loss, blurred vision, light and/or noise sensitivity, alteration in smell, anxiety, depression, personality change, sleep disorders, decreased libido, decreased appetite, memory loss, alteration in cognitive function, personality changes, and physical or cognitive decline. Symptoms usually subside with time; however, it can take months for total resolution.

Diffuse Axonal Injury (DAI)
Defined as a primary injury of diffuse white matter that results in tearing or shearing of axons and small blood vessels. Presentation of the patient with DAI is neurological compromise, possibly coma, with decerebrate or decorticate posturing. DAI lesions may be detected by magnetic resonance imaging (MRI). Treatment is determined by the neurological presentation of the patient and is usually supportive. Support of respiratory and hemodynamic functions may be warranted. DAI is classified as mild, moderate, and severe. Patients with mild DAI may have only mild long-term cognitive disabilities, whereas severe DAIs are associated with significant mortality and long-term disabilities.

Primary/Secondary Injuries
Refers to the mechanical injury to the brain. The injury is a direct result of the initial insult to the brain and may be localized, such as occurs with a laceration or contusion, or diffuse, such as with a concussion or DAI.

Secondary injury is a result of the body's response to the primary insult to the brain. It is caused by a flow-metabolism mismatch, which results in cerebral ischemia, which then triggers the ischemia cascade, which is a series of events that results in changes on the cellular level, which then results in cerebral infarction. It can be the result of a single event or a series of events. Deficits in cellular metabolism in the brain can cause cell death, leading to death of brain tissue, compromised neurological function, and poor patient outcomes. Causes of secondary injury are many, and include respiratory insufficiency, hypoxia, sepsis, hypotension, metabolic dysfunction, cerebral edema, and increased ICP. It has been estimated that 50% of patients with head trauma succumb to effects of secondary injury.

Nursing Management (General Traumatic Brain Injury)

The patient with TBI is one with multifaceted challenges. TBI patients require the collaboration of many specialists and ancillary services.

Critical Alert

Patients with a decreased level of consciousness are at risk for aspiration and respiratory compromise. Monitor respiratory status carefully, suction as needed, and ensure airway protection.

(See Appendixes #41 and #42.)

Cerebral Vascular Disorders
Stroke

Stroke is a brain attack that is caused by interruption of blood flow to a certain area of the brain. The cause is either an obstructed artery (ischemia) or an artery hemorrhage (hemorrhagic). Both methods cause ischemia, or a lack of oxygen to the brain cells. Cells that are deprived of oxygen for an undetermined amount of time begin to die, resulting in tissue death or infarction. The infarct tissues no longer function, resulting in neurological disabilities involving motor function, sensory function, speech, memory, and other cognitive mechanisms. Regardless of the type of stroke, the area of infarcted tissue is surrounded by tissue that is hypoperfused, the ischemic penumbra. This ischemic area is viable and can be saved if blood flow is restored quickly and cerebral edema is diminished. "Time is brain" is a strong statement exclaiming the importance of timely treatment before neurological deterioration.

Critical Alert

The onset of neurological symptoms indicating stroke is a medical emergency. Notify health care provider immediately for any new symptoms indicating possibility of a stroke. Stroke protocols must be initiated immediately.

Risk Factors for Stroke

- Hypertension
- Family history
- Atrial fibrillation
- Hyperlipidemia
- Diabetes mellitus
- Stress
- Excessive alcohol use
- Sedentary lifestyle
- Obesity
- Smoking
- Valvular disease
- Coronary artery disease

Ischemic Stroke

Ischemic stroke is the most common form of stroke.

Thrombotic Stroke

- Thrombotic stroke is often caused by thrombus (blood clots) formed around atherosclerotic plaques, further narrowing the lumen of the artery and causing severe stenosis.

Embolic Stroke

- Embolism results when a clot breaks off and travels to an area of decreased circulation, blocking off blood flow. Embolisms commonly occur from atrial fibrillation; however, any condition that can cause a reduction in systemic blood flow can cause an ischemic event.

Lacunar Stroke

- Caused by small artery occlusive disease. Hypertension is the predominant risk factor.

Transient Ischemic Attacks (TIAs)

- TIAs are episodes of neurological deficit resulting from ischemia that is temporary and resolves in minutes to hours. Resolution of accompanying neurological deficits occurs in less than 24 hours, often in less than 1 hour. TIAs are an important warning sign of impending stroke.

Hemorrhagic Stroke

Hemorrhagic strokes occur rapidly and without warning. The hemorrhage triggers a series of conditions, such as increased mass effect, decreased cerebral blood flow, and cerebral edema. It may further increase ICP and possibly lead to herniation. Hemorrhagic strokes may be intracerebral, intraparenchymal, or subarachnoid hemorrhage (SAH). Hypertension is most common cause of intracerebral hemorrhage.

Signs and Symptoms

Dependent on the Location of the Vessel Involved and the Extent of the Occlusion

- Sudden numbness, weakness of the face, arm, or leg, especially on one side
- Sudden confusion, trouble speaking or understanding
- Sudden trouble seeing in one or both eyes
- Sudden trouble walking, dizziness, loss of balance or coordination
- Sudden severe headache—*most common sign of hemorrhagic stroke*

Diagnostics

- Accurate history of events
- Presentation of symptoms
- Risk factors identification for stroke
- Noncontrast CT scan of the head
  - To rule out hemorrhagic stroke
  - CT will not immediately show infarcted tissue or presence of an occluded artery
- Carotid duplex sonography to diagnose carotid stenosis

Patient Care Management

Determine type of stroke—Ischemic versus Hemorrhagic

Consistent Neurological Evaluation to Follow Progression

- Use of a standard outcome grading scale by all health care providers

Ischemic Stroke

- Reprofusion—If symptom onset is within 3 hours
  - Tissue plasminogen activator (t-PA), which lyses the clot and restores blood flow
- Reduce and manage complications
  - Antiplatelet and antithrombotic therapy
  - Heparin
  - Warfarin with atrial fibrillation
  - Antihypertensive medications
  - Statins to lower lipids
  - Aspiration precautions
  - DVT prophylaxis
  - Seizure medications
- Carotid endarterectomy
- Percutaneous angioplasty with or without intervascular stenting
- Extracranial to intracranial bypass procedure

Hemorrhagic Stroke

- Careful monitoring in ICU for ICP
  - Placement of an external ventricular drain (EVD) may be necessary to monitor and treat elevated ICP.
- Blood pressure support
- Respiratory support
- Reduce and manage complications
- Craniotomy and evacuation of large hematomas

Nursing Management
Risk of Aspiration

- Maintain NPO status until swallow evaluation completed
- Follow guidelines on allowed foods

- Sit patient upright to eat
- Monitor food intake and ability to swallow

Risk of Complications—DVT, UTI, Fall Potential, Impaired Skin Integrity
- Initiate rehabilitation early
- Provide DVT prophylaxis
- Monitor for signs of infection, remove Foley catheters early
- Provide safety from falls
- Maintain skin integrity with turning and mobility

Knowledge Deficit
- Teach modification of stroke risk factors
- Instruct patient and family on the signs/symptoms of stroke
- Stress urgency of seeking care: "Time is brain"—call 911

Cerebovascular Malformations

Cerebral Aneurysms/Subarachnoid Hemorrhage (SAH)
A cerebral aneurysm is defined as a "saccular outpouching of a cerebral artery." Intracerebral aneurysms may occur singularly or in multiples. Familial intracranial aneurysms are defined as two or more family members with documented cerebral aneurysms. Rupture of an intracerebral aneurysm results in subarachnoid hemorrhage, defined simply as bleeding into the subarachnoid space. Though SAH can occur from other causes, such as trauma, or be idiopathic, SAH most often occurs from aneurysm rupture, incidence increases with age, and is higher in women than in men. The cause of cerebral aneurysms is not clear.

Risk Factors for Aneurysms
- Smoking
- Hypertension
- Previous aneurysms
- Family history of aneurysms
- Connective tissue disorder

- Age greater than 40 years
- Female
- Blood vessel injury or dissection

Signs and Symptoms

The location of cerebral aneurysms, their size, and whether or not they have ruptured are the most important factors in determining signs and symptoms of the patient.

Unruptured Aneurysms
- Localized headache
- Cranial nerve signs
  - Dilated pupil
  - Decreased mobility of the eye
  - Ptosis (drooping of the eyelid)
- Dizziness and balance difficulties

Subarachnoid Hemorrhage— Ruptured Aneurysms
- Headache described as the "worst headache of my life"
- Extreme vertigo and nausea and vomiting
- Neurological deterioration
- Seizures are not uncommon.
- Presenting sign may be death.

Diagnostics
- CT scan of the head
- Cerebral angiogram for the location of the ruptured aneurysm

Patient Care Management
- Surgical clip across the neck of the aneurysm to completely obliterate aneurysm to prevent re-bleeding
- Endovascular procedures such as coiling or stenting

- Aggressively manage medical complications associated with SAH
  - Rebleeding—The highest in the first 24 to 48 hours, continues for first 2 weeks
  - Vasospasm
  - Hyponatremia
  - Hypertension
  - Seizures
  - Hydrocephalus

Complications of SAH

Cerebral Vasospasm
Vasospasm decreases CBF causing cerebral ischemia, and infarction if left untreated. Peak incidence of vasospasm is from 3 to 14 days but may occur up to 21 days later.

Signs and Symptoms
- Completely asymptomatic
- Confusion
- Impaired level of consciousness
- Focal neurological impairment, such as hemiplegia, aphasia
- Fever
- Neck stiffness

Diagnostics
- Transcranial Doppler studies (TCDs)
- Cerebral angiography
- Serum Electrolytes
- CBC

Patient Care Management
Triple-H therapy to increase cerebral perfusion pressure and CBF, and reduce the risk of further neurological deficits

- Hypertension
  - Systolic blood pressure should be kept at no less than 160 mmHg, and may be kept as high as 180 to 200.
  - Induced with vasopressors, such as dopamine, phenylephrine, or dobutamine
- Hemodilution—increases CBF
  - Maintain hematocrit of 32% to 35%
  - Infusion of volume expanders, such as albumin
- Hypervolemia
  - Hemodynamic monitoring in ICU required
- Additional therapy for vasospasm
  - Calcium channel blockers, such as nimodipine
  - Hypothermia to decrease cerebral ischemia due to vasospasm

Hyponatremia

Hyponatremia in SAH is caused by either syndrome of inappropriate antidiuretic hormone (SIADH) or cerebral salt wasting. It is very important for the cause of hyponatremia to be determined, because the treatment strategies for SIADH and cerebral salt wasting are very different.

(See also Fluid and Electrolytes for Hyponatremia.)

Signs and Symptoms

- Decreased LOC
- Suddenly confused, restless, or lethargic
- Seizure

Patient Care Management
SIADH Treatment

- Fluid restriction (contraindicated with SAH, due to vasospasm)

Cerebral Salt Wasting Treatment

- Hypertonic saline, with oral salt supplements
- IV fluids, usually normal saline, administered at 100 to 150 mL/hr for the prevention of vasospasm

- Serum sodium levels monitoring frequently, every 6 hours if the patient is receiving hypertonic saline.
- Observe for vasospasm

Patient Care Management
Risk of Complications
- Monitor for neurological changes
- Monitor fluid intake and output carefully
- DO NOT discontinue IV fluids until ordered

> **Critical Alert**
> Fluid restriction in this setting is absolutely contraindicated.

- Monitor blood pressure at least hourly
- Do not administer antihypertensive medications without parameters for administration.
- Monitor Na levels

(See Stroke section.)

Arteriovenous Malformations
Arteriovenous malformations (AVMs) are a mass of abnormal blood vessels in which arterial blood flows directly into the venous system. AVMs contain blood vessels that are thin walled and do not have normal characteristics of blood vessels. AVMs are congenital, which implies a lifelong risk of hemorrhage. Hemorrhage may be the presenting symptom.

The AVM is a mass, which displaces normal tissue as it grows in size; even in cases where hemorrhage has not occurred, increased ICP may occur. Atypical shunting of arterial blood into the venous system results in an elevated intravascular pressure and aneurysm development, possible rupture and hemorrhage of vessels. The brain tissue surrounding the AVM may become ischemic. Neurological deficits may progress slowly without the presence of hemorrhage.

Signs and Symptoms
Most important variables are size, the location, and the presence of hemorrhage.

Unruptured AVM

- Related to the location of the lesion
- Slow growing, neurological symptoms may be slow in progressing.

Ruptured AVM

- Dramatic symptoms related to location and size of hemorrhage
- Severe neurological compromise
- Seizures
- Coma or death

Diagnostics

- CT scan
- MRI
- Cerebral angiography for determination of involvement of cerebral vasculature and presence of aneurysms

Patient Care Management

- Surgical resection
- Endovascular coiling or embolization
- Radiosurgery
- Conservative treatment
  - Management of symptoms (headaches or seizures)
  - Observation with serial MRI and/or cerebral angiograms

Nursing Management

(See Stroke section.)

Cavernous Malformations

Cavernous malformations are composed of clusters of enlarged capillary channels, separated by dense fibrous tissue, with little to no intervening normal brain tissue. These malformations grow and increase in size as a result of recurrent bleeding and thrombosis. Cavernous malformations usually are not diagnosed until they bleed, causing neurological deficits specific to the location of lesion. There are two types of cavernous malformations: sporadic and familial.

Signs and Symptoms

Dependent location, size of the lesion, and whether the lesion has bled.

- A cavernous malformation may produce neurological symptoms because it is a space-occupying lesion.
- First sign frequently is bleeding causing deficits based on its location.
- Seizures—the most common presenting symptom
- Focal neurological deficits
- Motor deficits
- Sensory deficits
- Cranial nerve deficits
- Repeated hemorrhages worsen the neurological deficits, especially if the lesion recovery from neurological deficits may occur, but it is rare to return to baseline.

Diagnostics

- MRI scan
- CT scan to determine the presence of a lesion, but is not specific to the type of lesion

Patient Care Management

- Surgical resection
  - Large lesion and accessible (curable if a completely resected) is possible
  - Refractory or worsening seizures, or neurological
- Observation for small lesion
  - Serial MRI
  - Seizures therapy

Nursing Management

(See Stroke section.)

Chronic Degenerative Neurological Disorders

Alzheimer's Disease

Alzheimer's disease (AD) is a chronic, progressive, irreversible brain disorder, characterized by deterioration of memory and cognition (dementia). Alzheimer's disease is found most frequently in adults ages 65 and older. The onset of AD begins with subtle lapses of memory, which gradually and progressively develop into a chronic loss of personality, recognition, reasoning, and independence. AD is marked by the profusion of amyloid plaques and neurofibrillary tangles, which form in the hippocampus and other parts of the brain critical to memory, that develop at a much greater rate and mass than in normal aging.

Risk Factors

- Growing old is the most significant risk factor for developing AD.
- Genetics/family history
- Atherosclerosis
- High cholesterol
- Elevated plasma homocysteine
- Diabetes
- Down syndrome
- Mild cognitive impairment (MCI)

Signs and Symptoms

Slow and insidious decline of cognitive function, ranging over 3 to 20 years. Stages corresponding to the area of the brain where degeneration is present.

Preclinical AD

The first symptom is likely to be an elusive, difficult-to-distinguish loss of memory. If the patient's memory loss appears to be greater than might be expected for his or her age, while other functions of cognition remain intact, then a diagnosis of mild cognitive impairment (MCI) may be rendered. In cases of MCI, the patient's experience of cognitive impairment may be uncorroborated by friends or family who do not notice the subtle behavior changes and memory anomalies of which the patient complains.

Mild AD

Escalating problems with memory and cognitive function become obvious. Friends and family who do recognize the patient's transitory condition corroborate these difficulties.

- Confusion about the location of familiar places
- Slow to accomplish simple tasks
- Difficulty handling money matters
- Loss of spontaneity and sense of initiative
- Mood swings and personality changes

Moderate AD

At this stage of the disease, neuronal degeneration expands to areas that control language and reasoning. The symptoms worsen as atrophy continues to spread. The patient may have a bout of wandering and can be easily agitated by the routines of daily living.

- Progressive memory loss and confusion
- Unable to recognize friends and family
- Language difficulties
- Difficulties with reading, writing, and simple math
- Problems learning new material, aligning thoughts, and thinking logically
- Hallucinations, delusions, paranoia

Severe AD

In the most advanced phase of AD, plaques and tangles have spread throughout the brain, causing generalized atrophy. The patient becomes completely dependent and is not able to recognize loved ones.

- Inability to communicate
- Weight loss secondary to difficulty eating and swallowing

- Bowel and bladder incontinence
- Increased sleeping
- Death usually occurs as a result of aspiration pneumonia or from other concurrent health conditions.

Diagnostics

- A definitive diagnosis of AD can be made only following a brain autopsy.
- Detailed medical history, physical examination, and neurological assessment, attention to the duration and progression of the patient's memory loss
- Cognitive status is often evaluated using the Folstein Mini-Mental Status Exam (MMSE).
- Laboratory and radiological tests are used to rule out other causes of dementia (metabolic imbalances, vitamin B_{12} deficiency, stroke, and brain tumor).
- MRI of brain to rule out other conditions (normal pressure hydrocephalus or subdural hematoma) and in later stages will show generalized atrophy.
- Positron emission tomography (PET) to detect significant alterations in brain metabolism

Patient Care Management

A comprehensive approach to patient and caregiver support throughout the course of the disease is important.

Medication Therapy to Slow Cognitive and Functional Loss

- Acetylcholinesterase Inhibitors
    - Galantamine (Reminyl)
    - Rivastigmine (Exelon)
    - Donepezil (Aricept)
- NMDA Receptor Antagonist
    - Memantine (Namenda)
- Behavioral Symptoms of Alzheimer's Disease Atypical Antipsychotics
    - Olanzapine (Zyprexa)
    - Quetiapine (Seroquel)

- Selective Serotonin-Reuptake Inhibitors
  - Sertraline (Zoloft)
  - Citalopram (Celexa)

Nursing Management

High Risk for Injury related to poor memory, insight, judgment, and self-control; unstable gait:

- Evaluate the environment to protect patient from injury
- Manage dysfunctional behaviors
- Provide safe ways for patient to complete ADLs

Disturbed Thought Processes (inappropriate reactions, dysfunctional behavior, delusions and paranoia) related to cognitive decline

- Reduce environmental stimuli
- Establishing predictable routines
- Simplifying tasks
- Using distraction and redirection
- Provide medication if needed for restlessness, agitation, anger, anxiety, wandering, or psychotic symptoms

Knowledge Deficit

- Teach safe, consistent medication administration
- Teach how to monitor for medication effectiveness and side effects
- Teach methods to reduce environmental stimuli and enhance safety in the home
- Refer to organizations for assistance with finding community resources, support groups, financial and legal advice, respite, and long-term care options

Amyotrophic Lateral Sclerosis (ALS)

Amyotrophic lateral sclerosis (ALS) is a degenerative disease involving upper and lower motor neurons. Degeneration of motor neurons in the spinal cord, brainstem, and cerebral cortex leads to the characteristic symptoms of weakness, muscular atrophy, and spasticity.

ALS, also known as Lou Gehrig's disease, is progressive, incurable, and fatal. The cause of ALS is unknown. Cognition, sensory function, vision, and hearing are spared. Aspiration, infection, and respiratory failure are usually the ultimate causes of death. Average disease duration is 3 to 4 years.

Signs and Symptoms

Initial complaints range from difficulty walking and problems with tripping and stumbling to trouble performing fine tasks. Symptoms are subtle at the onset and slow in progression.

- Painless muscle weakness and wasting
  - Spasticity
  - Cramping
  - Fatigue
  - Fasciculation (involuntary twitching) of the limb and tongue muscles
- Weakness and atrophy extend throughout the muscles
  - The arms and legs become severely impaired.
- Speech and swallowing muscles progressively deteriorate, increasing risk of aspirating food or saliva into the airway
  - Dysarthria
  - Dysphagia
  - Weight loss
- Respiratory muscle deterioration leads to dyspnea and respiratory failure.
- Cognitive functions remain intact, patients are highly aware of the disease and its progression.
  - Anxiety or depression

Diagnostics

- No definitive tests, diagnostic tests are used to rule out other conditions
  - MRI brain and spinal to r/o other conditions

- EMG may show denervation, muscle wasting and atrophy.
- CPK indicates muscle breakdown.
- Medical history
- Neurological examination and symptoms

Patient Care Management

With no cure, the focus of care is on slowing the progression and on symptom management.

Medication Therapy

- Riluzole (Rilutek), a benzothiazole, is the only drug known to slow the progression of ALS.
- Diazepam or dantrolene for spasticity
- Quinine sulfate or baclofen for muscle cramping

Nursing Management

Management of ALS requires a multidisciplinary approach to meet the needs of both the patient and family. Treatment goals should focus on providing symptom relief and on preserving comfort and dignity, because disease progression renders the patient to a completely dependent state. They will be faced with making difficult decisions regarding artificial feeding, ventilation, and end-of-life desires.

Ineffective breathing pattern related to muscle failure:

- Evaluate respiratory status frequently—report changes to health care provider
  - Work of breathing
  - Oxygen saturation
  - Signs of hypoxia
- Provide supportive therapy
  - Optimal patient positioning
  - Oxygen
  - Ventilator support, BiPap

Risk of Aspiration and Nutritional Deficit

- Monitor swallowing function
- Observe for coughing and signs of aspiration
- Assist with nutritional needs

Anticipatory Grieving

- Encourage verbalization
- Need to make proactive decisions regarding mechanical ventilation, artificial hydration and nutrition.
- Referrals for counseling, community support, and national ALS Association

Knowledge Deficit

- Teach patient and family disease progression and when to notify health care providers for assistance
- Instruct on proper use of equipment—ventilatory devices, feeding tubes, etc.
- Teach aspiration precautions
  - Avoid large meals
  - Sit upright during and following meals
  - Sleep with head elevated 15–30 degrees
  - Appropriate food selection

Multiple Sclerosis

Multiple sclerosis (MS) is a chronic and progressive neuroimmunologic disease characterized by multiple areas of demyelination in the white matter of the brain and spinal cord, often striking young adults. The subsequent scarring leads weakness, spasticity, visual difficulties, and paresthesias. Demyelination results from an inflammatory process and also leads to irreversible axonal injury and permanent loss of nerve function. Although viruses and environmental factors are suspect for their role in MS, the cause is still unknown.

Main Types of MS

- *Relapsing-remitting MS* is the most common type. It is known for its acute attacks followed by complete or partial remission. It makes up about 85% of initial diagnoses.

- *Primary-progressive MS* progresses without remission, although plateaus or minor improvements can happen. Approximately 10% to 15% of the diagnoses are for this form of the disease.
- *Secondary progressive MS* begins as relapsing-remitting, but then it develops into the primary-progressive course.
- *Progressive-relapsing MS* intersperses the progression of the disease with acute attacks. Both age and duration of the disease have the greatest influence on the rate of relapse.

Signs and Symptoms

Symptoms vary from patient to patient and within the same patient overtime based on the area of the CNS affected.

The most common initial signs:

- Fatigue
- Nystagmus
- Vertigo
- Gait disturbances
- Sensory loss
- Lower extremity weakness, spasticity
- Bladder disturbance
- Optic neuritis

   Other symptoms that may present at any time:

- Cognitive changes such as euphoria or depression
- Physical conditions such as muscle cramping and sexual dysfunction

Diagnostics

- Comprehensive medical history and neurological exam
- MRI to detect plaques

- Cerebrospinal fluid (CSF) tests—Elevated IgG index or presence of oligoclonal bands
- Visual evoked potentials (VEP)—slow conduction

Patient Care Management

Treating MS relies on medication therapy, relapse management, and symptom management.

Medication Therapy

- Immunomodulator/Interferons
  - Interferon beta-1a (Avonex)
  - Interferon beta-1b (Betaseron)
  - Interferon beta-1a (Rebif)
- Immunomodulator
  - Glatiramer acetate (Copaxone)
- Antineoplastic/Immunosuppressive
  - Mitoxantrone (Novantrone)
- Monoclonal Antibody
  - Natalizumab (Tysabri)
- CNS Stimulants
  - Pemoline
  - Modafinil
- Genitourinary Antispasmodics
  - Oxybutynin (Ditropan)
  - Tolterodine tartrate (Detrol)
- Skeletal Muscle Relaxant
  - Oral or intrathecal baclofen
  - Benzodiazepines
  - Diazepam
  - Clonazepam

Relapse Management

A relapse is a new sign or a worsening of neurological symptoms with a duration that is greater than 24 hours. Symptoms gradually resolve and patients fully or partially recover. Several conditions are known to precipitate symptoms or relapses. These include, but are not limited to, excessive exertion, extreme temperatures, infections, hot baths, fever, emotional stress, and pregnancy.

Relapses often are treated with an orally or intravenously administered glucocorticoid, such as methylprednisolone. Detailing the history of relapse and the consequential symptoms becomes the basis of care and treatment of the MS patient.

Symptom Management
Fatigue Management

- Evaluation of sleep habits, current and former medications, experiences of depression, and applied coping strategies
- Patient education
- Avoid hot ambient temperature
- Use of air conditioning, cool drinks, and ice packs can help
- Energy conservation strategies for ADLs
- Light exercise
- Scheduling rest times between activities
- Using labor-saving tools and appliances

Medications Therapy

- Amantadine
- Pemoline
- Modafinil
- Low-dose antidepressants

Nursing Management

Nursing care needs of the patient with MS are multifaceted and complex, encompassing both inpatient and outpatient care, best addressed by a multidisciplinary team approach. Symptom management is a major area of focus, with nursing care concentrating on nonpharmacologic management, patient education, and support.

Risk of Injury Related to Muscle Weakness, Ataxia, Decreased Sensory Perception

- Ambulate patient to evaluate gait, ataxia, potential for falling
- Consult with physical therapist use of assistive devices and safe use
- Consult with occupational therapist to provide instruction to compensate for sensory deficits while accomplishing ADLs

Fatigue Related to Disease Process

- Provide rest periods between physical activity
- Avoid prolonged exposure to hot ambient temperatures, hot baths or showers
- Encourage light exercise regime to increase endurance and minimize fatigue

Impaired Urinary Elimination Related to Spastic or Flaccid Bladder

- Careful intake and output
- Assess for signs of urine retention—bladder distention, monitor post void residual
- Observe for signs of urine infection (appearance, color, clarity)

Knowledge Deficit

- Instructed to avoid extreme temperatures and exposure to infections
- Stress management techniques should be emphasized
- Encourage exercise to manage fatigue, spasticity, and bowel and bladder problems
- Teach bladder management, signs and symptoms of urinary tract infection and ways to avoid problems
- Increasing fluids and fiber for bladder problems and constipation
- Encourage proper nutrition to aid in resistance to infection

Myasthenia Gravis (MG)

Myasthenia gravis (MG) is an uncommon chronic, autoimmune neuromuscular disorder in which acetylcholine receptors at the neuromuscular junction are destroyed. The two major clinical forms of MG are ocular and generalized. The hallmark feature is fluctuating weakness and fatigability of voluntary muscles. Cause is unknown, but there is increasing evidence that the thymus might play an important role.

Muscle weakness varies over the course of weeks or months, with exacerbations and remissions. As MG progresses, symptom-free periods decrease, and muscle weakness fluctuates from mild to severe. Myasthenic crisis (lack of acetylcholine) and cholinergic crisis (excess of acetylcholine) can progress to extreme weakness and respiratory insufficiency requiring mechanical ventilation.

Signs and Symptoms
Ophthalmic
- Ptosis and diplopia

Nonophthalmic
- Oropharyngeal muscle disturbances—swallowing, talking, and chewing
- Dysarthria and dysphagia, and a nasal quality to the voice
- Limb and trunk weakness
- Respiratory muscles which may lead to symptoms of respiratory insufficiency, and even respiratory failure, an emergency known as myasthenic crisis

Diagnostics
- History and physical assessment, including a neurological examination
- Tensilon test
- EMG
- Computerized tomography (CT) or MRI scan to evaluate the thymus gland and to rule out mass lesions

- Laboratory studies
- Immunologic assays to detect AChR antibodies
- Thyroid function tests to rule out associated Graves' disease or hyperthyroidism

Patient Care Management

Rapid assessment of crisis and ventilation support

Medication Therapy

- Cholinesterase inhibitors (neostigmine, pyridostigmine, or ambenonium)
- Immunotherapeutics (corticosteroids, azathioprine, and cyclosporine)
- Plasmapheresis—Circulating AChR antibodies are removed from the patient's circulation by removing whole blood, extracting the plasma from it, and returning the blood along with fresh or frozen plasma to the patient.
- Intravenous immunoglobulin therapy—an alternative to plasmapheresis
- Ptosis is treated best by lid crutches; diplopia is treated with the use of Fresnel prisms.
- Surgical treatment includes thymectomy, strabismus surgery, and blepharoptosis.

Nursing Management

Risk of Respiratory Depression Related to Neuromuscular Weakness

- Evaluate respiratory status, especially during ADLs
- Assess work of breathing and patient level of anxiety
- Breath sounds and breathing pattern
- Vital signs—monitor for hypoxia

Risk of Aspiration and Diminished Nutritional Health

- Evaluate integrity of gag/swallow reflex
- Assess ability to chew and swallow
- Assist with food selections, monitor intake

Knowledge Deficit

- Teach about muscle weakness related to eating and respiratory functions

- Importance of avoiding respiratory infections and to report any signs and symptoms

- Teach patient and family early signs of impending crisis and when to seek medical attention

- Emphasize risk of aspiration, teach proper safety techniques while eating

- Promote rest period between activities

Parkinson's Disease

Parkinson's disease (PD) is the most common movement disorder; it is characterized by tremor, rigidity, bradykinesia, and postural instability. Although the cause of PD is not known, both genetic and environmental factors have been implicated. PD is not considered a fatal disease, but the degrading effect it has on the patient's ability to carry out basic daily functions can cause susceptibility to more threatening conditions such as pneumonia or traumatic injury. The chronic and progressive nature of PD can significantly impact older, spousal caregivers, who may not have the physical strength to handle the weight of a patient with limited mobility.

PD is a disease of the basal ganglia, a structure deep in the brain that includes the corpus striatum and globus pallidus. Neurons begin to degenerate and die, resulting in a lack of dopamine production causing difficulty with movement, tremor, rigidity, and difficulty maintaining posture. Acetylcholine, another neurotransmitter, also is believed to be involved in the pathology. The lack of dopamine upsets the delicate balance between these two neurotransmitters.

Critical Alert

Drug-induced Parkinson symptoms can occur with the following drugs—Antiemetics: prochlorperazine (Compazine), metoclopramide (Reglan); Neuroleptics: chlorpromazine (Thorazine); haloperidol (Haldol). These drugs are contraindicated in Parkinson's disease.

Signs and Symptoms

Primary Symptoms

- Resting tremor
- Muscle rigidity, bradykinesia, and postural instability may combine to produce gait abnormalities, like a shuffled walk, difficulty turning while walking, and stooped posture
- Bradykinesia
- Postural instability
- Hypokinetic dysarthria (soft muffled speech) due to face and neck muscle dysfunction
- Dysphagia
- Micrographia, or small, cramped handwriting

Autonomic Symptoms

- Constipation (medications may exacerbate)
- Orthostatic hypotension
- Sexual dysfunction
- Excessive sweating
- Urinary incontinence

Neuropsychiatric Symptoms

- Cognitive impairments including dementia occur in 30% of patients.
- Depression

Diagnostics

- Definite diagnosis by autopsy only
- Laboratory or radiological tests are used to rule out other causes of presenting symptoms.
- Neurological exam and clinical history
- Bradykinesia and either resting tremor or rigidity
- Positive response to levodopa

Patient Care Management

Treatment focuses on decreasing symptoms, supporting mobility and improving quality of life.

Medication Therapy

- Dopaminergic drugs—effective for 4 to 6 years; after that time, patients will develop motor fluctuations and/or dyskinesia as effectiveness wears off
- COMT inhibitors—in conjunction with levodopa to counteract wearing-off responses
- Dopamine agonists
- Anticholinergics
- Antiviral
- MAO-B inhibitors
- Tricyclic antidepressants
- Selective serotonin reuptake inhibitors (SSRIs)
- Atypical antipsychotics
- Glucocorticoid
- Vasopressor
- Genitourinary antispasmodic

Surgical procedures for advanced, cases—ablative procedures, deep brain stimulation, and cell transplantation.

Nursing Management
Risk for Malnutrition and Dehydration

- Evaluate dysphagia
- Monitor food and fluid intake
- Dietary consultation for appropriate food selection
- Monitor for nausea, vomiting, and loss of appetite due to medications

Impaired Physical Mobility

- Assist patient to ambulate and perform ADLs to coincide with optimum medication benefit
- Instruct patient to stand straight and walk with a wide-based gait while swinging arms to help maintain balance and momentum
- Perform range of motion to all joints to counteract the effects of rigidity

- Consult with physical therapist. Can prescribe and tailor appropriate gait assistive devices and also exercises to counteract stiffness and rigidity.
- Consult with occupational therapist. Can assess need for adaptive aids for ADLs such as specialized eating utensils or button hook for dressing.

Knowledge Deficit
- Teach patient and family medication administration and side effects
    - Take as directed, usually starting with low dose and titrating upward
    - Do not abruptly stop medications unless directed by health care provider
- Teach fall prevention strategies
    - Remove throw rugs, clear walking paths
    - Install railings along hallways and stairways, and grab bars in bathrooms

Spinal Cord Injuries

Spinal cord injury (SCI) occurs when a mechanical force is applied to the spinal cord, causing either a temporary or permanent loss of sensory, motor, or autonomic function below the level of injury. The majority of SCIs occur because of trauma to the spinal column. Morbidity and mortality after SCI is generally affected by age at the time of injury as well as the level and severity of the injury.

Young male adults are primarily affected with more than 50% in the cervical spine. The thoracolumbar juncture is the second most common site for injury because of the relative mobility of the spine at this level. Spinal cord injuries are classified according to the degree of loss of motor and sensory function below the level of injury. Rehabilitation goals and degree of independence after recovery are dependent on the type of SCI.

Complete Spinal Cord Injury

Results in complete and irreversible loss of voluntary motor and sensory functions below the level of injury.

Functional Loss After Complete Spinal Cord Injury

Level of Injury	Motor Function	Deep Tendon Reflexes	Sensory Function	Bowel and Bladder Function
C_1–C_4	Tetraplegia (quadriplegia) *Lost:* All motor function below the neck	All reflexes lost	*Lost:* All sensation from the neck down	Lost
C_5	Tetraplegia *Lost:* All function below the shoulders *Intact:* Sternocleidomastoid Cervical paraspinal muscles Trapezius	C_5, C_6 Biceps	*Lost:* Sensation below the clavicles Most of the arms Hands Chest Abdomen Lower extremities *Intact:* Sensation to head	Lost

(continued)

Functional Loss After Complete Spinal Cord Injury (*continued*)

Level of Injury	Motor Function	Deep Tendon Reflexes	Sensory Function	Bowel and Bladder Function
			Shoulders Deltoid Clavicle Lateral aspect of the forearm	
C_6	Tetraplegia *Lost:* All function below the shoulders and upper arms *Intact:* Deltoid Biceps Rotator muscles of the shoulder	C_5, C_6 Brachio-radialis	*Lost:* Sensation below the clavicles Chest Abdomen Lower extremities *Intact:* Sensation to the head Shoulders Arms Palms of hands Thumbs	Lost

C$_7$	Tetraplegia *Lost:* Function in portions of the hands and arms *Intact:* Shoulder depressors Shoulder abductors Shoulder internal rotators Radial wrist extensors	C$_7$,C$_8$ Triceps	*Lost:* Sensation below the clavicles Chest Abdomen Lower extremities *Intact:* Sensation to the head Shoulders Most of the arms and hands	Lost
C$_8$	Tetraplegia *Lost:* Function in portions of the hands and arms *Intact:* Elbow extensors Wrist Finger extensors and flexors		*Lost:* Sensation below the chest Portions of the hands *Intact:* Sensation to the head Shoulders Part of the upper chest	Lost

(continued)

467

Functional Loss After Complete Spinal Cord Injury (*continued*)

Level of Injury	Motor Function	Deep Tendon Reflexes	Sensory Function	Bowel and Bladder Function
T_1–T_6	Paraplegia *Lost:* Function below the midchest including the muscles of the trunk *Intact:* Shoulders Upper chest Arms Hands		*Lost:* Sensation below the midchest *Intact:* Everything above the midchest T_1, T_2 provide sensation to the inner arm T_4 provides sensation to the nipple area	Lost
T_6–T_{12}	Paraplegia *Lost:* Function below the waist		*Lost:* Sensation below the waist	Lost

	Intact: Shoulders Arms Hands Long trunk muscles		*Intact:* Shoulders Arms Hands T_{10} provides sensation to the umbilicus T_{12} provides sensation to the groin	
L_1–L_3	Paraplegia *Lost:* Most control of the legs and pelvis *Intact:* Shoulders Arms Hands Torso Hip rotation	L_2–L_4 Knee jerk	*Lost:* Lower abdomen Legs *Intact:* Some sensation to the inner and anterior thigh L_3 supplies the knee	Lost

(continued)

Functional Loss After Complete Spinal Cord Injury (*continued*)

Level of Injury	Motor Function	Deep Tendon Reflexes	Sensory Function	Bowel and Bladder Function
L_3–L_4	Paraplegia *Lost:* Portions of the lower legs Ankles Feet *Intact:* Increased knee extension		*Lost:* Sensation to portions of the lower legs Ankles Feet *Intact:* Sensation to the upper legs	Lost
L_4–S_5	Incomplete paraplegia L_4–S_1: Abduction and internal rotation of the hip Ankle dorsiflexion Foot inversion	S_1–S_2 Ankle jerk	L_5: Medial aspect of the foot S_1: Lateral aspect of the foot S_2: Posterior aspect of the thigh/calf	Possibly spared S_2–S_4: Urinary control S_3–S_5: Bowel control

		Lower sacral nerves: Perineum
	L_5–S_1: Foot inversion	
	L_4–S_2: Foot eversion	
	S_1–S_2: Plantar flexion	
	S_2–S_5: Bowel and bladder control	

Adapted from Hickey, J. V. (Ed.). (2003). *The clinical practice of neurological and neurosurgical nursing* (5th ed., pp. 424–425). Philadelphia: Lippincott Williams & Wilkins.

Incomplete Spinal Cord Injury

Will have some preservation of sensory and/or motor function below the level of injury. Sparing of some of the spinal cord tracts, allows neurotransmission to occur.

Five main syndromes are associated with incomplete SCI:

Central Cord Syndrome

This is the most common incomplete SCI. Seen most frequently in older patients who have degenerative bony changes in the cervical spine resulting in narrowing. It most often is caused by a hyperextension injury resulting in damage to the center of the spinal cord. Greater loss of motor and sensory function occurs in the upper extremities than in the lower extremities. Bladder dysfunction is variable. The overall prognosis for recovery from this injury is generally favorable. The typical pattern of recovery is return of lower extremity function first followed by return of bladder function. Recovery of hand intrinsic function is variable and often the last to return.

Anterior Cord Syndrome

This is caused by direct injury to the anterior portion of the spinal cord or disruption of the anterior spinal artery resulting in ischemia and infarction of the anterior two-thirds of the spinal cord This is often due to compression from either an acute disk herniation or from a hyperextension injury resulting in fracture-dislocation of the vertebra. Paralysis and loss of pain and temperature sensation are evident below the level of injury. Light touch, vibration, and proprioception are preserved because these tracts are located in the dorsal columns of the spinal cord, which are perfused by the posterior spinal arteries. The prognosis for recovery from this injury is variable, although generally not favorable.

Brown-Séquard Syndrome

This is rare and results from a penetrating injury causing transverse hemisection of the spinal cord. Paralysis and loss of proprioception are seen on the ipsilateral side of the injury, and pain and temperature sensation are lost on the contralateral side. Functional recovery from this type of injury is variable, although it can be quite favorable.

Cauda Equina Syndrome

This is caused by compression of the lumbar nerve roots below the level of L_1. Commonly seen with large disk herniations at the L_4/L_5 level affecting the nerve roots as they descend through the spinal canal. The deficits related to this syndrome are variable, but can involve motor and sensory functions of the pelvic organs and lower extremities. Weakness, sensory deficits, loss of the Achilles reflex, and bowel and bladder dysfunction including bowel incontinence, urinary retention, and overflow urinary incontinence can be seen. Recovery is variable.

Spinal Cord Injury Without Radiographic Abnormality (SCIWORA)

SCIWORA is defined as spinal cord injury following a traumatic event without signs of fracture, dislocation, or ligamentous injury on plain radiographs, computed tomography (CT), or myelography. Patients who have experienced a SCIWORA type injury often will demonstrate abnormality of the soft tissue structures or spinal cord on MRI that is not evident on standard radiography.

Causes of Spinal Cord Injury

- Hyperflexion injuries occur when there is a sudden deceleration in motion such as can occur in a head-on motor vehicle collision or diving accident. The injury results in fracture of the anterior portion of the vertebral body as well as fracture and dislocation of the facets in the posterior aspect of the spinal column. The posterior spinal ligament and the intervertebral disk also may be disrupted. The presence of fracture and dislocation of the facet joints increases the probability of injury to the spinal cord.

- Hyperextension injuries occur when the spine is extended backward as can occur in rear-impact collisions when the head and neck are forcefully extended back, or in forward falls in which the chin or forehead is struck. The spinal cord can be stretched and degenerative changes of the spinal column including the presence of bone spurs and hypertrophy of the ligaments can cause excessive compression of the spinal cord resulting in an SCI.

- Rotational injuries occur when there is extreme lateral flexion or rotation and flexion of the spine, most commonly in the neck. The posterior ligaments may rupture and fracture and dislocation of the facets may occur, resulting in spinal instability. If the facets on both sides of the spine are affected, the incidence of SCI is increased.

- Compression injuries occur because of axial pressure or loading of the spine. A vertical force is applied to the spine causing fracture of the vertebral body. These injuries typically occur as a result of landing on the feet or buttocks after a fall from a significant height or from extreme flexion of the spine. A compression fracture also can occur because of weakening of the vertebral body due to infection, malignancy, or osteoporosis. Bone fragments from the fracture can cause compression or mass effect on the spinal cord.

- Penetrating injuries occur as a result of a projectile such as a bullet or sharp object entering the spinal column. The spinal cord can suffer a contusion (bruising) or even a partial or complete transection (severing of the cord). Damage to the bony structures of the spine can also occur resulting in bone fragments in the spinal canal, which can cause additional compression of the spinal cord. The degree of injury to the spinal cord is related to the velocity of the object as it enters the spinal canal.

Types of Spinal Cord Injury

The spinal cord may sustain one or a combination of several types of injuries as a result of the above mechanisms of injury:

- Concussion—Usually occurs as a result of a blow to the spinal column. The spinal cord is jarred or shaken. A temporary loss of function can be seen for a period of hours or days.

- Contusion—Often caused by fracture, dislocation, or direct trauma to the spinal cord. The spinal cord is bruised, resulting in hemorrhage and edema into the cord. Necrosis of spinal cord tissue may occur because of compression from bleeding or edema or because of direct damage of neural tissue. The degree of neurological dysfunction is dependent on the severity of the contusion.

- Compression—Occurs as a result of squeezing or pressure on the spinal cord. The pressure can last momentarily as in a hyperextension injury or can be prolonged because of mass effect from bone fragments, neoplasm, hemorrhage, or disk herniation. The spinal cord may also suffer contusion, concussion, laceration, or transection as a result.

- Laceration—A tear or cut in the spinal cord. Neurological deficits resulting from this type of injury are permanent.

- Transection—Severing of the spinal cord.

- Hemorrhage—Bleeding that can occur either within the spinal cord or the surrounding tissues. This can result in compression on the spinal cord or irritation to the neural tissues.

- Infarction—Ischemia of the spinal cord as a result of interruption of blood flow. This type of injury can occur because of compression or injury to the vessels that perfuse the cord.

Primary Injury is a result of the insult to the spinal cord resulting in physical damage. The degree of damage to the spinal cord is dependent on the amount of force applied to the cord at the time of the initial injury and may range from mild cord concussion resulting in a transient loss of function to severe injury resulting in complete and permanent loss of function. As a result of the initial trauma, the neural elements of the spinal cord, including nerve cells and the ascending and descending spinal tracks, will be disrupted at the level of the injury. The vasculature of the spinal cord also can be affected, resulting in hemorrhage and ischemia of the spinal cord.

Spinal Shock   is a state of areflexia in which there is a loss of all motor, sensory, and reflex activity at the level of the injury and below as a result of the primary injury. The duration is variable, lasting as little as a few hours or as long as several weeks after injury. During this state, it is impossible to determine the extent of the SCI.

Secondary Injury   is a cascade of complex events that can worsen the extent of the primary injury by causing damage to the adjoining neural tissues. The secondary process begins almost immediately after the initial trauma to the spinal cord. Ischemia within the spinal cord at the time of the primary injury leads to additional vascular changes, which worsen the disruption of the normal perfusion of the spinal cord. Current treatment strategies for SCI are directed at reducing the damage caused by this secondary process.

Neurogenic Shock   occurs due to disruption of autonomic regulation by the sympathetic nervous system, most commonly seen in patients who have had an SCI at T6 or above and should be differentiated from spinal shock. Neurogenic shock occurs when the normal impulses from the brainstem, which contribute to the reflexive control of heart rate and blood pressure, are disrupted. Vagal tone is left unopposed causing bradycardia, peripheral vasodilation below the level of injury resulting in decreased systemic vascular resistance, hypotension, and decreased cardiac output are evident. The resulting hypotension and diminished cardiac output are thought to contribute to ischemia of the spinal cord at the site of injury.

Critical Alert

With a trauma patient it is important to distinguish between neurogenic shock and hypovolemic shock to ensure appropriate treatment strategies. Hypotension is a hallmark sign for both types of shocks. In neurogenic shock patient will be warm, hyperemic, bradycardic, and requiring vasopressors. The hypovolemic shock patient will be tachycardic, cool to touch, and requiring volume replacement.

Autonomic Hyperreflexia occurs as a result of a noxious stimulus below the level of the SCI. Common causes include urinary tract abnormalities such as a distended bladder, abnormalities of the lower intestinal tract such as constipation or fecal impaction, and pressure ulcers. A sympathetic response is triggered, resulting in vasoconstriction below the level of the SCI. Blood volume is shifted from the vasculature below the SCI to the vasculature above the injury, causing elevation of blood pressure, slowing of the heart and vasodilation. These sympathetic impulses are blocked at the level of the SCI and vasoconstriction continues unchecked below the level of injury. This response will continue until the noxious stimulus is removed.

Critical Alert

Autonomic hyperreflexia is a medical emergency that could lead to serious complications if left untreated. When the patient exhibits symptoms of autonomic hyperreflexia, it is important to institute measures to treat the blood pressure and to identify and correct the cause.

Signs and Symptoms

Spinal cord injury assumes systemic effects causing dysfunction of multiple organ systems depending on the level and severity of the injury.

Cardiovascular

- Neurogenic shock is most evident in the patient who has sustained an SCI at T_6 or above

  - Sympathetic innervation is lost leaving vagal tone unopposed
  - Bradycardia, peripheral vasodilation below the level of injury
  - $\downarrow$ Systemic vascular resistance
  - Hypotension
  - $\downarrow$ Cardiac output

- Orthostatic hypotension due to loss of sympathetic vascular tone. If left unchecked, cerebral ischemia is possible.

- Deep venous thrombosis (DVT) due to pooling of blood in the peripheral vascular system, flaccidity of the extremities, and immobility

- Pulmonary embolus (PE)

Pulmonary

Patients with SCI above T_{12} have potential for impairment of respiratory function. Generally, higher level injuries have more significant impairment.

- Atelectasis and pneumonia can contribute to decompensation in respiratory function.

- Diaphragm impairment—injuries at C_4 or higher will cause paralysis of the diaphragm, necessitating intubation and ventilation.

- Loss of use of accessory muscles—injuries involving the lower cervical spine, thoracic spine, or lumbar spine usually will not require immediate intubation, but warrant close monitoring for signs of respiratory decompensation.

Gastrointestinal

- Gastroparesis, loss of intestinal peristalsis, and ileus. The resulting abdominal distention places the patient at risk for vomiting. and aspiration

- Placement of a nasogastric or oral gastric tube necessary in the acute phase of SCI for decompression of the stomach and minimization of these risks
- Gastric stress ulceration
  - Prophylactic medication regimen needed in all SCI patients
- Decreased sensory and motor function of the bowel
  - Above T_{12}
    - Decreased intestinal peristalsis, absent rectal sensation, and an increase in anal sphincter tone
    - Anal reflex activity may be preserved, patients are prone to chronic constipation.
  - L_1 and below
    - Loss of tone throughout the colon and rectal sphincters
    - Likely to experience bowel incontinence

Genitourinary

The spinal tracts responsible for bladder control are disrupted resulting in loss of the normal bladder reflexes and control of urination.

- Atonic bladder
  - Urinary retention and bladder distention
  - Urinary incontinence from a distended bladder
  - Overdistension of the bladder
    - Urinary tract infection (UTI)
    - Hydronephrosis
    - Decline in renal function
    - Renal calculi

Integumentary

Patients with SCI are at high risk for development of pressure ulcers because of impairment in sensory and motor functions as well as impairment of tissue perfusion due to hypotension and pooling of blood in the lower extremities. Factors that contribute:

- Fever
- Infection
- Poor nutrition
- Prolonged immobilization on the firm spinal board

> **Critical Alert**
> Prevention is the best strategy to deal with pressure ulcers; they can be very difficult to heal and can increase the risk of infection.

Diagnostics

- X-rays of the entire spinal axis
- CT scan
- MRI

Patient Care Management

Pre-Hospitalization

Evaluation and management of SCI begins at the scene of the trauma and is carried throughout the acute care hospitalization and rehabilitation phases. Early assessment and management are vital for determining the extent of injury and minimization of secondary injury to the spinal cord.

- Rapid assessment of the victim
- Spinal precautions
- Evaluation and management of the ABCs (airway–breathing–circulation)
- Stabilization and control of life-threatening injuries
- Rapid transport to an appropriate facility for continuation of care

In-Hospital

- Expedite diagnostic testing to facilitate early identification of spinal cord compression or spinal instability

- Stabilize the spine at the level of injury, optimize neurological outcome, and prevent neurological deterioration
- Prevent spinal cord ischemia
  - Maintain oxygenation
  - Support blood pressure and heart rate
- Evaluation and support of pulmonary function
  - Supplemental oxygen and monitored continuously with pulse oximetry
  - Baseline arterial blood gas (ABG)
  - Lung sounds assessment repeated periodically
  - Monitor for apnea, stridorous respirations, use of accessory muscles, rapid, shallow respirations and decline of oxygen saturation
  - Prepare for ventilatory support and intubation if necessary. Care should be taken to ensure the spine remains in alignment and extension or flexion of the neck is avoided
- Evaluation and support of circulatory function
  - Evaluate and support circulatory function
  - Monitor heart rate, rhythm, and blood pressure
  - Observe for neurogenic shock verses hypovolumic shock
  - Vigilant assessment for signs of other organ injury
- Baseline neurological examination is crucial prior to administering pain medication, sedatives, or paralytics.
  - Glasgow Coma Scale (GCS) score
  - Detailed assessment of motor function of all major muscle groups
  - Initially and hourly with vital signs for the first 48 to 72 hours
  - The strength of each major muscle group is tested individually and compared with the corresponding muscle group on the contralateral side

- Sensory examination in all dermatomes using a sequential side-to-side manner
  - Evaluation of the deep tendon reflexes (DTRs) and rectal sphincter tone
  - Reflex activity is lost below the level of injury when spinal shock is present. As spinal shock abates, reflexes will generally return
- Physiological support
- Minimization of secondary injury
- Prevention of complications
- Optimization of existing function

Medication Therapy

- Steroids—Methylprednisolone
- Cardiac med—Atropine, dopamine/dobutamine
- Anticoagulants—Low-molecular heparin, warfarin
- Gastrointestinal—Proton pump inhibitors; stool softeners; bowel stimulants; osmotic laxatives
- Psychological—Anxiolytics; antidepressants

Surgical Management

- Decompression of the spinal canal and/or fusion to provide structural stability for spine fractures or dislocations (laminectomy; spinal fusion)

The patient with an SCI will require a multidisciplinary team approach to treatment throughout the continuum of care. Nurses are an integral part of the multidisciplinary team, providing a common link for all team members as well as providing education and support to the patient and family through all phases of treatment.

Nursing Management

The focus is accurate, ongoing assessment of the patient and prevention of complications.

Monitor and urgently report these findings:

- Respiratory complications
  - ↑ respiratory rate
  - ↑ work of breathing

- • ↑ heart rate
- • ↑ anxiety
- • ↓ oxygen saturation
- • Change in character of secretions
- Cardiovascular complications
  - • ↓ heart rate
  - • ↓ blood pressure
- Neurological complications
  - • Changes in mental, motor, and sensory status

Risk for Autonomic Hyperreflexia

- Prevent noxious stimulus
  - • Distended bladder
  - • Constipation or fecal impaction
  - • Pressure ulcers
- Recognize symptoms
  - • ↑ Blood pressure
  - • ↓ Heart rate
  - • Vasoconstriction below the level of the SCI
  - • Vasodilation above the level of SCI—skin flushing, piloerection, and nasal congestion
- Initiate treatment
  - • Place patient upright to lower blood pressure
  - • Eliminate causative factor
  - • Notify MD, antihypertensive medication may be needed

(See Appendix #39, Nursing Process: Patient Care Plan for Spinal Cord Injury and Appendix #40, Patient Teaching & Discharge Priorities for Spinal Cord Injury.)

Renal and Genitourinary Disorders

There are multiple diseases of the kidney, all of which cause loss of filtration capacity. Some are rapidly reversible and others cause permanent damage to the kidneys. When approximately two-thirds of filtration capacity is lost, symptoms of renal failure appear with end-stage renal disease being the loss of approximately seven-eighths of filtration capacity. The goal of care for all the disease processes is to stop the source of damage to the kidneys and preserve what filtration capacity remains.

Glomerulonephritis

Glomerulonephritis is the inflammation of the glomerular capillary membranes, which alters the structure and function of the glomerulus ending in a change in filtration.

Acute Glomerulonephritis

A degenerative inflammation of the glomeruli can occur at any age but is more common in young males. As neutrophils collect in the inflamed loops of the glomeruli, the blood flow to the nephrons is reduced resulting in less filtration into Bowman's capsule and less urine production. The glomeruli begin to degenerate along with the nephron and the kidney tissue.

Causes
- Previous streptococcal infection usually of the respiratory tract.
- IgA nephropathy
- Thin basement membrane disease
- Hereditary nephritis (Alport syndrome)

- Systemic lupus erythematosus
- Mesangial proliferative glomerulonephritis
- Goodpasture's syndrome (anti-GBM antibody)

Signs and Symptoms

- Mild edema
- Oliguria
- Decreased urine output of less than 400 mL in a 24-hour period
- Proteinuria
- Azotemia
- Hematuria
- Fatigue
- Hypertension

Diagnostics

- Health history and physical examination
- Laboratory
  - Urinalysis
  - Urine creatinine
  - Complete blood count (CBC)
  - Serum creatinine
  - Throat culture

Patient Care Management

Overall goals address relief of symptoms and prevention of complications

- Fluid restriction
- Bed rest
- Dietary modifications
  - Nutritional Services Consult
    - High caloric
    - Low protein
    - Low sodium
    - Low potassium
- Correction of electrolyte imbalances

- Diuretics to reduce extracellular fluid
- Anti-hypertensives if needed

Chronic Glomerulonephritis

Slow progressive disease caused by inflammation of the glomeruli that result in sclerosis and scarring. The result is the remaining glomeruli do all of the filtration and the patient develops hypertension.

Causes

- Membranoproliferative glomerulonephritis
- Membranous glomerulopathy
- Focal glomerulosclerosis
- Rapidly progressive glomerulonephritis
- Systemic lupus erythematosus
- Goodpasture's syndrome
- Diabetes mellitus

Signs and Symptoms

The manifestations may not be exhibited for several years. Eventually, the patient enters the progressive phase and the following symptoms are common:

- Hypertension
- Proteinuria
- Hematuria
- Azotemia
- Nausea and vomiting
- Pruritus
- Dyspnea
- Fatigue
- Mild to severe edema
- Anemia
- Heart failure due to hypertension-induced hypertrophy

Diagnostics

- Health history and physical examination

- Laboratory
  - Urinalysis
  - Serum creatinine
  - Blood urea nitrogen (BUN)
- Imaging
  - Ultrasound to determine kidney size
- Procedural
  - Renal biopsy

Patient Care Management
The Goals of Treatment

- Antihypertensives
- Sodium restrictive diet
- Correction of electrolyte imbalances through dietary restrictions and supplements
- Diuretics for edema and possible heart failure
- End-stage glomerulonephritis:
  - Antibiotics for urinary tract infections
  - Dialysis for renal failure
  - Kidney transplantation

Nursing Management

The nursing responsibilities for both acute and chronic glomerulonephritis are similar with the goal being to preserve renal function and assist patient in a full recovery.

- Fluid Volume Excess
  - Assess for ↑ BP, HR, and RR
  - Assess lung sounds for crackles
  - Monitor of intake and output
  - Daily weight
  - Assess for presence of edema
  - Monitor serum creatinine, blood urea nitrogen (BUN) levels, electrolytes, and urine creatinine clearance

- Low sodium diet
- Fluid restriction
- Infection
  - Monitor for ↑T
  - Monitor white cell count (WBC)
  - Meticulous invasive line and catheter care
- Knowledge Deficit
  - Explain importance of keeping follow-up examinations so renal function can be monitored.
  - Instruct patient regarding purpose of dietary modifications.

Hydronephrosis

Hydronephrosis is an obstruction in the ureter, bladder, or urethra that causes the kidney to become extremely dilated with urine.

Causes
- Enlarged prostate gland
- Urethral strictures
- Renal calculi
- Stricture or stenosis of the bladder outlet or ureter
- Tumors of the abdomen, ureter, and bladder
- Blood clots
- Neurogenic bladder
- Congenital abnormalities

Signs and Symptoms
- Mild to severe colicky flank pain
- Slightly decreased urine flow
- UTI symptoms

Diagnostics
The finding of hydronephrosis is often accidental, occurring when a radiograph or ultrasound of the abdomen is ordered for another reason.

- Laboratory
  - Blood urea nitrogen (BUN)
  - Serum creatinine
  - Creatinine clearance
- Imaging
  - IVP
  - Renal ultrasound

Patient Care Management
- Health history and physical examination
- Removal of the obstruction:
  - Dilation of stricture in the urethra
  - Prostatectomy for prostatic hypertrophy
  - Surgical removal of calculi or tumor
  - Inoperable obstructions may require drainage of the kidney using a nephrostomy tube.

    (See Procedures & Therapies, Nephrostomy Tube)

Nursing Management
- Refer to the nursing management section of glomerulonephritis.

Renal Calculi (Nephrolithiasis or Kidney Stones)
Renal and ureteral calculi are formed when substances in the urine come out of solution and form a precipitate that accumulates and grows in size.

- Composed of calcium oxalate
- Form most commonly developed in the renal pelvis or calyces of the kidneys are commonly referred to as *kidney stones.*
- Vary in size and may be single or multiple
- Staghorn Calculus: calculus that remains in the renal pelvis and becomes so large it is unable to pass leading to hydronephrosis, renal parenchyma damage, or pressure necrosis

Predisposing Factors

- Infection
- Dehydration
- Metabolic factors:
  - Hyperparathyroidism
  - Renal tubular acidosis
  - Gout (due to the elevated uric acid levels)
  - Defective metabolism of oxalate
  - Genetic defect in the metabolism of cystine
  - Excessive intake of vitamin D or dietary calcium
- Obstruction
- Hereditary diseases:
  - Renal tubular acidosis
  - Cystinuria
  - Hyperoxaluria
  - Hypercalciuria

Signs and Symptoms

- Pain
  - Severe and colicky
  - Travels from the costovertebral angle to the flank, and then to the suprapubic area and external genitalia
  - Constant and dull if the calculi remain in the renal pelvis and calyces
- Nausea and vomiting
- Signs of UTI (fever, dysuria, frequency, urgency)
- Hematuria from damage by the calculi

Diagnostics

- Health history and physical examination
- Laboratory
  - Urinalysis to detect hematuria and presence of UTI
  - Calculus analysis to determine composition of stone

- Imaging:
  - Kidney/ureter/bladder radiograph (KUB)
  - CT of kidney, ureter, bladder
  - Renal ultrasonography to determine hydronephrosis

Patient Care Management

Goal of treatment focuses on promoting the passage of the renal calculi.

- Hydration
- Pain control:
  - Antispasmodics relax tense muscles and reduce reflex spasms.
  - Analgesics
- Diuretics may be given to prevent urinary stasis and continuing calculus formation.
- Surgical Interventions:
  - Cystoscope to retrieve calculi from the ureter
  - Ureteroscope to remove calculi from the kidney
  - Lithotripsy:
    - The use of acoustic shock waves travel through soft tissues to shatter the calculi into fragments, which can then pass normally. The procedure may be performed with the patient immersed in a tank of water, and is then called hydrolithotripsy.

Nursing Management

- Pain, Acute
  - Administer analgesics
  - Assess pain using a numeric scale and self-report of pain characteristics to determine effectiveness of therapy.
- Impaired urinary elimination
  - Monitor for presence of hematuria

- Monitor for signs of UTI (dysuria, fever, urgency, frequency)
- Monitor intake and output (may indicate obstruction)
- Strain all urine and send all solid material obtained to the lab for analysis
- Knowledge Deficit
  - Encourage intake of fluids to maintain output of 3–4 liters per day
  - Encourage the patient to ambulate to facilitate passage of calculi
  - Encourage patients with a history of renal calculi to avoid dairy products and food with high levels of calcium
  - Encourage patients to avoid antacids that have a calcium base
  - Instruct patient to modify diet based on composition of calculi (e.g., calcium oxalate or uric acid)
  - Explain routine postoperative care for lithotripsy (e.g., catheter care, pain, incision care, wound drainage, urine output)

Polycystic Kidney Disease

Polycystic kidney disease is a congenital anomaly that is characterized by multiple clusters of fluid-filled cysts that grossly enlarge the kidneys. As the cysts enlarge and fuse, they usually become infected. The cysts compress and gradually replace the functioning renal tissue leading to fatal uremia. The disease appears in two forms, infantile or adult, with both types affecting males and females equally.

Signs and Symptoms

- Infantile:
  - By age 2, signs of renal, respiratory, and cardiac failure develop.
  - Often fatal

- Adult:
  - Symptomatic between ages 30 and 50
  - Initial Nonspecific:
    - Hypertension, polyuria, and urinary tract infections
  - As disease progresses:
    - Lumbar pain
    - Swollen or tender abdomen
    - Abdominal pain that is exacerbated by exertion and relieved by lying down
  - Advancing disease:
    - Recurrent hematuria
    - Retroperitoneal bleeding from a ruptured cyst
    - Proteinuria
    - Abdominal pain caused by ureteral passage of clots or calculi
  - Without treatment fatal within four years

Diagnostics
- Health history and physical examination
- Imaging
  - Ultrasound, CT scan (determine size of kidneys and presence of cysts)
- Laboratory
  - Urinalysis (presence of protein and red blood cells indicate impaired filtration)
  - Serum creatinine and blood urea nitrogen (BUN) (determines renal function)

Patient Care Management
The goal of treatment is to preserve renal function and prevent infectious complications.
- Anti-hypertension medications (to slow deterioration of renal function)
- Dialysis and/or transplantation

Nursing Management
- Risk for imbalanced fluid volume
  - Assess for ↑ BP, HR, and RR
  - Assess lung sounds for crackles
  - Monitor of intake and output
  - Daily weight
  - Assess for presence of edema
  - Monitor serum creatinine, blood urea nitrogen (BUN) levels, electrolytes, and urine creatinine clearance
  - Low-sodium diet
  - Fluid restriction
- Anticipatory grieving
  - Young adult patients should be encouraged to seek genetic counseling.
  - Comprehensive patient teaching and emotional support are extremely important.
- Knowledge Deficit
  - Instruct patient and family of importance to keep medical appointments so kidney function and presence of complications can be monitored on a regular basis

Renal Failure

Renal failure is the inability of the kidneys to clear the blood of the waste products of protein metabolism, urea and creatinine. If the body is unable to excrete the urea, azotemia develops which produce signs of toxicity. Renal failure is either acute (rapid decline in renal function, which is usually reversible) or chronic (progressive deterioration of filtration).

Acute Renal Failure

Acute renal failure develops suddenly and can usually be reversed with treatment. If the condition causing the failure is not treated, the patient will progress to end-stage renal disease, uremic syndrome, and death.

Classifications
- Prerenal
  - Hypoperfusion to kidneys (dehydration, hypotension, poor cardiac output)
- Intrinsic
  - Acute tubular necrosis (ATN) (due to nephrotoxic medications, infections, renal thrombosis)
- Postrenal
  - Obstruction (benign prostatic hyperplasia [BPH], renal calculi, and tumors)

Phases
- Oliguric
  - Decrease in urine output (< 30 mL/hr) leading to increase in urine output
  - Elevated serum creatinine electrolyte imbalances
- Diuretic
  - Increase in urine output leading to improved renal function
  - Serum creatinine normalize, electrolyte imbalance remains
- Recovery
  - Healing of renal parenchyma
  - May last several months

Signs and Symptoms
Early Signs
- Oliguria
- Azotemia
- Anuria

As Disease Progresses
- Headache
- Irritability and confusion
- Nausea and vomiting
- Diarrhea

- Pruritus
- Pallor
- Purpura
- Hypotension leading to hypertension
- Fluid overload, anasarca (total body edema)
- Altered clotting mechanisms and bleeding
- Kussmaul's respirations
  - Due to acidosis
  - Deep sighing respirations
  - Odor of ammonia on breath
- Electrolyte imbalances
  - Hyperkalemia
    - Muscle weakness
  - Hyperchloremia
  - Hyponatremia

Chronic Renal Failure

Chronic renal failure is generally not reversible and often gets progressively worse. The symptoms of renal failure usually appear when approximately two-thirds of filtration capacity is lost, usually requiring the patient to be placed on maintenance dialysis or kidney transplantation. At this point the patient is said to have end-stage renal disease (ESRD). If the patient continues without treatment, uremic toxins accumulate and cause potentially fatal physiological changes in all of the major organ systems.

Signs and Symptoms
Initial
- Fatigue
- Loss of sense of well-being
- Muscle cramps (calf)
- Loss of appetite
- Nausea and vomiting

Late
- Worsening nausea and vomiting
- Weakness, lethargy
- Confusion

System Changes
- Cardiovascular changes
  - Hypertension
  - Cardiomyopathy
  - Uremic pericarditis
  - Pericardial effusion
  - Heart failure
  - Peripheral edema
  - Arrhythmias
- Respiratory changes
  - Pulmonary edema
  - Pleural effusions
  - Uremic pleuritis
  - Uremic pneumonitis
  - Dyspnea
  - Kussmaul's respirations
- Gastrointestinal changes
  - Inflammation and ulceration of gastrointestinal mucosa
  - Ulceration and bleeding gums
  - Uremic colitis
  - Pancreatitis
  - Uremic fetor: ammonia smell to breath
  - Anorexia, nausea, and vomiting
- Neurological changes
  - Peripheral neuropathy:
    - Pain, burning, and itching in the legs and feet
    - Paresthesia and foot drop from motor nerve dysfunction

- Muscle weaknesses and gait disturbances
- Shortened memory and attention span
- Drowsiness, fatigue, insomnia
- Irritability
- Confusion
- Coma
- Seizures
- Endocrine changes
  - Stunted growth in children
  - Infertility and decreased libido in both sexes
  - Amenorrhea
  - Impotence and decreased sperm production in men
  - Increased aldosterone secretion
  - Increased blood glucose levels
  - Increased triglyceride levels
- Hematopoietic changes
  - Anemia
  - Decreased red blood cell survival time
  - Blood loss from dialysis and gastrointestinal bleeding
  - Mild thrombocytopenia
  - Platelet defects
  - Increase in bleeding and clotting disorders
- Skeletal changes
  - Calcium–phosphorus imbalance and parathyroid imbalance cause:
    - Skeletal pain
    - Skeletal demineralization
    - Pathologic fractures
    - Calcifications in the brain, eyes, gums, joints, myocardium, and blood vessels
- Cutaneous changes
  - Skin appears yellowish bronze, dry, and scaly

- Itching and pruritus
- Purpura, petechiae
- Uremic frost: crystallized deposits of urea on the skin
- Ecchymosis
- Thin, brittle fingernails with lines
- Dry, brittle hair that may fall out easily

Diagnostics

A thorough health history and physical examination is necessary to determine the likely cause of acute renal failure. The diagnosis of chronic renal failure is made through clinical assessment and a history of progressive debilitation with gradual deterioration of renal function. Additional diagnostic studies are identified in the following tables.

Diagnostic Tests for Acute Renal Failure

Test	Expected Abnormalities	Rationale
Blood urea nitrogen (BUN)	Increased	Impaired glomerular filtration
Serum creatinine	Increased	Impaired glomerular filtration
Serum electrolyte levels	Increased	Impaired filtration
Potassium	Decreased	Dilutional
Sodium	Increased	Impaired filtration
Phosphorus	Decreased	Response to increased phosphorus
Calcium		

(*continued*)

Diagnostic Tests for Acute Renal Failure (*continued*)

Test	Expected Abnormalities	Rationale
Urinalysis	Presence of red blood cell casts, proteinuria Low specific gravity (1.010) Low osmolality (less than 400 mOsm/kg)	Impaired filtration Decreased ability to concentrate urine
Imaging: Renal ultrasound Computed tomography (CT scan) without contrast Retrograde pyelography Isotopic renal scan	Identification of size of the kidneys. Characterization of the parenchyma and collecting systems. Identifies urinary tract obstruction Assess renal perfusion and function	Determine degree of renal impairment Determines cause of ARF

Diagnostic Tests for Chronic Renal Failure

Test	Expected Abnormalities	Rationale
Serum electrolytes Urea nitrogen Creatinine Potassium Sodium	Increased Increased Increased Increased	Impaired glomerular filtration
Hemoglobin and hematocrit	Decreased	Insufficient production of erythropoietin

Test	Expected Abnormalities	Rationale
Arterial pH and bicarbonate levels	Decreased	Impaired glomerular filtration
Urinalysis	Presence of red blood cell casts, proteinuria Low specific gravity (1.010) Low osmolality (less than 400 mOsm/kg)	Impaired filtration Decreased ability to concentrate urine
Imaging: Renal ultrasound Computed tomography (CT scan) without contrast Isotopic renal scan	Reduced kidney size Characterization of the parenchyma and collecting systems. Reveals decreased function. May show decreased perfusion.	Permanent damage to the kidney Permanent damage to the kidney
Kidney biopsy	Histological identification of underlying pathology	Identifies pathology

Patient Care Management
Acute Renal Failure

The goal of treatment is to identify and treat reversible causes. Supportive measures include:

- Dietary Modifications:
  - Protein restriction

- Caloric intake of > 400 kcal per day to reduce tissue catabolism
- Limit dietary potassium intake
- Correction of electrolyte imbalances:
  - Potassium:
  - Hypertonic glucose and insulin infusions
  - Administration of intravenous calcium
  - Oral or rectal administration of potassium exchange resin
  - Avoid nonsteroidal anti-inflammatory drugs (NSAIDs), and angiotensin converting enzyme inhibitors (ACE inhibitors)
  - Hemodialysis
- Prevention of fluid overload
  - Restrict free water intake to avoid water overload and hyponatremia
- Medications
  - Anti-hypertensive therapy
  - Avoid nephrotoxic agents
  - Adjust doses of all medications that are excreted by the kidneys
  - Avoid magnesium-containing drugs (antacids)
- Prevention of infection
- Intermittent hemodialysis or continuous renal replacement therapy (CRRT)
  - CRRT is a way to remove solute and fluids slowly and continuously in a patient that may be hemodynamically unstable.

Patient Care Management
Chronic Renal Failure

With chronic renal failure, management is aimed at slowing the progression of the disease to end-stage renal disease and avoiding complications. Treatment is aimed at treating any underlying condition that may be contributing to or causing the failure; treating specific symptoms; and minimizing complications. Collaboration with nutritionists, social workers, and psychiatry may be helpful as patient progresses into chronic phase of illness and treatment options begin to change.

- Medications
  - Antihypertensive therapy
    - Diuretic if needed
  - Avoidance of drugs or diagnostic contrast that adversely affects renal function
    - NSAIDs
    - ACE inhibitors
    - Aminoglycoside antibiotics
    - Radiographic contrast
- Dietary Modifications:
  - Nondialysis Patients:
    - Low-protein diet, high calorie
    - Nutritional supplements
  - Dialysis Patients:
    - Modified protein intake
- Dialysis

  (See Procedures and Therapies, Hemodialysis and Peritoneal Dialysis.)

  - Hemodialysis
  - Peritoneal Dialysis
- Transplantation

  (See Procedures and Therapies, Kidney Transplantation.)

Nursing Management
- Fluid Volume Excess
  - Monitor fluid and electrolyte balance
    - Daily weights, using same scale
    - Accurate intake and output

- Assess lung sounds for crackles and presence of edema
- Assess laboratory data trends (e.g., potassium, sodium, magnesium, phosphorus, creatinine, BUN)
- Impaired Tissue Perfusion
  - Monitor vital signs
  - $\uparrow$ BP, $\uparrow$ HR (signs of volume overload and uncontrolled HTN)
  - $\downarrow$ BP, $\uparrow$ HR (signs of bleeding)
  - Assess for signs of bleeding
    - Stools, emesis
    - Catheter insertion sites
    - Intracerebral: assess mental status

Critical Alert
Contact health care provider if patient is taking NSAIDS and/or ace-inhibitors as they impair renal function and will worsen current condition.

- Assess for drug toxicity due to impaired renal function

Critical Alert
Special consideration is given for geriatric patients, especially those taking digitalis since clearance may be slowed, resulting in digitalis toxicity.

- Assess dialysis access device for patency

Critical Alert
To prevent clotting of the access device, avoid performing blood pressure measurements, blood draws, and intravenous lines on the arm that has the access device.

- Risk for Infection
  - Hand washing
  - $\uparrow$ T (indicator of infection)

- Meticulous catheter and line care
- Monitor laboratory data (WBC, culture results)
- Imbalanced Nutrition, Less than Body Requirements
  - Consult with nutritional services for dietary modifications:
    - Acute Renal Failure
      1. Sodium approximately 20–40 mEq/day (2–3 grams/day)
      2. Protein approximately 0.25–0.5 gram/kg. If on dialysis, may increase protein to 1.2 grams/kg daily.
      3. Potassium approximately 25–40 mEq. Adjust when urine volume increases.
    - Chronic Renal Failure
      1. Nondialysis Patients:
         - Low-protein diet: 0.60 g/kg per day
         - 35 kcal/kg per day
         - Patients < 60 years: 30 to 35 kcal/kg per day
         - Nutritional supplements which are high energy density
      2. Dialysis Patients:
         - Protein intake of 1.2 g/kg per day with at least 50% of the protein being of high biologic value
  - Drug interactions
  - Phosphate binders are most effective when taken with meals to bind dietary phosphate to prevent hyperphosphatemia.
  - Offer small frequent meals
  - Antiemetics for nausea
- Knowledge Deficit
  - Instruct patient/family regarding disease process and signs and symptoms that should be reported immediately

- Encourage patient to discuss dietary modifications with nutritionalist
- Provide instruction related to changing treatment options (e.g., dialysis, transplantation)
- Provide patient/family with resources to assist them in coping with progression of chronic illness

Renal Infarction

An occlusion of a renal blood vessel results in renal infarction, and an area of necrosis in one or both kidneys. The location of the infarction depends on the site of the occlusion. In approximately 75% of infarctions, the vessel that becomes occluded is the renal artery.

Causes
- Cardiovascular disease
  - Mitral stenosis
  - Atrial fibrillation
  - Microthrombi in the left ventricle
  - Rheumatic valvular disease
  - Endocarditis
  - Myocardial infarction
- Atherosclerosis of the renal vasculature (e.g., thrombus from flank trauma, sickle cell anemia, and scleroderma)
- Renal vein thrombosis (RVT)

Signs and Symptoms
- Severe upper abdominal pain
- Constant flank pain with tenderness
- Fever
- Nausea and vomiting
- Renovascular hypertension

Diagnostics
- Health history and physical examination
- Laboratory

- Urinalysis
- Serum LD, alkaline phosphatase, and aspartate aminotransferase
- Imaging
  - Renal vascular angiography or venogram

Patient Care Management

The goal for the patient is to remove the occlusion and restore renal function.

- Medications
  - Intra-arterial streptokinase
  - Heparin therapy
- Surgical
  - Catheter embolectomy
  - Surgical repair of the occlusion
  - Removal of the kidney

Nursing Management

- Impaired Urinary Elimination
  - Monitor intake and output
  - Daily weights
  - Monitor electrolytes, BUN, and creatinine (to determine renal function)
- Pain, Acute
  - Assess pain using a numeric scale and self-reported characteristics
  - Administer analgesics and reassess within 30–60 minutes.
- Knowledge Deficit

  Encourage the patient to schedule follow-up appointments to monitor return of renal function

Neurogenic Bladder

Difficulty with bladder control occurs when the nerves that control the release of urine are not functioning normally.

Common Causes

- Diabetes: autonomic neuropathies
- Cerebral disorders: stroke, brain tumor, dementia
- Vaginal childbirth
- Infections or trauma to spinal cord or brain
- Multiple sclerosis, Parkinson's disease
- Heavy metal poisoning
- Collagen diseases: systemic lupus erythematosus
- Herpes zoster

Signs and Symptoms

Urinary Retention

- Hydronephrosis
- Stagnant urine leading to infection
- Overflow incontinence

Poor Control of Sphincter Muscles

- Leakage due to loose muscles
- Retention due to tight muscles

Overactive Bladder

- Urinary frequency and urgency
- Urinating eight or more times a day or two or more times a night
- Urge incontinence

Diagnostics

- History and physical examination
- Urinalysis and urine culture
- Radiographic examination if nerve damage suspected (bladder scan)

Patient Care Management

The goals for managing patients with neurogenic bladder include: protect the kidney and upper urinary tract; prevent infection; and prevent urinary incontinence by evacuating the bladder.

Urinary Retention

- Credé's method
- Valsalva's maneuver
- Intermittent or indwelling catheterization
- Medications:
  - Baclofen (Lioresal)
  - Diazepam (Valium)
  - Alpha-adrenergic blockers terazosin (Hytrin) and doxazosin (Cardura)
- Surgery:
  - Urethral stents
  - Sphincterotomy (Sphincter resection)
    - Complications of the surgery can include bleeding, infection, and problems obtaining an erection.
  - Urinary diversion via an ileal conduit

Sphincter Control

- Electrical stimulation of the nerves that control the bladder and sphincter muscles
- Medications:
  - Anticholinergics
  - Oxybutynin chloride (Ditropan)
  - Hyoscyamine (Levsin)
  - Propantheline bromide (Pro-Banthine)
  - Tolterodine (Detrol)
- Surgery:
  - Augmentation cystoplasty

Overactive Bladder

- Bladder training

Nursing Management

Nursing care for patients with neurogenic bladder varies depending on the underlying cause and the method of treatment.

- Urinary elimination, impaired
  - Credé's method: the application of manual pressure over the lower abdomen to promote emptying of bladder

> **Critical Alert**
> Take special caution with patients with spinal cord injury due to incidence of causing autonomic dysreflexia.

  - Valsalva's maneuver: performing a forced exhalation against a closed glottis to promote emptying of bladder
  - Monitor intake and output
  - Encourage fluid intake
  - Document residual urine via bladder scan
  - Intermittent or indwelling catheterization
  - Bladder training
    - Maintain log to include fluid intake, times of voiding, and any episodes of urine leakage. Helps identify any urinary patterns and how to avoid incontinence.
    - The patient plans to void at certain times of the day and as they gain more control, may increase the interval of time between voiding.
    - Kegel exercises for women
  - Monitor side effects of medications
    - ↓ BP, ↑ HR, dizziness, dry mouth, constipation
- Pain, Acute
  - Alpha-adrenergic blockers
  - Anti-spasmodics
- Risk for infection
  - Monitor for signs of UTI
  - ↑ T, foul smelling urine, cloudy urine
  - Dysuria

- Knowledge Deficit
  - Explain use of Kegel exercises
  - Instruct patient and family regarding bladder training, including maintaining log and establishing voiding patterns
  - Instruct patient regarding postoperative care, including use of urinary catheter
  - Explain importance of maintaining adequate fluid intake and avoiding stimulants such as caffeine and nicotine

Urinary Tract Infections: Cystitis, Urethritis, Pyelonephritis

Urinary tract infections (UTIs) include those infections that occur in the upper and lower urinary tract. The bladder, ureters, urethra, and kidneys are the most common sites of infection. Eighty percent of hospital associated UTIs are catheter-associated urinary tract infections (CAUTIs) estimated to cost $650–$3,800 per case.

Cystitis

Cystitis is an inflammation of the urinary bladder and is more common in women than in men due to women's urethra being shorter.

- Introduction of *Escherichia coli* from fecal material into the urethra
- The bacteria then travel up to the bladder
- May also develop following sexual intercourse when organisms around the vaginal opening enter the urethra
- Sexually transmitted infections

Urethritis

Urethritis is an inflammation of the urethra.

- Causative microorganism is *Escherichia coli,* followed by *Klebsiella*, *Enterobacter*, *Proteus*, and *Pseudomonas*
- Sexually transmitted infections

- Acute nongonococcal urethritis (NGU) is one of the most common sexually transmitted infections affecting men.

Pyelonephritis

Pyelonephritis is a sudden inflammation of the kidney and renal pelvis caused by bacteria. The bacteria are normal intestinal and fecal floras that grow readily in urine.

- More common in women due to shorter urethra and the proximity of the meatus to the vagina and rectum
- Can be introduced by instrumentation such as catheterization, cystoscopy, or urologic surgery; bacteria translocated by the blood as in septicemia or endocarditis; and from lymphatic infections
- Most common causative bacteria are *Escherichia coli,* followed by proteus, pseudomonas, staphylococcus aureus, and streptococcus faecalis

Risk Factors
- Inability to empty the bladder
  - Neurogenic bladder
  - Urinary obstruction (tumor, kidney stone, prostatic hyperplasia)
  - Urinary stasis
- Gender, Women:
  - Sexually active women due to the increased risk of bacterial contamination from intercourse
  - Pregnancy
- Diabetes:
  - Development of neurogenic bladder, which causes incomplete emptying and urinary stasis
  - Glucose in the urine may support bacterial growth
- Compromised renal function from other renal diseases

Signs and Symptoms
- Urinary urgency, frequency, and burning
- Dysuria, nocturia, hematuria

- Urine may appear cloudy and have the odor of ammonia or fish
- High fever, chills, flank pain (costovertebral angle), and fatigue (Pyelonephritis)

Diagnostics
- Health history and physical examination
- Urinalysis reveals bacteria, pus, and casts in the urine
- X-ray films of the kidneys, ureters, and bladder may reveal cause (e.g., obstruction, calculi, tumor)

Patient Care Management
- Identification of the infecting organism
- Intravenous antibiotic therapy
- Phenazopyridine for urinary urgency and frequency
- Surgical intervention for obstruction (pyelonephritis)

Nursing Management
Nursing goals are to treat the infection and associated symptoms and provide patient teaching that will help prevent further infections.
- Pain, Acute
  - Administer urinary analgesics
- Risk for fluid volume deficit
  - Encourage fluids to maintain a urine output of more than 2,000 mL/day to empty the bladder of contaminated urine
  - Avoid drinking more than three liters of fluid as that may decrease the effectiveness of the antibiotics
- Hyperthermia
  - Administer antipyretics, cooling measures if needed
- Knowledge Deficit
  - Instruct patient about disease process and risk factors to prevent further episodes
  - Instruct patient to continue with full course of antibiotic therapy

- Inform the patient that the phenazopyridine will turn urine a bright orange color that will stain clothing
- Instruct patient to allow for rest periods to prevent fatigue
- Explain the importance of cleansing the female genital area from front to back to avoid contamination by fecal material
- Encourage the female patient to void as soon as possible after having sexual intercourse
- Encourage male patients to have protected sex

SEXUALLY TRANSMITTED INFECTIONS

Pelvic Inflammatory Disease

Sexually transmitted infections (STIs) are those that are passed from person to person during sexual contact. Hepatitis and HIV infections will not be discussed in this section.

Chlamydia

This bacterial infection is caused by *Chlamydia trachomatis,* which involves the cervix, urethra, anus, and pharynx. Women who do notice symptoms often complain of burning urination, vaginal discharge, and mild lower abdominal cramps.

Gonorrhea

This infection is caused by the bacterium *Neisseria gonorrhoeae,* which infects the warm, moist environment of the reproductive tract, along with any other mucous membranes in the body, such as the oral mucosa and the mucosa of the eye in a newborn. Symptoms in women include burning with urination, a vaginal discharge, vaginal bleeding between periods, pelvic pain, and fever.

Syphilis

Syphilis is a complex sexually transmitted infection that can lead to serious systemic illness, and even death, if untreated. It is caused by the *Treponema pallidum* bacterium, is a systemic infection and is referred to as the "great imitator" because its symptoms often mimic those of other STIs. Transmission occurs through sexual contact, contact with a genital ulcer, or with syphilis-infected blood. Initially the patient notices a painless chancre (genital ulcer) and if untreated the infection progresses to the secondary stage, where a rough rash will appear on various parts of the body, but in particular on the soles of the feet and the palms of the hands. Without treatment, the infection progresses to the latent and final state of the disease. The infection remains in the body for years and slowly damages the brain, nerves, eyes, heart, blood vessels, liver, bones, and joints. Symptoms, which typically progress to what is termed *neurosyphilis,* include muscle weakness, difficulty coordinating muscle movements, paralysis, numbness, blindness, dementia, and eventual death.

Genital Herpes

Herpes is caused primarily by the herpes simplex virus (HSV). Once a person is infected, HSV becomes a chronic, lifelong viral infection. Generally, a person can get HSV type 2 only by sexual contact with someone who has the infection. Unfortunately, the infected person does not have to have open lesions to transmit the virus to a partner. This makes it very difficult to prevent transmission between partners because many people infected with HSV-2 are not aware of their infection. Herpes presents as painful multiple vesicular or ulcerative lesions found on the labia, perineum, and vaginal areas.

Human Papillomavirus (HPV)

The human papillomavirus (HPV) infection, also referred to as genital warts, is the most common sexually transmitted viral infection in the United States. Patients experience genital warts that appear as cauliflower-like growths in the genital, anal, and vaginal areas. They can be raised or flat, single or multiple; some are small and some are large. Additionally, itching, increased vaginal discharge, and abnormal vaginal bleeding after intercourse are also noted.

Pelvic Inflammatory Disease

Pelvic inflammatory disease (PID) is an infection of the uterus, fallopian tubes, and ovaries. It is a common and a serious complication of many sexually transmitted infections, with up to 80% of cases being related to chlamydia and gonorrhea infections.

Signs and Symptoms
- Lower abdominal pain
- Fever
- Foul-smelling vaginal discharge
- Painful intercourse and urination
- Irregular menstrual bleeding
- ↑ white blood count (WBC)
- Pain with palpation of the adnexal areas and/or the cervix

Diagnostics
- Health history and physical examination
- Laboratory
  - Culture (vaginal, cervical, lesion)
  - Pap smear
- Imaging
  - Pelvic ultrasound (rule out a fallopian tube or ovarian abscess and ectopic pregnancy)

Patient Care Management
- Medical
  - Antibiotics
  - Antiviral medications (HPV)
  - Topical medications (for genital warts)
- Other
  - Protected sex using condoms

Nursing Management
- Infection, actual
  - Monitor for signs of infection
  - ↑ T, ↑ HR, ↑ WBC
  - Worsening drainage
  - Worsening pain
- Pain, Acute
  - Assess pain using numeric scale and patient self-reported descriptors

- Administer analgesics and reassess pain accordingly
- Position for comfort, offer baths, loose fitting clothing
- Knowledge Deficit
  - Instruct patient to avoid sexual contact until infection is cleared (drainage and lesions disappear)
  - Encourage patient to use condoms during sexual contact
  - Encourage partner to be evaluated for STIs
  - Inform patient regarding option of HPV vaccination

Upper Respiratory Disorders

Nasal Fractures

Nasal fractures typically are caused by a traumatic injury to the bone or cartilage of the nose. Although most of the nasal structure is made up of cartilage, the nasal bones usually are fractured in injury. Fights and sports injuries account for most nasal fractures in adults, followed by falls and vehicle crashes.

Signs and Symptoms

- Deformity
- Tenderness
- Nasal hemorrhage, ecchymosis
- Edema
- Instability of nose
- Crepitation
- Combination of above

Diagnostics

Diagnosing nasal fractures is done by facial x-rays and a thorough physical examination. Additional neurological assessments to determine cognition and response may need to be done if damage to the ethmoid bone is suspected.

Patient Care Management
Uncomplicated (Nondisplaced)

- Analgesics
- Rest
- Elevate head and ice application

Displaced Fracture
- Surgery
  - Reduction of fracture
  - Drainage of septal hematomas to prevent nasal obstruction
  - Between the 5th and 10th day after the injury, before the nasal bones start to fixate
  - If needed, reconstructive surgery at later date

Nursing Management
- Pain, Acute
  - Assess pain using numeric scale, 0–10
  - Provide analgesics and reassess for effectiveness
  - Reduce swelling with ice packs
  - Elevate head of bed
- Body Image, Disturbed
  - Encourage patient to view face, provide mirror
  - Allow patient to express fear and anxiety related to altered body image and injury
  - Explain purpose of nasal packing (postoperative), allow for patient to visualize
- Knowledge Deficit
  - Explain to patient and family expected postoperative care
  - Instruct patient and family in use of ice pack

Peritonsillar Abscess

Tonsillitis is an inflammation of the tonsils, most commonly caused by a virus, and mainly occurs in children. Tonsillitis usually is self-limiting and treated symptomatically; however, if a throat culture reveals the cause as Group A beta-hemolytic streptococci, then an antibiotic such as penicillin will be prescribed. Complications such as sinusitis, mastoiditis, rheumatic fever, or peritonsillar abscess may occur with tonsillitis.

A peritonsillar abscess (Quinsey tonsillitis) is a rare complication of tonsillitis in which infection spreads to the tissue around the tonsillar capsule.

Signs and Symptoms

- Severe throat pain
- Mouth breathing
- Drooling
- Muffled voice

Diagnostics

Physical examination reveals a large unilateral fullness of the affected tonsillar pillar and soft palate, and deviation of the uvula to the unaffected side. Throat culture is also considered in some cases.

Patient Care Management

A peritonsillar abscess is treated with incision and drainage of the abscess and use of antibiotics. Four to six weeks after recovery a tonsillectomy may be necessary to prevent recurrent infections and allows for removal of scar tissue from the tonsillar area.

Nursing Management

- Risk for Infection
  - Monitor for ↑ temperature, HR, RR
  - Administer antibiotic therapy
- Pain, Acute
  - Assess pain thoroughly using numeric scale and patient self-report
  - Instruct patient to inform the nurse when pain begins and if the pain is not relieved after interventions
  - Advise patient to use cool liquids and frequent gargling with salt water
- Ineffective Breathing Pattern
  - Monitor RR, respiratory effort, lung sounds (e.g., stridor, wheezes)
  - Elevate head of bed at least 30 degrees

> **Critical Alert**
> Tonsillectomy: Monitor for oral cavity bleeding. Notify health care provider if excessive bleeding occurs as patient's airway may be compromised.

- Knowledge Deficit
  - Explain to patient and family of importance to maintain adequate fluid hydration and nutritional intake

Pharyngitis

Pharyngitis is an inflammation of the pharynx. Group A beta-hemolytic streptococci (GABHS) is the most common bacteria known to cause pharyngitis. Transmission is from person to person via respiratory droplets.

Complications
- Rheumatic heart disease
- Glomerulonephritis

Signs and Symptoms
- Severe sore throat, especially with swallowing
- Pharynx and tonsils are red with purulent drainage
- Enlarged lymph nodes
- Fever

Diagnostics
- Health history and physical examination of throat
- Laboratory
  - Throat culture
  - Rapid antigen test

Patient Care Management
- Medical
  - Antibiotics if bacterial cause
  - Analgesics
  - Antipyretics
  - Hydration

Nursing Management

- Pain, Acute
  - Encourage use of warm salt water gargle
  - Assess pain on a numeric scale, 0–10
  - Administer analgesics and monitor effectiveness
  - Warm compresses to neck
- Knowledge Deficit
  - Instruct patient and family regarding complications associated with disorder
  - Encourage patient to refrain from social interaction (work, school) until 24 hours of antibiotics have been taken
  - Advise patient to take entire course of antibiotics

Sleep Apnea

Sleep apnea is a disorder in which a person stops breathing for more than 10 seconds, typically more than 20 to 30 times in an hour. The three main types of sleep apnea are central, obstructive, and a combination of central and obstructive.

Central Sleep Apnea

- Impairment in the respiratory center such that the brain fails to send the appropriate signal to the breathing muscles to initiate respirations
- Less common form

Obstructive Sleep Apnea (OSA)

- Caused by physical obstruction from tissues in the upper airway
- Approximately 12 million Americans have obstructive sleep apnea and of those, more than half are overweight or obese

Combination Sleep Apnea (Mixed)

- Starts as central sleep apnea, quickly followed by thoracoabdominal movements and upper airway obstruction
- Second most common form of sleep apnea

Risk Factors

- Obesity or being overweight
- High blood pressure
- Decreased airway size in the nose, throat, or mouth. Caused by the shape of these structures or by medical conditions causing congestion in these areas, such as hay fever or other allergies
- Family history of sleep apnea

Signs and Symptoms

- Recurrent sleep interruptions
- Loud snoring
- Choking and gasping spells on awakening
- Daytime drowsiness
- Loss of memory and concentration caused by the lack of normal sleep

Diagnostics

- Health history and physical examination (full ENT examination recommended)
- Imaging
  - Fiber-optic endoscopy
  - An x-ray or CT scan of the head and neck (helpful in identifying obstructive structures and checking the position of the tongue in relation to the jaw; the majority of patients)
- Other
  - Polysomnography (sleep study)

Patient Care Management

- Medical Management
  - Weight loss
  - Avoid the use of alcohol, tobacco, and sleeping pills
  - Sleeping devices (e.g., pillows) that help them sleep in a side-lying position

- Dental device that moves the tongue or mandible forward (mild cases)
- Continuous positive airway pressure (CPAP)
  - Opens the airway and prevents airway collapse
  - Blows air into the respiratory tract with just enough pressure to prevent the tissue collapse during sleep
  - Reduces the number and severity of apneic episodes and significant oxygen desaturation
  - Side effects: claustrophobia, dry mouth, rhinitis, and sinus congestion (Humidification and antihistamines effectively treat these side effects.)
- Surgery
  - Uvulopalatopharyngoplasty (UVPPP)
    - Resection of the uvula and soft palate (shortens and stiffens the palate)
    - 40% effective
  - Tracheostomy
    (See Procedures & Therapies.)

Nursing Management

- Ventilation, Impaired Spontaneous
  - Continuous pulse oximetry (monitor oxygen saturation level)
  - Assess lung sounds for crackles
  - Monitor for signs of flash pulmonary edema (caused by surgical relief of elevated pulmonary pressure)
    - Dyspnea, respiratory distress
    - ↓ O_2 sat
    - Crackles in lungs
- Fatigue
  - Encourage weight loss
  - Encourage no alcohol, tobacco, or sedative use

- Knowledge Deficit
  - Explain purpose of CPAP therapy along with techniques to improve tolerance
  - Explain importance of refraining from alcohol, tobacco, and sleeping aids
  - Explain importance of compliance since development of medical complications due to OSA is common

Vocal Cord Paralysis

Vocal cord paralysis is a disorder that occurs when one or both of the vocal cords (or vocal folds) do not open or close properly. It may occur at any age from birth to advanced age and is seen equally in males and females from a variety of causes. It can be the result of an infectious process, trauma to the neck or chest area, neurological disorders, and cancer. In addition, transection of the recurrent laryngeal nerve during thyroidectomy remains a common cause.

Signs and Symptoms

The severity of the patient's symptoms (breathy voice, ineffective cough, and dysphagia) is dependent on the position of the paralyzed cord, the degree of injury to the cord (paresis versus paralysis), and the ability of the opposite cord to compensate.

- Change in the voice
  - Hoarse
  - Croaky or rough
  - Breathy
- Shortness of breath
- Noisy breathing
- Choking or coughing while swallowing food, drink, or saliva
- The need to take frequent breaths while speaking
- Inability to speak loudly
- Inability to "bear down" while lifting

Diagnostics

- Endoscopy to directly visualize the vocal cords.
- Imaging studies (CT scans, x-rays, MRI) to determine if damage is due to other causes.
- Referral to a neurologist may be necessary to rule out damage to nerves other than those to the vocal cords.

Patient Care Management

Effectively managing aspiration is the priority of the medical team. This requires placement of a permanent enteral feeding tube (gastrostomy tube) and, often times, a tracheostomy.

(See Procedures and Therapies, Tracheostomy.)

Nursing Management

The nursing process guides the management of patients with vocal cord paralysis. It is essential that the assessment begins with the identifying risk for aspiration. The expected outcome is prevention of aspiration and the evaluation parameters include the following:

- Ineffective Airway Clearance
  - Position patient upright in a chair to eat
  - Remain with the patient to observe for coughing or frequent throat clearing after swallowing
  - Assess lung sounds, work of breathing, and oxygen saturation (maintain at 95% or baseline)
  - If difficulty occurs, remove food and fluids and notify health care provider
- Altered Role Performance
  - Assess for signs of depression (e.g., withdrawing, altered sleep patterns, inability to concentrate)
  - Consult psychiatry or social worker to discuss issues related to changes in basic social functions (e.g., relationships, employment) due to difficulty speaking
  - Consult with speech therapist, who will provide skills to maximize function and vocal cord,

decrease risk of aspiration, and improve communication skills

- Knowledge Deficit
    - Instruct patient and family regarding complications of vocal cord paralysis (e.g., aspiration) and need for recommended treatment

Vascular Disorders

Vascular disorders are abnormalities of the arterial, venous, and lymphatic systems of the body. Peripheral arterial disease includes occlusive, aneurysmal (dilated), and vasospastic disorders affecting the arterial system of the neck, abdomen, and extremities. Peripheral venous disease predominantly involves the legs and is usually due to thrombosis or insufficiency of the veins. Lymphatic disease leads to abnormal fluid collection, edema, and fibrosis. These peripheral vascular diseases may cause serious complications such as loss of limb or even loss of life.

Peripheral Arterial Disease

PAD is a vascular disease caused primarily by atherosclerosis and thromboembolic processes affecting the aorta, its visceral arterial branches, and the arteries of the lower extremities. The prevalence of peripheral arterial disease increases with age.

Signs and Symptoms

- Intermittent claudication—burning, throbbing pain
- Muscle/limb weakness with use
- Absent or diminished pulses
- Poor hair growth
- Cool skin
- Paresthesia
- Poor healing of sores
- Gangrene and infection
- Resting limb pain—sign of severe ischemia

Diagnostics

- Health history and physical examination
- Imaging
  - Duplex ultrasound angiography
  - Computed tomography (CT)
  - Magnetic resonance imaging (MRI) and magnetic resonance angiography (MRA)
- Other
  - Resting ankle-brachial index (ABI)
  - Treadmill exercise arterial studies
  - Segmental arterial pressures

Patient Care Management

The goal of treatment is to prevent complications and increase quality of life. Patients with PAD should be evaluated for other vascular disorders.

- Medical
  - Antiplatelet therapy
- Surgical and Procedural
  - Endovascular treatment
  - Percutaneous transluminal angioplasty (PTA); stents
  - Arterial bypass
  - Amputation for uncontrolled infection, uncontrolled pain, and extensive tissue loss

Nursing Management

(See Appendix #1, Nursing Process: Patient Care Plan for the Postoperative Patient Following General Surgery.)

- Impaired tissue perfusion, risk of
  - Obtain bilateral blood pressure (differences may indicate aortic coarctation or subclavian artery lesion)
  - Assess for bruits (carotid, abdomen, flank area)
  - Palpate abdomen to assess for signs of a pulsatile abdominal mass, indicating abdominal aortic aneurysm
  - Assess peripheral pulses for presence, rate, equality, regularity, and strength
  - Assess skin color, temperature, and integrity of the skin, including any ulcerations
  - Assess skin color with the patient in various positions
  - Inspect the lower extremities for pallor, cyanosis, hair loss; thin, smooth, shiny skin; thick, brittle nails with or without fungal infection; tapering of toes or fingers—and any skin breakdown
  - Frequent and careful assessment of circulation to the leg and foot is essential.
  - Pulselessness distal to the graft site indicates decreased or no blood flow and requires immediate health care provider notification.

> **Critical Alert**
> Acute arterial ischemia is an emergency. Notify the heath care provider immediately. Assessment findings in acute arterial ischemia include the "six Ps": pain, pallor, pulselessness, poikilothermia (coldness), paresthesia, and paralysis of the affected extremity.

- Altered skin integrity and infection, risk of
  - Assess hands and toes for the presence of ulcers and gangrene
  - Provide daily skin care
  - Monitor for signs of infection and sepsis

- Pain
  - Assess pain using numeric scale (0–10) to quantify pain
  - Provide a supportive environment where patient is able to express pain level
  - Use pain control measures before the pain becomes severe to intervene early and with less medication
  - Teach nonpharmacologic methods of pain control; that is, guided imagery and breathing exercises to augment other treatments
  - Encourage periods of rest when walking for pain relief
- Knowledge Deficit
  - Explain the importance of smoking cessation to promote understanding and compliance—provide resources for smoking cessation
  - Importance of glucose control for diabetic
  - Importance of blood pressure control
  - Encourage patient to keep legs in dependent position to enhance arterial perfusion
  - Encourage patient to walk regularly and progressively to promote conditioning and blood flow
  - Teach about prescribed medications and exercise programs
  - Teach patient to avoid trauma, heat, and sunburn to feet/legs to prevent wounds and infection
  - Teach patient about foot care: Keep feet and toes clean, mild soap only; dry well between toes; use lanolin emollient; inspect feet daily; clip toenails straight; wear proper fitting shoes; avoid walking barefoot
  - Avoid extremes in temperature to the extremities (hot baths, heating pads, cold water) because sensation may be diminished
  - Teach patient about good nutrition to promote healing
  - Teach patient signs and symptoms of infection

- Teach signs and symptoms that must be reported to health care provider

Aortic Aneurysm

A diseased segment of the aortic artery that has become thin and dilated. Aneurysms are caused by atherosclerosis and degeneration of the vessel from congenital weakness, trauma, and disease. The aneurysm will grow larger as the tension on the vessel wall increases, putting pressure on the adjacent organs interrupting blood flow. If growing and left untreated it may rupture. Factors that can increase the risk of rupture include hypertension, smoking, and family history of ruptured aneurysm.

Signs and Symptoms
Thoracic Aneurysms
- Substernal, back, and neck pain
- Dyspnea, stridor, and brassy cough due to pressure on the trachea
- Hoarseness, if the laryngeal nerve is compressed

Abdominal Aortic Aneurysms (must exceed 3 centimeters in diameter)
- Typically asymptomatic

Diagnostics
- Discovered during routine physical exam or x-ray
- Visual inspection may reveal a pulsatile abdominal mass.
- Auscultation of this mass reveals a bruit.
- Abdominal ultrasound
- CT scan
- Abdominal angiography
- MR angiography
- Serial diagnostic tests to evaluate growth

Patient Care Management
- Ongoing surveillance for stable aneurysms with ultrasound
- Smoking cessation

- Blood pressure control
- Lipid management
- Surgical and endovascular repair—Immediate repair for expanding aneurysm or rupture

Nursing Management

Prior to surgery, the nurse needs to monitor the patient closely for signs and symptoms of impending rupture:

- Restlessness
- Abdominal pain and tenderness
- Hypotension
- Shock

Critical Alert

Spontaneous rupture of an aortic aneurysm causes sudden onset of abdominal and back pain accompanied by signs of hypotension, shock, and collapse. The unstable patient who has experienced rupture of an abdominal aortic aneurysm (AAA) requires immediate fluid and blood resuscitation, blood pressure control with propranolol (Inderal) or nitroprusside (Nipride), and pain management while being prepared for emergency surgery.

Postoperative Care of the Patient Undergoing Aortic Aneurysm Repair

(See Appendix #1.)

- Hemodynamic instability, risk of—immediate post-operative phase

  - Invasive monitoring with arterial line/central venous catheter and/or pulmonary artery catheter
  - Urine output
  - Postoperative bleeding
  - Hypothermia
  - Hypovolemia
  - Third spacing of fluid
  - ECG monitoring to assess for arrhythmia
  - 12-lead ECG to monitor for myocardial ischemia or infarction

- Altered tissue perfusion, risk of
  - Impaired renal function—monitor urine output, BUN, serum creatinine
  - Gastrointestinal disturbances—assess for nausea, vomiting, abdominal pain/tenderness, distention, presence/ absence of bowel sounds, blood in stools, and diarrhea
  - Spinal cord ischemia—assess for sensory and motor deficits
  - Neurological function
- Knowledge Deficit
  - Teach importance of blood pressure control and compliance with their medication regime
  - Provide information on smoking cessation
  - Teach wound care
  - Teach activity restrictions
  - Teach reportable symptoms, such as changes in sensation to the legs, which may indicate thrombosis of the graft, or gastrointestinal bleeding, which may indicate erosion of the graft into the duodenum

Aortic Dissection (AD)

Aortic dissection is a life-threatening condition whereby the intimal layer of the aorta separates, creating a tear in the lumen of the aorta. The disruption of the aorta can cause life-threatening complications or death if not rapidly recognized and treated.

Ascending Aorta (most common)— Stanford Type A or DeBakey Type I

- Requires immediate surgical repair

Descending Aorta—Stanford Type B or DeBakey Type III

- Does not generally require immediate surgery and are stabilized medically

Causes

- The exact cause of AD is unknown.
- Chronic stress from hypertension may play a significant role in the deterioration of the aortic wall.

Signs and Symptoms

- Pain
  - Sudden, sharp, shifting chest or back pain
  - Describe it as "ripping" or "tearing"
  - Not affected by position changes
  - May wax and wane
  - Can mimic acute myocardial infarction, pulmonary embolus, or ruptured AAA
- Signs of ischemia from blood flow obliterated by the dissection
  - Syncope or altered level of consciousness
  - Stroke
  - Anuria
  - Mesenteric and/or extremity ischemia

Critical Alert

Rapid identification of aortic dissection is key in preventing death. Signs and symptoms of aortic dissection (AD) can mimic other disorders such as acute myocardial infarction and pulmonary embolus, making the diagnosis difficult. The most classic symptom of AD is the abrupt onset of severe, tearing chest pain that may radiate to the back. Patients may also present with sudden onset aortic insufficiency, neurological changes, and cardiac tamponade.

Diagnostics

- Health history and physical examination
  - Risk factor identification
- Imaging
  - Aortic angiography
  - Transesophageal echocardiography
  - CT scan

- MRI studies
- Chest x-ray
- Other
  - ECG

Patient Care Management
Ascending Aorta
- Requires immediate surgical repair
  - Aortic valve may need to be replaced and the coronary arteries reimplanted.
  - Surgical complications include myocardial ischemia or infarction, arrhythmias, pulmonary atelectasis, renal failure, ischemic bowel, prolonged ileus, and leg ischemia.

Descending Aorta
- Aggressive control of blood pressure
  - Endovascular repair
  - Surgical repair

Nursing Management
- Rapid recognition (1 to 2 days in the intensive care unit for careful monitoring)
- Careful management of medication regime to control blood pressure
- Observing for complications related to ineffective tissue perfusion
- Knowledge deficit
  - Explain the importance of careful blood pressure control for the rest of their lives
  - Compliance with their medication regime is essential

Carotid Artery Disease
Carotid artery disease occurs when there is atherosclerotic plaque buildup, causing an obstruction to blood flow to the carotid and vertebral arteries supply blood to the brain resulting in stroke.

Transient Ischemic Attack (TIA)

TIA is a "warning stroke" or "mini-stroke" that produces stroke-like symptoms but no lasting damage, which usually disappear within 1 to 5 minutes. TIA may precede a stroke.

Causes
- Hypertension
- Smoking
- Diabetes
- Atrial fibrillation
- Hyperlipidemia
- Physical inactivity
- Obesity
- Illicit drugs, such as cocaine

Signs and Symptoms

Neurological deficits are dependent on location of damage to the brain.

- Numbness or weakness in the face, arm, or leg, especially on one side of the body
- Confusion
- Difficulty in talking or understanding speech
- Trouble seeing in one or both eyes
- Difficulty with walking, dizziness, or loss of balance and coordination

Diagnostics

- Health history and physical examination
  - Bruit is auscultated over the artery
- Imaging
  - Duplex ultrasound
  - Magnetic resonance imaging and/or computed tomography angiography (CTA) —gold standard for defining anatomy
  - Contrast angiography (less common)

Patient Care Management

- Medical therapy
  - Antiplatelet therapy with aspirin
- Surgical and procedural therapy
  - Carotid endarterectomy (CEA)
  - Endovascular therapy (Carotid artery balloon angioplasty and stenting with cerebral protection devices to decrease the risk of complications.)

Nursing Management

(See Appendix #1.)

- Injury, risk for
  - Monitor for complications (carotid artery occlusion, cerebral embolization, cranial nerve damage)
  - Neurological assessment to evaluate cranial nerve function and assess for perioperative stroke
    - Facial symmetry
    - Ability to swallow
    - Tongue deviation
    - Shoulder strength
    - Mental status
    - Level of consciousness
    - Pupillary responses
    - Motor/sensory changes on the contralateral side of the body
    - Reportable conditions—change in neurological status, agitation, lethargy, visual disturbances, slurred speech, and paresthesias or paralysis
- Impaired gas exchange, risk of
  - Have emergency equipment available, suction supplies and tracheostomy tray
  - Careful monitoring for respiratory obstruction from edema or expanding hematoma at the surgical site

- Oxygen saturation levels
- Arterial blood gases
- Stable work of breathing
- Emergency nursing interventions include:
  - Administering oxygen
  - Elevating the head of bed
  - Loosening the neck dressing if it appears to be constricting the neck
  - Immediate intervention required for stridor or deviation of the trachea from midline
  - Suction supplies/equipment and a tracheostomy tray is indicated
- Alterations in blood pressure related to stimulation of the carotid sinus
  - Frequent blood pressure monitoring
  - Hypotension can occur as a result of surgery.
  - Hypertension can lead to bleeding or damage the arterial reconstruction.
- Knowledge Deficit
  - Teach patients and their families to report signs and symptoms of stroke, new onset fever, signs of wound infection
  - Follow-up care and activity instructions
  - Teach about daily aspirin, adequate blood pressure control, and risk factor modification
  - Teach patients reportable signs and symptoms of TIA/stroke
  - Teach patients importance of risk factor modification

Raynaud's Disease (RD)
An arterial vasospastic disorder caused by emotional distress or cold. Abnormalities of the endothelium initiating vasospasm resulting in a decreased blood flow to the affected extremity.

Causes

- Precise pathophysiology unclear
- Associated with many diseases:
  - Connective tissue diseases, such as rheumatoid arthritis, scleroderma, and systemic lupus erythematosus (SLE)
  - Myeloproliferative diseases, such as leukemia and polycythemia rubra vera
- Triggers include smoking, alcohol use, caffeine intake, cocaine, and amphetamines

Signs and Symptoms

- Numbness, tingling, pain due to decreased perfusion
- Joint pain
- Skin lesions
- Malaise
- Light sensitivity

Diagnostics

- Cold stimulation challenge to induce symptoms
- Nail-fold capillaroscopy—distinguishes between primary and secondary Raynaud's disease

Patient Care Management

Complete history of the patient's past medical history is important to identify other connective tissue disorders, such as SLE and scleroderma.

- Medical
  - Avoiding known stressors (cold, emotional stress); controlling exposure to extremes in climate; dressing warmly in cold weather; and limiting tobacco, caffeine, and alcohol intake
  - Relaxation techniques
  - Regular physical exercise to improve circulation and warm the body temperature

- Calcium channel blocking agents (nifedipine, isradipine, amlodipine, and nicardipine)
- Prazosin (Minipress)
- Surgical therapy
  - Surgical sympathectomy, removal of the sympathetic ganglia, for severe symptoms

Nursing Management

Nursing care for Raynaud's Disease patients focuses on minimizing episodes and limiting complications.

- Altered skin integrity and infection, risk of
  - Assess hands and toes for the presence of ulcers and gangrene
  - Provide daily skin care
  - Monitor for signs of infection and sepsis
- Knowledge Deficit
  - Instruct patient to carefully assess hands and toes, notify health care provider if sores develop
  - Instruct patient in ways to minimize episodes
  - Avoid exposure to cold and tobacco
  - Wear warm clothes and gloves, mittens, and/or hand warmers when in cold environments. Avoid oral contraceptives, beta-adrenergic blockers, and ergot preparations. Always tell health care provider all medications taken
  - Provide information on smoking cessation
  - Provide information on behavioral modification therapy, which may help decrease the emotional components

Renovascular Disease

Disorders of the arteries of the kidneys resulting in systemic hypertension and kidney dysfunction. Two disorders primarily affect the renal arteries—atherosclerotic renal artery stenosis (AS-RAS) and fibromuscular dysplasia (FMD).

Causes
AS-RAS

is progressive abnormal narrowing of the renal artery, which can eventually lead to total blockage resulting in shrinkage of the kidney. The resulting hypertension is caused by reduced renal blood flow and activation of the renin-angiotensin-aldosterone mechanism.

FMD is a noninflammatory, nonatheroclerotic disorder seen almost exclusively in women, which leads to obstruction of blood flow, yet rarely leads to total renal artery blockage. The cause of FMD is unknown; a genetic predisposition, smoking, hormonal factors, and disorders of the blood supply to the renal artery itself are some of the causal theories associated with the disease.

Signs and Symptoms
- No family history of HTN
- Onset before age 50
- Recent onset of significantly elevated blood pressure
  - Frequently higher than 180/100 mmHg and resistant to two or more medications

Diagnostics
- Imaging
  - Duplex ultrasonography
  - CTA
  - Magnetic resonance angiography (MRA)
  - Contrast angiography

Patient Care Management
- Medical
  - Blood pressure control
  - Antiplatelet therapy
  - Lipid management
  - Smoking cessation

- Weight reduction
- Angiotensin-converting enzyme (ACE) inhibitors may be indicated for renal stenosis
- Monitor for decline and complications
  - Severely elevated blood pressure
  - Stroke
  - Renal insufficiency and failure
  - Heart failure
  - Retinopathy
  - Death
- Surgical Therapy
  - Endovascular therapy (renal angioplasty, percutaneous ballooning and stenting of renal artery)
  - Aortorenal bypass, (the most common surgery)
  - Renal artery thromboendarterectomy
  - Renal artery reimplantation

Nursing Management
Nursing Care for Patients Following Endovascular Therapy
- Impaired tissue perfusion, risk of
  - Monitor blood pressure
  - Monitor distal pulses following percutaneous arterial access and stenting
- Impaired renal function, risk of
  - Monitor urinary output
  - Monitor blood urea nitrogen (BUN) and creatinine levels
- Complications at percutaneous site, risk of
  - Assess vascular access site for hematoma, bleeding
  - Observe for back pain, which may indicate retroperitoneal bleed

Subclavian Steal Syndrome

A form of a transient ischemic attack caused by an obstruction of an extracranial artery that impairs blood flow to the vertebrobasilar arterial system

Signs and Symptoms

- Dizziness
- Syncope
- Vertigo
- Arm claudication

Diagnostics

- Difference in blood pressure between right and left arm; difference greater than 20 mmHg suggests subclavian stenosis
- Carotid bruit may be audible

Patient Care Management

- Surgical therapy
  - Repair of the subclavian stenosis
    - Balloon angioplasty and stenting
    - Carotid-subclavian bypass
    - Axilloaxillary bypass

Nursing Management

(See Appendix #1.)

- Monitor coronary artery bypass patients for this condition
  - Difference in blood pressure between right and left arm; difference greater than 20 mmHg suggests subclavian stenosis, report findings

Thoracic Outlet Syndrome (TOS)

Rare disorder characterized by compression of the nerves and arteries of the arm in the thoracic outlet from repetitive activities that require the arms to be held overhead

Signs and Symptoms
- Pain
- Paresthesias
- Muscular weakness
- Fatigue
- Swelling, and coldness in the arm and hand

Diagnostics
- Health history and physical examination, identification of an accident or trauma
- Imaging
  - Elevated arm stress test (EAST)
  - Cervical and chest x-ray
  - Color flow duplex scanning
  - MRI
  - Ulnar nerve conduction or electromyography
  - Arteriogram
  - Venography

Patient Care Management
- Medical therapy
  - Physical therapy
    - Exercises to strengthening the supporting muscles of the thoracic outlet structures.
  - Pain management
    - Muscle relaxants
    - Nonsteroidal anti-inflammatory drugs such as aspirin or ibuprofen
    - Moist heat and massage
    - Analgesics
    - Steroids
- Surgical therapy
  - Decompression of the thoracic outlet to remove the point of compression

Nursing Management
- Pain management
  - Assess pain using numeric scale (0–10) to quantify pain
  - Provide analgesics and reassess for effectiveness
  - Medicate prior to physical therapy sessions
  - Ease discomfort with moist heat
- Knowledge deficit
  - Explain proper use of prescribed medications
  - Explain to patient the importance of physical therapy regime

Thromboangiitis Obliterans (TAO)—Buerger's Disease

Inflammatory vascular disease causing recurrent thrombus formation and occlusion bilaterally of the small vessels of the feet and hands. It is thought to be an autoimmune disease and is most common in young men who are heavy cigarette smokers.

Signs and Symptoms
- Foot claudication
- Paresthesias of the feet and hands
- Distal toe and/or finger ischemia
- Ulcerations and gangrene of the fingers and toes in late stages
- Superficial thrombophlebitis

Diagnostics
- Based on clinical findings and history

Patient Care Management
- Medical therapy
  - Smoking cessation and avoidance of secondhand smoke
  - Steroids
  - Antiplatelet agents
  - Anticoagulants

- Surgical revascularization
  - Sympathectomy
  - Amputation if required for nonhealing wounds, and gangrene

Nursing Management

Nursing care focuses on supportive care and limiting complications.

- Decreased tissue perfusion
  - Assess for abnormal findings such as pale or cyanotic skin, diminished or absent pulses, or skin ulcerations
  - Interventions to improve circulation to the affected areas
- Altered skin integrity and risk for infection
  - Assess hands and toes for the presence of ulcers and gangrene
  - Provide daily skin care
  - Monitor for signs of infection and sepsis
- Knowledge Deficit
  - Provide information on smoking cessation
  - Teach to avoid cold environments and medications that may cause vasoconstriction
  - Teach the patient to protect the limbs from injury
  - Instruct patient to carefully assess hands and toes, monitor for infection and notify health care provider

Peripheral Venous Disease

Venous disease is more likely to affect the lower extremities. The patient may experience intermittent swelling, tightness, and discomfort in one or both lower extremities due to a venous disorder.

Chronic Venous Insufficiency (CVI)

A complication of varicose veins and acute deep vein thrombosis

Signs and Symptoms

- Pain in legs—cramping, heaviness, or aching

- Skin changes—hyperpigmentation, dependent edema, dermatitis, ulcerations, or scarring from healed ulcerations

Patient Care Management

The primary goal is prevention of CVI by the use of elastic compression stockings for at least 2 years following an acute DVT episode.

- Medical
  - Treatment of wounds and prevention of infection
    - Compression therapy (if peripheral arterial disease not present)
    - Topical steroids, topical zinc oxide, topical antimicrobial (silver sulfadiazine)
    - Wound cleansing/debridement and dressing changes
    - Adhesive hydrocolloid dressings
    - Appropriate systemic antibiotic (initiated after cultures obtained)

Nursing Management

- Impaired healing
  - Accurate assessment and documentation of venous ulcers
  - Maintain adequate nutritional status—dietary consultation
  - Minimize edema through activity and positioning
  - Monitor glycemic control with diabetic patients
- Pain management
  - Use pain scale (0–10) to quantify pain
  - Provide pain medication prior to dressing changes/ debridement
  - Encourage walking or elevating legs which may decrease pain sensation; avoid dependent position of extremity
  - Use pain control measures before the pain becomes severe to intervene early and with less medication

- Knowledge Deficit
  - Provide factual information about diagnosis, treatment, risk factor modification, medications, and treatment plan to ensure compliance
  - Explain all procedures and allow patient to ask questions

Lymphangitis/Lymphedema

Lymphangitis is an acute inflammation of the lymphatic channels most commonly caused by an infection in one of the extremities resulting in enlarged and tender lymph nodes. Primary lymphedema is inherited as an autosomal dominant trait. Secondary lymphedema occurs as a result of an acquired disorder, such as a malignancy, radiation, surgical removal of a component of the lymphatic system, trauma, or infection.

Signs and Symptoms
- Interstitial accumulation of lymph fluid
- Affected limb(s) become edematous with thickened skin.
- Patients may complain of heaviness or fullness of the affected extremity.

Diagnostics
- Health history and physical examination—previous surgeries, radiation treatment, trauma, and infection
- Imaging
  - Lymphoscintigraphy

Patient Care Management
- Medical therapy
  - Control fluid accumulation
  - Maintain skin integrity
  - Prevent infections

- Prevent complications
  - Cellulitis and/or lymphangitis
  - Deep venous thrombosis
  - Severe functional impairment
  - Cosmetic embarrassment
  - Amputation (rare)

Nursing Management

- Altered skin integrity, risk of
  - Provide good hygiene
  - Observe for signs of skin alterations and sign of infection
  - Encourage activities to decrease fluid accumulation
    - Bedrest, limb elevation
    - Compression therapy
    - Manual lymphatic drainage
    - Short stretch compression wrapping
- Knowledge Deficit
  - Teach to inspect regularly extremities for signs and symptoms of infection and to report them promptly
  - Teach patient the importance of excellent skin hygiene
  - Teach activities to decrease fluid accumulation
    - Bed rest, limb elevation
    - Compression therapy

Critical Alert

The prevalence of peripheral arterial disease, abdominal aortic aneurysm, deep venous thrombosis, and chronic venous insufficiency increases with age.

Varicose Veins

Varicose veins are subcutaneous veins that remain dilated when the patient is standing or sitting. Dilated, tortuous veins occur as a result of incompetent valves of the deep and superficial venous system leading to valve reflux.

Risk Factors
- Older age
- Family history
- Female gender
- Pregnancy
- Occupations that require standing
- Obesity
- History of phlebitis or clot
- Constipation/low-fiber diet
- Smoking
- Hypertension
- Injury

Complications
- Increased risk of DVT
- Chronic venous insufficiency (CVI) leading to hyperpigmentation and ulceration of the feet and legs
- Increased susceptibility to injury and infection

Signs and Symptoms

Symptoms vary greatly, and may intensify by end of the day, especially after standing for long periods of time.

- No symptoms
- Leg symptoms
  - Heaviness
  - Tiredness
  - Itching
  - Burning
  - Aching

Diagnostics
- Physical examination and the patient's report of clinical manifestations
- Imaging
  - Doppler ultrasound
  - Angiography

Patient Care Management

- Procedural
- Nonsurgical (interventional therapy)
  - Sclerotherapy
- Surgical therapy, reserved for more severe varicose veins
  - Ligation
  - Stripping
  - Laser therapy
  - Radiofrequency ablation of the saphenous vein

Nursing Management

(See Appendix #1.)

- Pain, Acute
  - Assess pain using numeric scale 0–10
  - Provide analgesics and reassess for effectiveness
  - Medicate prior to ambulation
  - Limit venous pooling
    - Compression stockings
    - Bed rest for 24 hours, foot of bed elevated
    - Progressive ambulation every 2 hours
- Knowledge Deficit
  - Teach patient to avoid activities that cause venous pooling, such as sitting for long periods of time and standing in one position for long periods of time
  - Encourage patient to develop a walking program and to maintain an ideal weight
  - Demonstrate the proper method for applying and wearing compression

Venous Thromboembolism (VTE)

Consists of two conditions: deep venous thrombosis and pulmonary embolism. Virchow's triad—venous stasis, damage of the endothelium, and hypercoagulability remains the theory behind the thrombus formation of VTE.

Risk Factors

- Major abdominal, thoracic, gynecologic, and/or urologic surgeries
- Major orthopedic surgeries such as total hip or total knee procedures
- Spinal cord injuries; paresis
- Fracture of the pelvis, hip, or long bones
- Multiple trauma; burns
- Malignancy
- Myocardial infarction, heart failure, respiratory failure, sepsis, ulcerative colitis
- Intensive care unit admission; presence of central venous catheters
- Previous DVT/ pulmonary embolism (PE)
- Age > 40 years
- Obesity
- Prolonged immobility of 3 days or more
- Varicose veins
- Pregnancy/postpartum
- Oral contraceptive use
- Acquired and inherited disorders of coagulation

Pulmonary Embolism (PE)

(See Respiratory Disorders, Lower.)

Deep Venous Thrombosis (DVT)

A DVT is when a clot forms in the deep veins, usually those of the lower extremities and pelvis, but can also occur in the upper extremities.

Risk Factors

- Venous stasis
- Hypercoagulability
- Immobility

Signs and Symptoms

Signs and symptoms of DVT are variable, and the presence of a DVT may not be known until the patient develops a pulmonary embolism.

- No discomfort
- Unilateral extremity discomfort and pain, edema, warmth, tenderness, and redness
- Palpable vein cord along the vein
- Homans' sign
  - Pain in the calf when the foot is dorsiflexed (Not a reliable indicator of DVT)

Diagnostics

- Laboratory
  - D-dimer
- Imaging
  - Duplex ultrasound (most common)
  - Venography
  - CT scan (pelvic and abdominal thrombus)
  - MRI
  - Venous duplex imaging
  - Photoplethysmography

Patient Care Management

The goals for managing patients with DVT is to prevent mobilization of the clot and pulmonary embolism

- Medical therapy
  - Anticoagulants
    - Intravenous or subcutaneous unfractionated heparin
    - Subcutaneous low molecular weight heparin
    - Intravenous or subcutaneous direct thrombin inhibitors
    - Oral warfarin for 3 to 6 months

Surgical

Indicated for patients who have a contraindication to anticoagulation for DVT prophylaxis and treatment, such as the trauma patient or patients who have failed therapy by developing a clot while on anticoagulation

- Venous thrombectomy
- Vena cava filters

Nursing Management

Nursing must take an active role in DVT prevention, prophylaxis, and monitoring for treatment effectivenss.

(See Appendix #13, Patient Teaching & Discharge Priorities for Use of Anticoagulant Medications.)

- Tissue perfusion, impaired
    - Early ambulation whenever possible
    - Active and passive range of motion exercises
    - Extremity elevation
    - Mechanical methods of prophylaxis (graduated compression stockings, intermittent pneumatic devices, and venous foot pumps)
    - Observe for changes in oxygenation
    - Monitory for signs of PE
        - Dyspnea, $\uparrow$ RR, $\downarrow$ O_2 sat
        - Anxiety and apprehension
        - $\uparrow$ HR, chest pain, shock, and cardiac arrest

---

Critical Alert

Right ventricular failure is the cause of death in patients who die of PE. The nurse must be monitoring for these important findings.

- Pain, Acute
    - Assess pain using numeric scale, 0–10
    - Provide pain relief measures and re-assess for effectiveness

- Knowledge Deficit
  - Instruct to avoid prolonged immobility, standing for long periods of time, car/airline flights > 6 hours; avoid constrictive clothing.
  - Encourage patient to wear properly fitting and applied graduated compression stockings
  - Instruct patient to notify health care provider if experiencing increase in pain, tenderness, swelling of affected extremity
  - Instruct patient to notify health care provider if experiencing a new onset pain, tenderness, swelling in another extremity, new onset shortness of breath, chest pain, anxiety, restlessness, new onset bleeding, headache, mental status changes

---

Critical Alert

Peripheral arterial disease, stroke, and myocardial infarction are the principal causes of death and disability in patients over age 50. Elderly patients with acute and chronic venous disease are at higher risk of pulmonary embolus and death.

VISUAL DISORDERS

Diabetic Retinopathy (DR)

Diabetic retinopathy (DR) is the leading cause of legal blindness among young adults and working-age Americans, those persons under the age of 60, typically affecting individuals in their most productive years. Retinopathy generally refers to degenerative changes in the retina. Diabetic retinopathy results in edema from leaking capillaries that hemorrhage.

Major Risk Factors
- Diabetes for many years
- Family history
- Hyperglycemia
- Hypertension
- Hyperlipidemia
- Smoking
- Anemia
- Renal disease

Signs and Symptoms
- Floating spots
- Streaks
- Lines
- Scattered lights
- Distortion
- Hazy and cloudy view
- Darkness
- Poor color vision

Diagnostics

- Baseline dilated eye examination and evaluation once diagnosed with diabetes

- An annual evaluation is encouraged unless retinopathy is present, then frequency will be determined by the health care provider.

- Fluoresein angiography: Scans reveal microaneurysms, blot and dot hemorrhages, areas of nonperfusion, and evidence of collateral vessels that do not leak

Patient Care Management

- Controlling diabetes and maintaining the HbAIc level in the 6–7% range are the overall goals.

- Managing hypertension and hyperlipidemia helps prevent the development (or worsening) of diabetic retinopathy.

- Laser photocoagulation: The laser is applied to diffuse areas of leakage and thickening.

A multidisciplinary team approach, which consists of health care providers: family practitioner, internist, or endocrinologist, and ophthalmologist, and ophthalmic advance nurse practitioner, nurses, nutritionist, and optometrist serves to provide comprehensive care to patients with diabetic retinopathy.

Nursing Management

Nursing management of patients with diabetic retinopathy can be complex and multifaceted.

(See Glandular section.)

Glaucoma

Glaucoma includes a group of conditions that feature an optic neuropathy accompanied by optic disk cupping and visual field loss. It generally is associated with an increase in intraocular pressure; however, some people with normal intraocular pressure may develop characteristic optic nerve and visual field changes.

Primary Glaucoma

Develops when any sequence of the production of aqueous humor or the drainage of aqueous humor does not function properly. This causes the intraocular pressure to increase in the eye, thus putting pressure on the optic nerve and causing it to atrophy, which can lead to permanent blindness if left untreated.

Chronic Open-Angle Glaucoma

Elevated intraocular pressure occurs due to the increase of aqueous production or the decrease in aqueous drainage due to trabecular meshwork obstruction, canal of Schlemm's obstruction, or degenerative changes of the drainage tissue.

Acute Angle Closure Glaucoma

Occurs when the angle in the anterior chamber closes suddenly due to shallow or narrow anterior angle (which is between the iris and cornea) by iris blockage, thereby preventing aqueous flow through the trabecular meshwork and into the canal of Schlemm.

Secondary Glaucoma

Is the result of another preexisting ocular condition

- Vascular changes due to diabetes mellitus
- Infection
- Hemorrhage into anterior chamber
- Trauma
- Surgery
- Long-term steroid use

Signs and Symptoms
Open-Angle Glaucoma

- Bilateral involvement
- "Silent blinder" or "thief in the night" because patients experience no symptoms in the early stages
- First recognized due to noticeable vision loss
- Side vision loss usually comes later in the course of the disease

Closed-Angle Glaucoma

- Patients seek medical care due to sudden onset of pain in one eye and other noticeable symptoms
- Extreme eye pain and pressure
- Blurry vision
- Fixed mid-dilated pupil
- Corneal edema
- Hyperemia
- Photophobia
- Light halos
- Epiphora
- Frontal headaches that can be accompanied by nausea, vomiting, and abdominal ache

Diagnostics

- Pachometry: to measure central corneal thickness. Normal is about $545 \pm 20 \, \mu m$.
- Tonometry: to measure intraocular pressure
- Physical examination and health history

Patient Care Management

The treatment goal is to lower intraocular pressure and preserve vision as quickly as possible, with systemic medications orally or intravenously, as well as topical ophthalmic drops that are ordered by the health care provider.

- Anti-glaucoma eye drops
  - Beta-adrenergic blocking agents (Timolol): to reduce aqueous humor production and increase outflow
  - Epinephrine: to reduce aqueous humor production
  - Miotics (Carbachol, Pilocarpine): for pupil contraction and assist with aqueous humor outflow
- Oral medications
- Laser or surgery intervention
  - YAG laser (neodymium: yttrium-aluminum-garnet) for peripheral iridectomy or iridoplasty

- Laser trabeculoplasty (LTP), laser trabeculectomy, visco canalostomy, ciliodestructive procedure, or trabeculotomy and trabeculectomy filtering procedure

The best results for patients with glaucoma are achieved through a multidisciplinary team approach, including the ophthalmologist, ophthalmic advance nurse practitioner, nurse, and optometrist. Management of glaucoma may include medical controls with the continuous use of eye drops or surgical intervention by the ophthalmologist. The nurse practitioner or nurse can provide the necessary education and follow-up monitoring of patients' progress to ensure compliance with the glaucoma regimen.

Nursing Management

- Disturbed Sensory Perception: Visual
  - Use patient's name with each interaction
  - Explain the purpose of interaction
  - Orient to time, place, person, and situation as needed
  - Orient to the environment
  - Provide visual aids (books, clocks, telephone) keeping them near patient where he/she can reach them
  - Assist with meals, arrange food items and explain location to patient
- Risk for Injury
  - Assist with ambulation
  - Assess ability to care for self
  - Provide safe environment; remove furniture and other objects that could cause a fall
  - Side rails up as appropriate

Critical Alert

Assess for new onset of hazy cornea, vision loss, eye pain, headache, nausea, and vomiting. These signs indicate a worsening condition and the health care provider must be alerted immediately.

- Knowledge Deficit
  - Explain disease along with risk factors
  - Instruct the patient/family regarding correct use of eye drops. Return demonstration of drop installation. Provide list of medications along with scheduled administration times.
  - Explain common side effects of eye drops
  - Explain importance of regular eye examinations

Macular Degeneration

Macular degeneration is defined as the deterioration of the macula, the area of central vision in the posterior pole or retina, causing central acuity loss. Age-related macular degeneration (ARMD or AMD) is the most common cause of vision loss in those aged 60 and above.

Major Types

- Dry Age-Related Macular Degeneration
  - Light-sensitive cells in the macula slowly break down, gradually blurring central vision in the affected eye.
  - Early sign:
    - Drusen: yellowish, round, slightly elevated, different-sized subretinal pigment epithelial deposits in the macula.
- Wet Age-Related Macular Degeneration
  - Exudative, serous, or neovascular changes in the macula.
  - Occurs when abnormal blood vessels behind the retina start to grow under the macula. The new blood vessels are very fragile and often leak blood and fluid, which raise the macula from its normal place at the back of the eye.
  - Damage to the macula occurs rapidly and loss of central vision can develop quickly.
  - Early sign:
    - Straight lines appear wavy

Risk Factors

- Aging
- Hypertension
- Atherosclerosis
- Cardiovascular disease
- Smoking
- Lung conditions
- Diabetes
- Hyperlipidemia
- Hyperopia
- Light colored iris
- Ultraviolet light exposure
- Heredity

Signs and Symptoms

- Difficulty seeing with the affected eye while doing close-up work or have trouble seeing at a distance, especially with driving
- Metamorphopsia:
  - Visual distortion (e.g., straight lines such as doorframes or posts look crooked or irregular)
- Loss of contrast sensitivity:
  - Difference in the sizes and colors of objects between eyes
- Difficulty completing tasks that require looking directly at some object

Diagnostics

Physical examination including visual acuity testing is the most common diagnostic tool used when evaluating for macular degeneration. The Amsler grid, a self-testing tool, can be used by the patient to help recognize early macular changes from macular degeneration.

Patient Care Management

- Antioxidant eye vitamins
- Dietary supplements
  - Dark green, leafy vegetables
  - Orange/yellow vegetables and fruits
  - Precautions are needed if patient is on anti-coagulants
- Specific for Wet Macular Degeneration
  - Nonsteroidal anti-inflammatory medications
  - Laser photocoagulation
  - Photodynamic therapy
  - Vitrectomy with choroidal neovascularization removal
  - Intravitreal injection of anti-Vascular Endothelial Growth Factor (anti-VEGF) antigen binding drugs

To achieve potential vision restoration and return to society as before, patients with wet macular degeneration need a multidisciplinary team approach, including the ophthalmologist, ophthalmic advance nurse practitioner, nurse, social worker, and optometrist or low vision rehabilitation specialist.

Nursing Management

- High risk for injury or falls
  - Educate on visual defects and provide the necessary safety skills and management to prevent injury or falls
- Self-care deficit
  - Provide resources for normal daily activities, self-care needs and tools, and support system information
  - Encourage self-care in keeping compliant and proactive in maintaining vision health
  - Provide resources to patient so they have means to keep an adequate supply of antioxidant eye vitamins when indicated

> **Critical Alert**
>
> Antioxidant eye vitamins should not be used for patients taking anticoagulants as they will speed the clotting process.

- Knowledge Deficit
  - Provide education and resources about vision loss, means of treatment and management, and role in self-care and alternative devices in assisting
  - Instruct patient and family of importance of regular eye examinations
  - Educate and promote normalization with enhancement skills in self-esteem and socialization, and means to access support systems

Procedures and Therapies

Bladder Surgery and Ileal Conduit

A urinary diversion is created using the intestinal tract and is usually an ileal conduit. A segment of ileum is separated from the small intestine and formed into a tubular pouch with the open end being brought to the skin surface, forming a stoma. The ureters are then connected to the pouch and the patient will need to wear an external pouch to collect the urine.

Nursing Management

- Impaired urinary elimination
  - Monitor urine output to determine functioning of surgical bladder
  - Self-catheterization
    - Done twice daily to remove residual urine and prevent infection
    - Irrigation of bladder done through the catheter to remove mucous on the neobladder wall
- Pain, Acute
  - Administer analgesics
  - Assess pain using numeric scale and self-reported characteristics
- Sexual Dysfunction
  - Penile implant for sexual intercourse without ejaculation (scheduled at later date)
  - Allow for patient to express concerns regarding change in customary sexual practices

- Knowledge Deficit
  - Instruct patient/family in stoma care once readiness to learn has been established
  - Referral to enterostomal therapist
  - Instruct patient to tighten the abdominal muscles (allows for normal voiding via urethra)

Bleeding Precautions

Although exact bleeding precautions vary among clinical sites, the following measures are widely implemented to minimize the risk of injury to patients:

- Avoid intramuscular and subcutaneous injections
- Hold firm pressure to venipuncture sites for a minimum of 5 minutes
- Minimize venipunctures and invasive procedures
- Provide a soft toothbrush or tooth sponges for mouth care
- Avoid rectal suppositories, thermometers, enemas, and other rectal/vaginal manipulation
- Prevent constipation and straining with stools
- Use electric razor only
- Maintain a safe environment to avoid injury
- Assist with ADLs and ambulation as necessary to avoid injury
- Avoid medications with antiplatelet activity (e.g., aspirin and aspirin-containing products, NSAIDs)

Nursing Management, Blood Administration Procedure

Purpose

- To administer blood products safely to patients with altered hematologic function
- To replace circulating blood volume
- To restore oxygen carrying capacity
- To stop and prevent bleeding

Equipment

- Y-type blood transfusion tubing
- 250- to 500-mL bag of normal saline (0.9% NaCl)
- Blood product from blood bank
- Blood administration record for vital sign assessment
- Nonsterile gloves
- Alcohol wipes
- Tape
- 18- to 20-gauge IV catheter
- IV pole

Assessment Parameters

- Size of IV catheter (18 to 20 gauge)
- Health care provider's order for type, amount, and rate of blood administration
- History of blood transfusion reactions
- Religious or other personal objections to receiving blood products
- Compatibility of blood product to recipient blood type
- Circulatory and respiratory status
- Vital signs before, during, and after transfusion
- Presence of rash prior to transfusion

Special Considerations

- No medications are to be piggybacked into a transfusion.
- The transfusion is never interrupted for medication administration.
- Only 0.9% NaCl is to be infused in the same line as the blood.

Planning for Blood Administration

- Obtain patient transfusion history (previous transfusions, transfusion reactions)
- Ensure the patient understands the need for blood administration and is willing to sign the informed

consent. Informed consent is obtained by the health care provider. The blood is not given without the consent

- Check health care provider's order for type of blood product to be administered
- Check size and insertion date of the IV catheter:
  - 18- or 20-gauge catheter, depending on the hospital protocol
  - If the catheter is more than 48 hours old, it should not be used for administration of blood products.

    (*Note:* Specific agency protocols supersede this procedure.)

Nursing Implementation, Administration Protocol

- Wash hands and assemble appropriate equipment
- Explain to patient/family the procedure and rationale, length of transfusion, as appropriate. Assess understanding.
- Instruct patient to report *any* unusual symptoms
- Follow hospital protocol for obtaining blood products from the laboratory
- Close all three clamps on the Y-type blood tubing with filter and attach the 0.9% NaCl (NS) bag, open the clamp to the NS, and purge the Y-tubing
- Make sure the filter chamber is completely filled with saline
- Using aseptic technique, connect tubing to IV catheter or to saline lock
- Check identification of blood product with two (2) *licensed staff nurses* and the patient:
  - Patient name and medical record number (in chart and on the blood product)

    (*Note:* It is often useful to check the birth date as well.)
  - Blood product type and unit number
  - Blood ABO group and Rh factor of both donor blood and patient

- Expiration date of blood product (may be given up to midnight on expiration day)
- Both nurse's sign and date blood bank slip that is attached to the blood bag
- Compare the above patient identification information with the patient's name band
- Obtain baseline vital signs (TPR, BP) and document on the chart. Follow hospital protocol for frequency of reassessing vital signs
- Prior to handling any blood products, put on non-sterile gloves and use standard precautions
  - Connect blood bag to the free arm of the Y-tubing and open the roller clamp on the same arm of the Y
  - Close the clamp on the NS side of the Y tubing before opening the clamp on the blood side of the Y tubing
  - Begin infusion of blood product by adjusting the roller clamp closest to the patient's IV site
  - Take vital signs prior to the infusion of the blood
  - The nurse must remain with the patient for this 15-minute period and observe the patient for transfusion reactions. Blood products should be infused very slowly for the first 15 minutes of the transfusion
  - Vital signs are taken after the first 15 minutes.
  - If there are no indications of a transfusion reaction, increase the infusion rate to the prescribed rate or the standard hospital infusion rate
- Continue observation for transfusion reactions until the blood product has completely infused
- Terminating the transfusion:
  - Flush the IV tubing with normal saline by closing the blood product roller clamp and opening the saline roller clamp.
  - Follow hospital protocol for discarding blood product bag and tubing.
  - Flush IV catheter after discontinuing blood tubing.

**Documentation in Patient Record
and Blood Administration Record**

- Date
- Time the infusion was started and completed
- Volume of blood product and normal saline infused (intake and output record)
- Blood product and number
- Signature of the two nurses who checked the blood product
- Baseline and continuing patient assessment

Special Equipment Used for Transfusion Therapy

- Blood warmers are used when blood is infused rapidly.
- Infusion pumps are used when blood needs to be given at a very specific rate to prevent fluid overload.

Nursing Evaluation

- Vital signs before, during, after the transfusion
- Lung assessment during and after the transfusion
- Hemoglobin and hematocrit
- Transfusion reaction
- Changes in fatigue levels
- Increased tissue perfusion
- Clinical manifestations of anemia

Cardiac Catheterization
**(See "Percutaneous Coronary Interventions"
for interventional procedure.)**

A procedure that is done in a special laboratory under sterile conditions. It consists of the insertion of a radiopaque catheter into the left or right side of the heart to provide anatomic and hemodynamic information about the heart and great vessels. This information is then utilized to assess the presence and severity of cardiac disease and assists to determine potential therapy and prognosis.

Care of Craniotomy Patients for Brain Tumor

(NATIONAL GUIDELINES American Association of Neuroscience Nurses)

Neurological

- Most complications occur within the first 6 hours postoperative
- ICU admission postoperative
- Frequent neurological assessments
  - Ask the neurosurgeon what complications or deficits are expected
- Incision care
  - Monitor incision for drainage
  - Keep incision dry
- Drains
  - Make sure the location of each drain is known; label clearly

Cardiovascular

- Cardiac arrhythmias
- Hypovolemic shock
- Monitor rate and rhythm
- Monitor blood pressure and maintain ordered parameters

Respiratory

- Related to decreased level of consciousness/inability to protect airway
- Especially relevant to surgery near brainstem
- Prevent atelectasis and pneumonia
- Maintain $SaO_2 > 94\%$
- Incentive spirometry unless contraindicated (transsphenoidal surgery)

Gastrointestinal

- Prevention of gastric ulceration (antacids, proton pump inhibitor, H2-blockers)
- Some drugs used in neurological treatment can contribute to gastric irritation (dexamethasone, phenytoin, some antibiotics)

Nutrition

- May require swallow evaluation
- May require enteral feedings

Serum Glucose

- Hyperglycemia may increase cerebral edema
- Hyperglycemia may result from steroid therapy
- Monitor blood glucose as ordered
- Maintain euglycemia

Serum Sodium

- Diabetes insipidus
  - Especially relevant to surgery involving or near the pituitary gland
  - Monitor intake/output and specific gravity
  - Notify health care provider for urine output > 200 mL/hr $\times$ 2 consecutive hours
- Syndrome of inappropriate antidiuretic hormone
  - Monitor sodium levels; treat as ordered

Activity

- Population at risk for DVT
  - Early ambulation
  - DVT prophylaxis, such as low-molecular-weight heparin, when ordered
  - Therapy consults
- Pain control
  - Assess per hospital protocol
  - Administer pain medication as ordered
  - Offer other techniques for pain management, such as deep breathing or music

Coronary Artery Bypass Graft Surgery (CABG)

Standard coronary artery bypass surgery is done via a median sternotomy using cardiopulmonary bypass (CPB), cold cardioplegia, and systemic hypothermia. CABG can provide more complete revascularization and show better long-term relief of symptoms than PCI. However, CABG patients also have more procedural-related pain, longer hospital stays, and more periprocedural myocardial infarctions.

Class 1 Recommendations for CABG for Stable Angina

- Significant left main coronary artery stenosis
- Significant (greater than or equal to 70%) stenosis of the proximal left anterior descending artery (LAD) and proximal left circumflex artery
- PCI not optimal or possible
- Ongoing ischemia not responsive to maximal non-surgical therapy
- Fail reprofusion therapy (thrombolytics or PCI)
- Surgical repair needed for post-infarction ventricular septal rupture or mitral insufficiency
- Cardiogenic shock in patients less than 75 years old with ST segment elevation or left bundle branch block who develop shock within 36 hours of MI and are suitable for revascularization that can be performed within 18 hours of shock
- Life-threatening ventricular dysrhythmias in the presence of greater than or equal to 50% left main stenosis and/or triple vessel disease

Class 1 Recommendations for CABG for Unstable Angina or Non–ST Segment Elevation MI

- Significant left main coronary artery stenosis
- Left main equivalent: significant (greater than or equal to 70%) stenosis of the proximal left anterior descending artery (LAD) and proximal left circumflex artery
- When percutaneous revascularization is not optimal or possible

- When ongoing ischemia not responsive to maximal nonsurgical therapy

The last group of patients would be those who are necessitating urgent intervention. Performing surgery amid an acute MI greatly increases the risks of perioperative complications.

Class 1 Recommendations for Urgent CABG for a Patient with ST Segment Elevation MI

- Failed angioplasty with persistent pain or hemodynamic instability

- Persistent or recurrent ischemia refractory to medical therapy in patients, who have a significant area of myocardium at risk, and who are not candidates for PCI

- During surgical repair of postinfarction ventricular septal rupture or mitral insufficiency

- Cardiogenic shock in patients less than 75 years old with ST segment elevation or left bundle branch block who develop shock within 36 hours of MI and are suitable for revascularization that can be performed within 18 hours of shock

- Life-threatening ventricular dysrhythmias in the presence of greater than or equal to 50% left main stenosis and/or triple vessel disease

Postoperative Considerations

The overall rate of mortality for CABG is between 1% and 3%, with the risk increasing according to the number comorbidities. Serious complications include stroke, myocardial infarction, bleeding, tamponade, renal failure, respiratory failure, dysrhythmias, wound infection, and both pericardial and pleural effusions. The amount of recovery time is individualized and is dependent on a patient's age and other health problems.

Nursing Management

In the immediate postoperative period, patients are typically taken directly from the operating room to a specialized intensive care unit (ICU) with nurses who are trained in close monitoring of the patient's hemodynamic status.

After initial recovery, patient is transferred to telemetry unit where cardiac monitor and standard postoperative care is delivered. Effective pain management is essential since aggressive mobilization and physical therapy must be a focus to limit complications and the zone of ischemia.

Dialysis (Hemodialysis or Peritoneal Dialysis)

- Analyze laboratory data for status of electrolytes, hematology, and blood glucose levels
- Assess for signs of peritonitis (abdominal pain, cloudy effluent, fever)
- Initiate good aseptic technique:
  - Hand washing
  - Gloves

The treatment regimen for dialysis is based on two factors: the restriction of certain nutrients and the removal of waste metabolites from the blood by regular dialysis. The management is effective only if the patient adheres closely with the therapeutic regimen.

Absolute Clinical Indications

- Pericarditis
- Volume overload or pulmonary edema that is refractory to diuretics
- Increasing hypertension that is minimally responsive to antihypertensive medications
- Progressive uremic encephalopathy or neuropathy
- Persistent nausea and vomiting
- Plasma creatinine concentration above 12 mg/dL or blood urea nitrogen greater than 100 mg/dL

Relative Clinical Indications

- Anorexia progressing to nausea and vomiting
- Decreased attentiveness
- Decreased cognitive tasking

- Depression
- Severe anemia that is unresponsive to erythropoietin
- Persistent pruritus or restless leg syndrome

Hemodialysis

Access

- Short-Term Access: Inserted at the bedside for acute hemodialysis treatment
  - Subclavian
  - Internal jugluar
  - Femoral
- Long-Term Access: Access to the arterial circulation and with return via the venous circulation
  - Arteriovenous fistula
  - Arteriovenous graft
  - Arteriovenous shunt

Complications of Hemodialysis

Complication	Cause
Hypotension	Rapid removal of vascular volume Decreased systemic vascular resistance Decreased cardiac output
Loss of blood	Residual blood not rinsed from the dialyzer Accidental separation of vascular tubing Dialysis membrane rupture Bleeding from access site after removal of needles
Muscle cramps	Rapid removal of sodium and water
Hepatitis	Blood transfusions IV drug abuse

Complication	Cause
Sepsis	Infection of the vascular access site Introduction of bacteria during dialysis due to poor technique or interruption of tubing
Disequilibrium syndrome (development of cerebral edema)	Rapid changes in the composition of the extracellular fluid due to removal of solutes from the blood more rapidly than from the cerebrospinal fluid and the brain

Nursing Management

The nursing implications for access devices are to protect the patency of the device and prevent infection.

Nursing Management for Hemodialysis

Complication	Nursing Responsibility
Grafts and Fistulas:	
• Infection	Hand washing Assess for redness, exudate, and fever Use aseptic technique when cannulating access
• Bleeding	Do not cannulate new access too early
• Thrombosis	**Critical Alert:** No Blood pressure on arm with access Teach patients not to wear anything constrictive on the accessed arm
• Pseudoaneurysm	Avoid multiple cannulations in the same area
• Pain from vascular steal syndrome	Apply warm compresses and administer analgesia

(continued)

Complication	Nursing Responsibility
Fistulas:	
• Inadequate blood flow	Palpate for thrill Auscultate for bruit Assess extremity for warmth and normal color Teach patients to develop blood flow through daily exercises such as squeezing a ball while applying slight impedance to the flow distal to the access point

Peritoneal Dialysis

Peritoneal dialysis is the infusion of sterile dialyzing fluid through an implanted catheter in the abdominal cavity. The dialysate fluid bathes the peritoneal membrane that covers the abdominal organs and overlies the capillary beds. Excess fluid and solutes travel via osmosis, diffusion, and active transport from the peritoneal capillary fluid through the capillary walls, through the peritoneal membrane, into the dialyzing fluid. After a prescribed amount of time, the fluid is drained from the abdomen by gravity.

Nursing Management

- Obtain baseline vital signs and weight
- Assess for fluid retention
  - Measure abdominal girth
  - Assess respiratory status
  - Assess for the presence of edema
  - Masks applied to all individuals in patient room
- Warm dialysate fluid to at least body temperature to provide comfort and enhance exchange
- Assess effluent (dialysis drainage)
  - Color and clarity

- Notify health care provider if fibrin strands or blood is present
- Compare outflow amount to infused amount to determine accurate I & O

Endoscopy

Endoscopy is the direct visualization of the mucosa in the esophagus, stomach, and duodenum using an endoscope. Tissue biopsies are obtained for further analysis.

Banding

Banding, or variceal ligation, involves the placement of tiny rubber bands on esophageal varices to occlude blood flow.

Sclerotherapy

Sclerotherapy is done by injecting esophageal varices with an agent that causes the vessel to become sclerotic thus stopping the uncontrolled bleeding.

- Preprocedure
  - Ensure informed consent procedures are followed and signed consent is in the chart
  - Ensure ID band is correct and on patient's wrist
  - Ensure NPO 8 to 12 hours prior to test
  - Have the patient remove any jewelry, dentures, or eyeglasses
  - Ensure the patient empties his bladder before the procedure
  - Take vital signs and start an IV for sedation
  - Answer any questions the patient has about the procedure, and explain that there may be a sensation of pressure as the endoscope is inserted and fullness in the stomach as air is injected to expand the stomach and allow for better visualization
- Postprocedure
  - Frequent vital signs
  - Check gag reflex
  - NPO until gag reflex returns

- Monitor for signs of complications: pain, dyspnea, tachycardia, or subcutaneous emphysema in the neck

Endotracheal Intubation

The indications for intubation include inability of the respiratory system to maintain oxygenation and/or ventilation. Other indications for intubation include airway protection and elective surgery. Assisting with intubation requires that the nurse know what equipment is necessary and the proper operation of that equipment. It also requires that the nurse anticipate the needs of the health care professional who is performing the procedure.

Prior to the Procedure
- Explain the procedure to the patient and the family
- Position patient on back with a small blanket under the shoulder blades to hyperextend the neck and open the airway
- Confirm that the equipment is working properly
- Using an MRB and mask, preoxygenates the patient
- During the procedure
  - Provide suction as necessary
  - Monitor pulse oximetry, heart rate, and blood pressure
  - Provide reassurance to the patient
- Documentation
  - Size of the endotracheal tube
  - Location of the tube in the airway, determined by the number of centimeters on the tube located at the teeth or gum line
  - Medication administered
  - Patient tolerance of the procedure

Equipment for Endotracheal Intubation
- Personal protective equipment
- Endotracheal tubes with intact cuff and 15-mm connectors

- *Adult female:* 7.5- to 8.0-mm tube
- *Adult male:* 8.0- to 9.0-mm tube
- Laryngoscope handle with fresh batteries
- Laryngoscope blades (straight or curved)
- Spare bulbs for laryngoscope blades
- Flexible stylet
- Self-inflating resuscitation bag with mask connected to 100% oxygen
- Oxygen source and connecting tubes
- Swivel adapter
- Nonsterile gloves
- Luer-Lok 10-mL syringe for cuff inflation
- Water-soluble lubricant
- Rigid pharyngeal suction tip catheter (Yankauer)
- Suction apparatus (wall or portable)
- Suction catheters
- Bite block or oropharyngeal airways
- Endotracheal tube securing apparatus or tape
- Stethoscope
- Anesthetic spray or jelly (for nasal approach)
- Sedating or paralyzing medication
- Magill forceps
- Ventilator

Endotracheal Intubation Complications

If the patient is not properly sedated

- Patient can occlude the tube with teeth or gums or remove the tube with her tongue.
- The tube can cause pressure ulcers and erode the lips.
- The tube can become kinked in the back of the throat.

The cuff of the ETT prevents most secretions from being aspirated into the lungs and prevents air from the ventilator from escaping from around the endotracheal tube into the upper airways instead of ventilating the lungs.

- Positioned too high, the ETT cuff can damage the vocal cords.
- The pilot balloon can leak and cause insufficient volumes to be delivered.
- The tip of the tube can be blocked with secretions, bacteria, or blood that prevent delivery of adequate tidal volumes.

Biofilm, a complex matrix of bacteria, develops on endotracheal tubes that are in place for any length of time. This biofilm has been associated with ventilator-associated pneumonia (VAP).

Kidney Transplantation

Kidney transplantation is the treatment of choice for end-stage renal disease because it improves the quality of life and reduces the mortality risk for most patients. The transplant donor can be living or cadaver. Success is dependent upon transplantation early in disease, accurate tissue typing, and post-transplant immunosuppression.

Complications

- Immediate:
    - Rejection
        - Signs: oliguria, sudden weight gain, fever, elevated BUN/Creatinine, hypertension, pain at graft site
- Long-term:
    - Infection
    - Hypertension
    - Chronic liver disease
    - Bone demineralization
    - CAD
    - Cancer
    - Cataracts
    - GI bleed

Nursing Management

The focus of nursing care is aimed at prompt recognition of signs of rejection and infection. Patients and their families need to alert their health care provider if they experience low grade fever, chills, or pain at the graft site.

Mechanical Ventilation

Modern ventilators are termed positive pressure ventilators because they provide an increased pressure on inspiration to the lungs. This is the most common type of ventilator used in the acute care setting. There are devices, such as the chest cuirass and iron lung, that create a negative pressure around the chest and assist with exhalation. These devices are sometimes used in the home. Finally, a combined type of ventilator using negative and positive pressure to deliver the gas is used in some situations. The high-frequency oscillator used in pediatric and adult patients with decreased lung compliance produces an oscillating wave of pressures to deliver the gas.

The ventilator circuit is connected to the patient and consists of a single plastic tube that fits directly onto the endotracheal tube or tracheostomy. The circuit divides at the wye into an inspiratory and expiratory circuit that connects directly to the ventilator. The ventilator monitors rates, pressures, and volumes, and delivers the set volumes or pressures or a combination of the two to the patient during the inspiratory cycle, by using microprocessors to synchronize and detect when the patient inspires and expires and to time the delivery of machine support.

Important Components of the System

- Humidification—Oxygen delivered without humidification can cause drying of the airways and solidification of secretions.

- Compressor—Compressed air is mixed with the percent of oxygen to deliver the ordered FiO_2.

- Waveform monitoring—Allows assessment of the lung mechanics and better adjustment of the ventilator to the patient's needs.

Providing nursing care to the patient on a ventilator has become increasingly complicated due to the complexities of ventilators and the variety and type of ventilators. The major resource for the nurse is the respiratory therapist who is responsible for the ventilator and for ensuring that the ventilator is meeting the respiratory needs of the patient. The nurse is responsible for knowing how the ventilator functions and the meaning of different modes to ensure that the patient receives an integrative approach and the best possible outcome. To ensure optimum care of a patient on a ventilator, the entire health care team must share a common goal, that is, to liberate the patient from the ventilator. But the respiratory therapist and the nurse have an added responsibility to work together in the care of the ventilated patient. The nurse and the therapist must ensure that they are communicating with each other with regard to changes in modes, sedation levels, and daily plans for weaning.

Nursing Management of the Ventilated Patient and Basic Modes of Ventilation

A mode describes the pattern of the breath delivery. The health care provider orders the mode that best meets the patient's needs. Different ventilator manufacturers use different names for the modes.

Complications of Mechanical Ventilation and Nursing Implication

As soon as a patient is intubated and mechanical ventilation is initiated, the next moment is when the nurse should be activating a plan to liberate the patient from the ventilator. An endotracheal tube and positive pressure ventilation expose the patient to an increased risk of morbidity and mortality. Coordination of the health care team to ensure timely extubation is important in decreasing the risks.

The nurse caring for a patient on a ventilator must recognize the possible complications and work diligently to prevent them if at all possible.

Complications

Cardiovascular—Variable and depends on the amount of pressure used to ventilate the lungs, the amount of PEEP, and the underlying heart and lung dynamics.

Common Ventilator Modes

Ventilator Mode	Key Features	Nursing Implications
Assist control (AC)	Each breath, whether patient or machine triggered, is a full pressure or volume breath.	You "get what you set." Patients can become tachypneic and the ventilator has no time to deliver a full breath. "Stacking breaths" can be a complication of this mode.
Synchronized mandatory ventilation (SIMV)	Machine (preset rate) breaths are interspersed with patient-initiated breaths. Patients set their own tidal volume when initiating breaths.	Standard mode used in most critical care units. Used in combination with PS.
Pressure support (PSV)	Used in combination with SIMV on patient-initiated breaths. PSV overcomes the resistance of the ETT and the ventilator tubing. Provides increased pressure on inspiration.	Only active when patient initiates a breath. If patient is too sedated and does not attempt to overbreathe the set rate, no PS is active. Can also be used in a stand-alone mode called PSV. Patient must have a reliable respiratory rate. The machine does not provide a rate.

(continued)

Common Ventilator Modes (*continued*)

Ventilator Mode	Key Features	Nursing Implications
Pressure control	A pressure-limited breath is delivered at a certain rate. This is a full control mode.	Usually used for patients who have restrictive disease and worsening lung function. This mode does not guarantee a set V_E (minute ventilation). This must be monitored.
Mandatory minute ventilation (MMV)	A pressure or volume breath that provides a minimum ventilation if the patient's spontaneous breaths do not achieve the set V_E.	Difficult to assess the amount of support the patient is receiving from the ventilator and how much effort is their own. Becomes problematic when attempting to liberate the patient from the ventilator.

Ventilator Mode	Key Features	Nursing Implications
Positive end-expiratory pressure (PEEP)	A pressure (usually 5 cm H_2O) that prevents the alveoli from returning to 0 pressure at the end of exhalation.	Increasing levels of PEEP can cause hypotension. All patients need some physiological PEEP.
Continuous positive airway pressure (CPAP)	The same as PEEP except that there is no rate set on the ventilator—the patient is spontaneously breathing.	Can be used with noninvasive ventilation as well as with an intubated patient.
Noninvasive positive pressure ventilation (NPPV)	Ventilation is provided without the benefit of an endotracheal tube.	Patient must be able to cooperate; must be alert and oriented and able to clear secretions.

- Hypotension related to decreased cardiac output, hypovolemia, and positive pressure delivered by the ventilator.
  - Assessment of heart failure and intervening with appropriate treatment in the patient on the ventilator is the primary role of the nurse in preventing cardiovascular complications.
- Cardiac dysrhythmias related to decreased cardiac output and decreased pH.
  - Careful attention to fluid and electrolyte replacement can help prevent this complication from occurring.

Gastrointestinal
- Gastric distention as a result of swallowed air from pressure ventilation
  - Routine use of a nasal or oral gastric tube to decompress the stomach
- Stress ulcer
  - Preventative interventions to prevent gastrointestinal bleeding

Psychological Complications
- Agitation, anxiety, and confusion are all complications of mechanical ventilation. Discomfort, lack of adequate sleep, and use of analgesics and sedatives may contribute.
  - Provide periods of uninterrupted sleep
  - Provide means of communication (speaking board, lip reading, or a special endotracheal tube that allows air through the vocal cords)
  - Sedate appropriately using a sedation scale and individualizing sedation

Pulmonary Complications
- Barotrauma: alveoli damage caused by increased pressure resulting from the ventilator
- Volutrauma: caused by increased volume that causes overdistention of alveoli

- Pneumothorax, pneumomediastinum, or subcutaneous emphysema
- Atelectasis: due to mucous plug or the result of tidal volumes that are too low to ventilate the entire lung
- Nasopharyngeal injury from high pressures, long-term ventilation
- Ulcerations of the lips, nose, and mouth from the endotracheal tube, the tape, or other devices used to secure the tube
  - Frequent changes of the device and assessment of underlying soft tissue is important
- Sinusitis produced by the increase in secretions and the inability of drainage
- Tracheal damage and tracheoesophageal fistulas
- Trachea-innominate artery rupture, although almost always fatal, is a unique and rare complication of tracheostomies
- Oxygen toxicity with FiO_2 levels greater than 50% for long periods of time
  - Careful monitoring of ABGs and keeping the PaO_2 to less than 50 mmHg whenever possible

Ventilated-Associated Pneumonia (VAP) is one of the most serious consequences of initiation of mechanical ventilation. VAP is the second most common hospital-associated infection after that of the urinary tract. The primary risk factor for the development of hospital-associated bacterial pneumonia is mechanical ventilation. Morbidity and mortality increase when an endotracheal tube is placed in a patient's airway.

The most common etiology for a VAP is aspiration of contaminated oropharyngeal secretions (saliva). The reason that the saliva is contaminated is multifactorial.

- Lack of appropriate mouth care
- Immune-compromised state that accompanies critical illness
- Relative xerostomia (dry mouth)

Prevention of Ventilated-Associated Pneumonia

- Use of endotracheal tube that allows continuous suctioning of secretions from above the cuff

- Hand hygiene using an alcohol-based antiseptic decreased the incidence of hand-transmitted infections

- Gloving helps prevent cross-contamination. Personnel should use gloves properly and decontaminate their hands after gloves are removed.

- Proper cleaning and sterilization or disinfection of reusable devices used for respiratory therapy, pulmonary diagnostic tests, or delivery of anesthesia helps prevent infection transmission.

- Maintaining head of bed elevated

- Decontamination of the oral cavity

  - Brush teeth, gums, and tongue at least twice a day using a soft pediatric or adult toothbrush

  - Provide oral moisturizing to oral mucosa and lips every 2 to 4 hours

  - Use an oral chlorhexidine gluconate (0.12%) rinse twice a day during the perioperative period for adult patients who undergo cardiac surgery. Routine use in other populations is not recommended at this time.

NATIONAL GUIDELINES for the Prevention of Health Care-Associated Bacterial Pneumonia

> I. Staff Education and Involvement in Infection Prevention
> Educate health care workers about the epidemiology of, and infection control procedures for, preventing health care-associated bacterial pneumonia.
> II. Infection and Microbiologic Surveillance
>   A. Conduct surveillance for bacterial pneumonia in intensive care unit (ICU) patients who are at high risk for health-care-related bacterial pneumonia (e.g., patients with

mechanically assisted ventilation or selected postoperative patients) to determine trends and help identify outbreaks and other potential infection-control problems. The use of the new National Nosocomial Infection Surveillance (NNIS) system's surveillance definition of pneumonia is recommended. Include data on the causative microorganisms and their antimicrobial susceptibility patterns. Express data as rates (e.g., number of infected patients or infections per 100 ICU days or per 1,000 ventilator days) to facilitate intrahospital comparisons and trend determination. Link monitored rates and prevention efforts and return data to appropriate healthcare personnel (IB).

B. In the absence of specific clinical, epidemiologic, or infection-control objectives, do not routinely perform surveillance cultures of patients or of equipment or devices used for respiratory therapy, pulmonary-function testing, or delivery of inhalation anesthesia (II).

III. Prevention of Transmission of Microorganisms

A. Sterilization or Disinfection and Maintenance of Equipment and Devices

1. Thoroughly clean all equipment and devices to be sterilized or disinfected.

2. Mechanical ventilators:
   - Do not routinely sterilize or disinfect the internal machinery of mechanical ventilators.

3. Breathing circuits, humidifiers, and heat-and-moisture exchangers (HMEs):
   - Do not change routinely, on the basis of duration of use, the breathing circuit (i.e., ventilator tubing and exhalation valve and the attached humidifier) that is in use on an individual patient. Change the circuit when it is visibly soiled or mechanically malfunctioning.

(*continued*)

- Periodically drain and discard any condensate that collects in the tubing of a mechanical ventilator, taking precautions not to allow condensate to drain toward the patient.
- Wear gloves to perform the previous procedure and/or when handling the fluid. Decontaminate hands with soap and water (if hands are visibly soiled) or with an alcohol-based hand rub after performing the procedure or handling the fluid.

4. Humidifier fluids:
   - Use sterile (not distilled, nonsterile) water to fill bubbling humidifiers.
   - Ventilator breathing circuits with HMEs.

5. Changing an HME:
   - Change an HME that is in use on a patient when it malfunctions mechanically or becomes visibly soiled.
   - Do not routinely change more frequently than every 48 hours an HME that is in use on a patient.
   - Do not change routinely (in the absence of gross contamination or malfunction) the breathing circuit attached to an HME while it is in use on a patient.

6. Oxygen humidifiers:
   - Follow manufacturers' instructions for use of oxygen humidifiers.
   - Change the humidifier-tubing (including any nasal prongs or mask) that is in use when it malfunctions or becomes visibly contaminated.

7. Small-volume medication nebulizers: in-line and handheld nebulizers:
   - Between treatments on the same patient, clean, disinfect, and rinse with sterile water.

- Use only sterile fluid for nebulization, and dispense the fluid into the nebulizer aseptically.
- Whenever possible, use aerosolized medications in single-dose vials. If multidose medication vials are used, follow manufacturers' instructions for handling, storing, and dispensing the medications.

8. Other devices used in association with respiratory therapy:
   - Respirometer and ventilator thermometer: Between their uses on different patients, sterilize or subject to high-level disinfection portable respirometers and ventilator thermometers.
   - Resuscitation bags: Between their uses on different patients, sterilize or subject to high-level disinfection reusable hand-powered resuscitation bags.

B. Prevention of Person-to-Person Transmission of Bacteria
   1. Standard Precautions
      - Hand hygiene: Decontaminate hands by washing them with either antimicrobial soap and water or with nonantimicrobial soap and water (if hands are visibly dirty or contaminated with proteinaceous material or are soiled with blood or body fluids) or by using an alcohol-based waterless antiseptic agent (e.g., hand rub) if hands are not visibly soiled after contact with mucous membranes, respiratory secretions, or objects contaminated with respiratory secretions, whether or not gloves are worn. Decontaminate hands as described previously before and after contact with a patient who has an endotracheal or tracheostomy

(*continued*)

tube in place, and before and after contact with any respiratory device that is used on the patient, whether or not gloves are worn.

- Gloving: Wear gloves for handling respiratory secretions or objects contaminated with respiratory secretions of any patient.

- Change gloves and decontaminate hands between contacts with different patients; after handling respiratory secretions or objects contaminated with secretions from one patient and before contact with another patient, object, or environmental surface; and between contacts with a contaminated body site and the respiratory tract of, or respiratory device on, the same patient.

- When soiling with respiratory secretions from a patient is anticipated, wear a gown and change it after soiling occurs and before providing care to another patient.

2. Care of patients with tracheostomy:
   - Perform tracheostomy under aseptic conditions.
   - When changing a tracheostomy tube, wear a gown, use aseptic technique, and replace the tube with one that has undergone sterilization or high-level disinfection.

3. Suctioning of respiratory tract secretions:
   - If the open-system suction is employed, use a sterile, single-use catheter.
   - Use only sterile fluid to remove secretions from the suction catheter if the catheter is to be used for reentry into the patient's lower respiratory tract.

IV. Modifying Host Risk for Infection
  A. Increasing Host Defense Against Infection: Administration of Immune Modulators
    1. *Pneumococcal vaccination:* Vaccinate patients at high risk for severe pneumococcal infections.
  B. Precautions for Prevention of Aspiration
    1. As soon as the clinical indications for their use are resolved, remove devices such as endotracheal, tracheostomy, and/or enteral tubes.
    2. Prevention of aspiration associated with endotracheal intubation:
      • Use noninvasive ventilation (NIV) to reduce the need for and duration of endotracheal intubation.
      • When feasible and not medically contraindicated, use noninvasive positive pressure ventilation delivered continuously by face or nose mask, instead of performing endotracheal intubation in patients who are in respiratory failure yet do not need immediate intubation (e.g., those who are in hypercapneic respiratory failure secondary to acute exacerbation of COPD or cardiogenic pulmonary edema).
      • When feasible and not medically contraindicated, use NIV as part of the weaning process (from mechanically assisted ventilation) to shorten the period of endotracheal intubation.
      • As much as possible, avoid repeat endotracheal intubation in patients who have received mechanically assisted ventilation.
      • Unless contraindicated by the patient's condition, perform orotracheal

(continued)

rather than nasotracheal intubation on patients.

- If feasible, use an endotracheal tube with a dorsal lumen above the endotracheal cuff to allow drainage (by continuous or frequent intermittent suctioning) of tracheal secretions that accumulate in the patient's subglottic area.
- Before deflating the cuff of an endotracheal tube in preparation for tube removal, or before moving the tube, ensure that secretions are cleared from above the tube cuff.

3. Prevention of aspiration associated with enteral feeding:
   - In the absence of medical contraindication(s), elevate at an angle of 30 to 45 degrees the head of the bed of a patient at high risk for aspiration (e.g., a person receiving mechanically assisted ventilation and/or who has an enteral tube in place).
   - Routinely verify appropriate placement of the feeding tube.

4. Prevention or modulation of oropharyngeal colonization:
   - Oropharyngeal cleaning and decontamination with an antiseptic agent: Develop and implement a comprehensive oral hygiene program (which might include the use of an antiseptic agent) for patients in acute care settings or residents in long-term care facilities who are at high risk for health care-associated pneumonia.
   - Chlorhexidine oral rinse: Use an oral chlorhexidine gluconate (0.12%) rinse during the perioperative period

on adult patients who undergo cardiac surgery.
- Oral decontamination with topical antimicrobial agents.

C. Prevention of Postoperative Pneumonia
  1. Instruct preoperative patients, especially those at high risk for contracting pneumonia, about taking deep breaths and ambulating as soon as medically indicated in the postoperative period.
  2. Encourage all postoperative patients to take deep breaths, move about the bed, and ambulate unless medically contraindicated.
  3. Use incentive spirometry on postoperative patients at high risk for pneumonia.

Source: Centers for Disease Control and Prevention. (2003). *Prevention of health care-associated bacterial pneumonia.* Retrieved May 9, 2008, from http://www.cdc.gov/mmwr/preview/mmwrhtml/rr5303a1.htm.

Assessment and Care of the Ventilated Patient

Many of the interventions that are provided by nurses in caring for a patient on a ventilator determine the success of weaning and the prevention of complications.

Inspection

- Use a standardized method of observation—Head-to-toe method
- Check endotracheal tube for size and depth of insertion
- Assess the method of securing the tube

Critical Alert

A tube that is loose can cause pressure ulcers or, worse, accidental extubation. Presence of an oral airway is noted.

- The ventilator circuit is inspected:
  - Ensure that it is not pulling on the endotracheal tube or creating tension on the tube
  - Circuit should be free of fluid to prevent lavage into the trachea
- Amount and color of secretions in the endotracheal tube, mouth, and nose are noted. Position of the head is assessed: Avoid torsion of the neck muscles because of keeping their heads turned toward the side of the ventilator
- Agitation is assessed:
  - Hypoxemia should be ruled out as a cause before administering medication for sedation and analgesia. Cyanosis present around the mouth and mucous membranes suggests central cyanosis and hypoxemia.
- Chest wall for symmetrical breathing pattern between the right and left side of the chest. Observe for unusual movements.
  - Tension pneumothorax or pleural effusion
  - Paradoxical breathing—On inspiration the chest rises and the abdomen is drawn in because the fatigued diaphragm cannot descend on inspiration
  - Trauma to the chest
  - Muscle fatigue of the diaphragm
  - Use of accessory muscles of ventilation and work of breathing
  - Phrenic nerve injury or paralysis can produce asymmetry in inspiration or paradoxical movement of the diaphragm
- Abdomen for distention and protruding into the chest, preventing adequate ventilation? Upper extremities edema common with ventilator use for a significant period
- Mottling present in the extremities
- Any noise of escaping air heard on expiration (could be caused by too low a volume in the endotracheal tube cuff)

Palpation

- Deviation of the trachea (tension pneumothorax, flail chest, pneumonectomies)
- Chest wall—Feeling for any abnormalities, bulging, or depressions
- Point of maximal impulse (PMI)
- Palpating for fremitus—Pleural friction, rhonchial
- Subcutaneous emphysema (produced when small pockets of air are trapped under the skin)

Auscultation

Frequency is patient specific and based on other assessment parameters.

Listen posteriorly and anteriorly, starting at the top of the thorax and moving down.

Compare Right Against Left Lung

- Normal lung sounds heard in abnormal locations can alert the nurse to certain abnormalities.
- Crackles occur first in the bases and without the posterior exam the majority of the lung fields cannot be assessed.
- Inspiratory or expiratory wheezes could be the result of a constriction of the bronchi. Gurgles or rhonchi should prompt suctioning the endotracheal tube.
- Diminished lung sounds can indicate pleural fluid accumulation or pneumothorax.
- When abnormal or absent sounds are observed, a portable chest x-ray is ordered.

Critical Alert

Tension pneumothorax is more common in patients who are receiving positive pressure ventilation. Air enters the pleural space through a defect in the lung parenchyma and is trapped in the pleural space. As the pressure in the pleural space increases from the trapped air, the lung collapses and the pressure displaces the trachea and great vessels to the opposite side. If not relieved, the remaining lung collapses. This can occur very rapidly. Successful treatment is a needle thoracostomy and placement of a chest tube.

Nutrition

- Preventing malnutrition is another important concern for care.

  - Enteral feeding via a nasogastric or oral gastric feeding tube is the preferred method. Small lumen feeding tubes are being used more often than larger bore feeding tubes because of increased patient comfort.

- Aspiration and other complications including malposition can be prevented by instituting standard protocols and by monitoring problems associated with these tubes at the unit level.

  - Interventions to prevent aspiration include keeping the head of the bed elevated and administering medications to assist with gastric motility.

Communication and Sleep

- Inability to communicate is a concern for the patient

  - Many devices are now available to provide some method for communication.

  - Speaking tracheostomy tube message board with an alphabet or symbols

- Lack of sleep

  - Periods of rest and uninterrupted sleep should be in the plan of care.

Weaning from Mechanical Ventilation

Patients who have been critically ill or "chronically critically ill" and required prolonged mechanical ventilation have difficulty being liberated from the ventilator.

Weaning is the process of discontinuation of a patient from the ventilator.

- The best process of weaning patients is by a multidisciplinary team approach.

- Successful weaning is important to patients in order to ensure continued recovery from their respiratory failure.

Noninvasive Positive Pressure Ventilation (NPPV)

Noninvasive positive pressure ventilation is the administration of pressure support and PEEP delivered via a face mask or nasal mask. NPPV avoids many of the complications of mechanical ventilation with placement of an endotracheal tube. Patients who are on NPPV can communicate, eat, and require very little, if any, sedation. Figure 36-11 illustrates one type of interface, an oronasal mask that is used to initiate NPPV.

- NPPV typically require more frequent assessments
  - Continuous heart rate, pulse oximetry (SpO_2)
- Complications
  - Potentially fatal complication is aspiration, because the airway is not protected
  - Facial trauma related to the tight-fitting mask
  - Abdominal distention

Contraindications to Noninvasive Positive Pressure Ventilation

- Cardiac or respiratory arrest
- Nonrespiratory organ failure
- Severe encephalopathy (e.g., GCS < 10)
- Severe upper gastrointestinal bleeding

- Hemodynamic instability or unstable cardiac arrhythmia
- Facial surgery, trauma, or deformity
- Upper airway obstruction
- Inability to cooperate/protect the airway
- Inability to clear respiratory secretions
- High risk for aspiration

Source: International Consensus Conferences in Intensive Care Medicine: Noninvasive Positive Pressure Ventilation in Acute Respiratory Failure. Organized jointly by the American Thoracic Society, the European Respiratory Society, the European Society of Intensive Care Medicine, and the Societé de Reanimation de Langue Française, and approved by ATS Board of Directors, December 2000. *American Journal of Respiratory and Critical Care Medicine, 163*(1), 288.

(See Appendix #37 Nursing Process: Patient Care Plan for Patient Receiving Noninvasive Positive Pressure Ventilation.)

Nasogastric Tubes

Nasogastric tubes are inserted to decompress the stomach, allow for gastric drainage, and provide a method to administer medications/nutrition when the patient cannot eat normally.

Nursing Management

- Maintain low intermittent suction
- Check placement every 4 hours.
  - Aspirate stomach contents and check pH
  - Insert 10 milliliters of air rapidly while listening with stethoscope over the stomach to hear the rush of air
- Monitor skin integrity of nostril of insertion and provide skin care
- Monitor bowel sounds (suction off)

- Irrigate tube with 30 milliliters NS every 4 hours or as needed to maintain patency
- Measure NG drainage at least every 8 hours
- Blue port
  - Never irrigate
  - If leaking, place it at the patient's shoulder
  - Do not plug the port unless ordered by the health care provider

Nephrostomy Tube

- Placed percutaneously under fluoroscopy or surgically
- Placed through the flank area into the renal pelvis and secured to a closed drainage system to allow drainage via gravity flow
- Preprocedure precautions:
  - Antibiotics to prevent infection
  - Coagulopathy corrected
  - Uncontrolled hypertension corrected

Nursing Management

- Assess the tube for kinks or clots that may impede drainage
- Assess for complications such as bleeding at and around the site, hematuria, fistula formation, and infection
- Assess insertion site for signs of inflammation, infection, bleeding, leakage of urine, and skin irritation
- Assess tube patency
  - Complaints of pain and pressure
- Use aseptic technique when replacing dressings
- Encourage oral intake of fluids to promote flushing of the kidney and nephrostomy tube
- Avoid clamping the nephrostomy tube
- Never irrigate a nephrostomy tube without specific orders

Paracentesis

Paracentesis involves removing fluid from the abdominal cavity to relieve dyspnea. A small-bore trocar is inserted into the peritoneal cavity and connected to vacuum tubing which allows fluid to be drained into a collection bottle. Daily removal of 500–1000 mL may be effective without increasing the risk of fluid and electrolyte imbalance. However, the removal of 4 to 6 liters of fluid may be needed to effectively relieve the respiratory symptoms.

Nursing Management

- Preprocedure
  - Weigh patient
  - Take vital signs and measure abdominal girth
  - Have the patient empty his bladder
  - Place sitting in an upright position, seated in a chair if possible
  - Assemble needed equipment
- During Procedure
  - Monitor blood pressure, pulse, and respiratory rate and effort
  - Reassure the patient and family
- Postprocedure
  - Monitor vital signs, especially blood pressure and respiratory effort
  - Monitor for bleeding or excessive drainage from the puncture site
  - Administer albumin if ordered
  - Send specimens to the laboratory for analysis if ordered
  - Change dressing as needed
  - Monitor for infection

Parenteral Nutrition

Parenteral nutritional support is indicated in the patient who is unable to tolerate adequate enteral nutrition for more than 1 week.

- Total parenteral nutrition (TPN) is delivered via a central line
  - Indicated in patients requiring support for at least 10 days
  - TPN is able to meet most patients' complete nutritional requirements
- Peripheral parenteral nutrition (PPN) is delivered via a peripheral vein
  - Used as short-term nutrition intervention to offset nutritional requirements until transition to alternative enteral nutrition is initiated
  - PPN is limited by the volume of fluid that can be tolerated peripherally and the lower concentration of nutrients that is required to maintain an isotonic concentration
  - May not provide complete nutrition for some patients and is only a short-term solution

Percutaneous Coronary Interventions (PCI)
(See "Cardiac Catheterization" for diagnostic procedure.)

Percutaneous coronary intervention (PCI) includes all devices used either to remove plaque or to alter its morphology in the catheterization laboratory. Such devices include intracoronary lasers, which can be used to open totally occluded coronary arteries; intracoronary balloons, intracoronary stents; and atherectomy devices, which shave the plaque and remove it. PCI angiographic success ranges from 96% to 99%, with MACE event rates from 0.2% to 3%, depending on the event measured. Long-term outcomes (5 to 10 years) are more difficult to measure, due to continuous changes in technology such as improved coronary stents, as well as clinical factors such as an increase in the number of elderly patients with poor left ventricular function undergoing PCI.

Patients undergoing PCI range from the stable person having an elective first procedure to the patient with an acute myocardial infarction (AMI) who is hemodynamically unstable, requiring ventilatory and inotropic support during the procedure. The clinical status of the patient and the planned procedure will dictate the exact patient management.

Class I Indications for Percutaneous Coronary Intervention (PCI)

Asymptomatic to Mild Angina

- Patients who do not have treated diabetes with one or more significant lesions in one or more coronary arteries and a high likelihood of successful PCI. The artery to be dilated must perfuse a large area of viable myocardium.

Moderate to severe symptoms, unstable angina, or non-ST segment elevation myocardial infarction

- Patients with one or more significant lesions in one or more coronary arteries suitable for PCI and a high likelihood of success. The artery to be dilated must perfuse a moderate or large area of viable myocardium.

Acute Myocardial Infarction (AMI)

- As an alternative to thrombolytic therapy in patients with ST segment elevation AMI or new left bundle branch block, if the patient can undergo PCI < 12 hours from the onset of ischemic symptoms or > 12 hours if symptoms persist and PCI can be performed quickly in a laboratory with experienced personnel and adequate equipment.
- In patients who are within 36 hours of an ST elevation AMI who develop cardiogenic shock, who are < 75 years old, and revascularization can be completed within 18 hours of the onset of shock in a laboratory with experienced personnel and adequate equipment.

Prior Coronary Artery Bypass Surgery

- Patients with ischemia within 30 days of surgery

Prior to Heart Catheterization and PCI

- Complete assessment, with special attention to the cardiovascular and peripheral vascular system, and renal function
- Indicate all medication taken, including warfarin, metformin, diuretics, or insulin
- Verify NPO status as ordered
- Review baseline laboratory values include serum chemistries, coagulation factors, and a complete blood count
- Teach patient and family about procedure and post-procedural care

Postprocedure

- Assessment includes:
    - Vital signs
    - ECG monitoring
    - Urine output
    - Pulses distal to the puncture site
- Physical examination of the vascular access site
    - Hemostasis
    - Presence of hematoma
        - Localized swelling, tenderness, discoloration
    - Presence of pseudoaneurysm or arteriovenous fistula
        - Bruit, a pulsatile mass
    - Presence of retroperitoneal hematoma
        - Flank or back pain
        - Nausea and vomiting
        - Hypotension and bradycardia—vaso-vagal response

Complications

- Myocardial infarction
- Neurological events

- Renal complications
- Dysrhythmias
- Vascular problems

Patient Care Management

Care of patients with CAD undergoing urgent PCI requires a collaborative approach among all members of the health care team in different areas of the hospital, such as the emergency department, the cardiac critical care unit, the pharmacy, the catheterization laboratory, the cardiovascular operating room, and the step-down units. Staff must be aware of the need for urgent identification and treatment of any patient presenting with AMI. Medications including antiplatelet and antithrombotic agents need to be started as soon as the diagnosis is confirmed.

Suctioning Procedure

Equipment
Sterile suction catheter
Sterile gloves
Sterile normal saline for irrigation, when indicated
Sterile disposable container

Technique
1. Perform routine procedures before suction. Administer medication, assemble equipment, explain the procedure to the patient, adjust bed to comfortable working position, prepare suction pressure, wash hands, and don gloves.
2. Hyperoxygenate the patient with 100% oxygen, using a manual resuscitation bag (MRB) or the ventilator. If the ventilator method is used, preoxygenation must last at least 3 minutes. Return to the previous oxygen setting after suctioning is completed. (Clinical research shows that the use of the patient's ventilator

for preoxygenation delivers higher oxygen concentrations and lower peak pressures than those generated with an MRB. In patients who do not tolerate suction with hyperoxygenation, a positive end-expiratory pressure (PEEP) attachment should be on the MRB at the appropriate setting, or in-line suctioning should be used to avoid loss of PEEP and desaturation.

3. Quickly, but gently, insert the catheter as far as possible into the artificial airway without application of suction.

4. Withdraw the catheter 1–2 cm, and apply intermittent suction while rotating and removing the catheter. Limit suction pressure to -80 to -120 mm Hg. Aspiration should not exceed 10 to 15 seconds. (Prolonged aspiration can lead to severe hypoxia, hemodynamic instability, and ultimately, cardiac arrest.

5. Hyperoxygenate the patient before and after each subsequent pass of the catheter for at least 30 seconds, and before reconnection to the ventilator.

6. Monitor heart rate and rhythm and pulse oximetry during and after suctioning. Discontinue the procedure if the patient does not tolerate it as evidenced by dysthymia, bradycardia, 9r a drop in Sao_2.

7. Remove equipment.

8. Perform oral hygiene.

9. Clean suction tubing.

10. Wash your hands.

11. Document procedure.

Source: Doering, L. V. (1993). The effect of positioning on hemodynamics and gas exchange in the critically ill: a review. *American Journal of Critical Care, 2,* 208–216. Used with permission; Morton, P. G., Fontaine, D. K., Hudak, C. M., & Gallo, B. M. 8th ed. (2005) Philadelphia, Lippincott, Williams & Wilkins.

Tracheostomy

Patients with severe facial injuries, edema in the head and neck area, infection, surgery, large obstructive tumors, or neurological changes to the larynx may require a tracheostomy. The tracheostomy tube is sutured into place to prevent inadvertent dislodgement. In addition, ties are placed through the faceplate of the tracheostomy tube and around the neck to further secure the tube. The tube remains sutured in place until the tract from the anterior neck into the trachea becomes well established. A post-tracheostomy tray is kept at the bedside or on the nursing unit for use in the event of early accidental decannulation or early tube obstruction.

Characteristics of Tracheostomy Tubes

- Usually made of silicone, plastic, stainless steel, or silver
- Contains the outer tube and inner cannula
  - Inner cannula
    - Disposable: Replaced with a new one as part of routine tracheostomy care to ensure patency of airway
    - Reusable: Removed, cleansed, and reinserted as part of routine tracheostomy care
    - The inner cannula serves as a safety device
- Tracheostomy face plate has openings to hold trach ties (or collar) which wrap around the neck to help secure tube in place
- Cuff tubes are used for patients on mechanical ventilation to seal the airway around the tube, but are not intended to hold it in place

Nursing Management

- Ineffective Airway Clearance
  - Auscultate lung sounds
  - Assess oxygen saturation
  - Monitor RR and work of breathing

- Suction as needed and note characteristics and amount of sputum
- Note presence of blood in sputum and notify health care provider accordingly
- Monitor for subcutaneous emphysema in the neck
- Provide humidification to tracheostomy as needed
- Perform tracheostomy care per facility policy
- Monitor skin integrity under and around tracheostomy face plate

Keep suction equipment, ambu bag, tracheostomy obturator, and additional complete tracheostomy tube set at bedside for emergency purposes.

Transplantation: Bone Marrow and Peripheral Blood Stem Cell

Bone marrow transplantation (BMT) offers patients the ability to receive intensive chemotherapy or radiation therapy when resistance to or failure of standard treatment occurs. BMT is the transfer of hematopoietic cells from the bone marrow of one person into another person and has been used to treat a variety of diseases. Peripheral blood stem cell (PBSC) transplantation is becoming more widely used in lieu of the traditional bone marrow transplantation. Indications for transplantation include malignant disorders, although success has been demonstrated for use in patients with nonmalignant diseases.

The types of BMT are based on where the donor cells originate, see following chart.

BMT Are Based on Donor Cells

Type	Origin
Allogeneic	• Syngeneic: identical twin • Related: blood relative, usually sibling • Unrelated: located by National Bone Marrow Registry or Cord Blood Registry
Autologous	• Patient

The Donor Process

Peripheral Blood Stem Cells

- Autologous PBSC
  - Mobilization
    - Stimulating the production of PBSCs with the administration of G-CSF or GM-CSF, possibly with chemotherapy.
  - Apheresis
    - Collection of PBSCs through a double-lumen central venous catheter that is placed into the patient.
    - Blood is run through a cell separator that is programmed to collect either lymphocytes or low-density leukocytes and return other blood components to the patient.
    - Apheresis usually takes one to three sessions each lasting 3 to 4 hours.
    - Collected stem cells are placed into a blood bag and cryopreserved and remain frozen at $-196°C$ until needed for transplantation.
- Allogeneic PBSC
  - Mobilization

    (See Autologous PBSC)
  - Apheresis

    (See Autologous PBSC)
    - Via a peripheral line inserted into the antecubital veins using the cell separator
  - Side effects (donor)
    - Bone pain, headache, fatigue, nausea, and insomnia
    - ↓ Platelet count (up to 50%)
      - Risk of bleeding

Bone Marrow Harvesting

- Autologous
  - Occurs in the operating room, likely under general anesthesia.

- Multiple punctures are made in the posterior or anterior iliac crest to obtain the necessary amount (500 to 700 mL) of marrow needed for transplant.
- Obtained marrow is obtained; it is mixed with heparin, filtered to remove bone fragments and fat, and placed into a blood bag.
- Bone marrow is purged (the process of removing any remaining malignant cells from the marrow) then placed into blood bag and frozen until needed.
- Allogeneic
  - Same as autologous harvesting minus the purging
  - Immediately transfused into the recipient

Umbilical Cord Blood

Collection and storage of umbilical cord blood (UCB), which is rich in stem cells, is the newest innovation in transplantation. Cord blood is obtained by withdrawing blood via the umbilical vein immediately after the umbilical cord has been clamped. The blood is then cryopreserved similar to that of PBSCs or bone marrow.

The Transplantation Process

Selection of the appropriate donor and recipient is crucial so graft rejection and other serious complications are avoided.

Criteria for Donor

- Histocompatibility as measured by HLA and mixed lymphocyte culture (MLC).
- The donor's health status is evaluated.
- The donor's psychosocial profile is evaluated.
- The donor's age is taken into consideration due to the amount of marrow needed for transplantation.

Recipient Preparation

- Initial evaluation
  - Multidisciplinary approach (to determine the recipient's physical and psychosocial status)
    - Laboratory tests and procedures
    - Consultations

- Conditioning (preparing the patient to receive bone marrow or stem cells)
  - High-dose chemotherapy (HDCT) with or without radiotherapy (results in severe myelosuppression)
  - Develops space in the marrow cavity for the transplanted stem cells as they begin reproducing
- Transplantation
  - Rapid IV push using syringes or by hanging the bag of cells and infusing over 20 to 30 minutes (autologous)
  - Infused slowly over 1 to 5 hours (allogeneic marrow or stem cells)
  - Engraftment: establishment of new bone marrow
    - Bone marrow engrafts within 3 weeks
    - Stem cells engraft within 11 to 16 days
    - Cord blood engrafts in 26 to 42 days

Complications of Transplantation
- Bleeding
- Infection
- Nausea, vomiting, and diarrhea
- Mucositis
- Graft-versus-host disease (GVHD)
  - Occurs after allogeneic transplants
  - Result of an immune-mediated reaction of the new stem cells reacting to the body of the recipient (antibodies attack the host tissues)
  - Sites: skin, liver, intestines, and the recipient's immune system cells
  - Chronic GVHD (several months to several years after transplant)
    - Avascular necrosis (AVN)
    - Osteoporosis
    - Cataracts

- Gonadal dysfunction
- Growth failure
- Hypothyroidism
- Secondary malignancies
- Need for revaccinations

Nursing Management

(See Appendix #36: Nursing Process: Care Plan for the Oncology Patient.)

T-Tubes

A T-tube is placed if stones are located in the common bile duct to maintain patency, allowing bile to pass from the liver into the duodenum until the edema from surgery diminishes.

Nursing Management

- Attach tube to sterile gravity drainage
    - Place patient in Fowler's position to maximize gravity drainage
- Monitor drainage and record the amount every 8 hours
    - Usual 500 and 1,000 mL on the first day, decreasing to about 200 mLs by day three.
    - Drainage may be blood tinged at first but becomes green-brown.
    - Drainage in excess of 500 mL by day three is excessive, and the surgeon must be notified.
- Monitor color of the stools
    - Pale stools indicate obstruction of flow of bile to duodenum.
- Clamp the T-tube as ordered, and monitor the patient's response to clamping
- Keep skin clean and free from bile drainage
    - Skin can be protected with zinc oxide, karaya, or other barrier.

- Teach the patient how to care for the tube during activities of daily living
    - Instruct on the signs of infection, such as fever, redness, swelling, or drainage from the site, as well as care for the tube, avoiding any direct pulling or traction on the tube. Showers only, no bathing.

Tube Feedings

The purpose of a gastrostomy tube or a jejunostomy tube is to provide complete nutrition through the alimentary system. It is safer and has fewer side effects than total parenteral nutrition (TPN), particularly when the patient is to have feedings at home.

Tube Feedings, Nursing Management

Problem	Intervention
Potential for foodborne illness	• Wash hands before handling formula and equipment. • Wipe off top of formula container before opening. • Label, cover, and store open formula in refrigerator for not >24 hours. • Limit "hang time" to 4 hours if water or other additions made to formula. Otherwise 8- to 12-hour hang time allowed if canned formula w/no additives is being used.
Aspiration	• Check gastric residuals. Hold feeding for large volume (>150 mL but treat individually and according to health care provider's order). • Elevate head of bed to at least a 30-degree angle. • Avoid bolus feedings. • Consider smaller bore or longer tube if nasally intubated. Routinely confirm tube placement. • Consider G-tube or J-tube if long-term feeding is required.

Problem	Intervention

Clogged tube	• Administer feeding with pump vs. gravity drip.
	• Administer room temperature feeding. High-temperature storage or heating of formula will cause protein content to coagulate.
	• Follow guidelines for medication administration:
	  1. Flush tube with 20 to 30 mL water before, between, and after each single medication.
	  2. Consult pharmacist regarding suitability of crushing medication with a small amount of water and availability of medication elixirs.
	
	Note: If using longer feeding tubes, ensure medication absorption site is not bypassed by tube.

Diarrhea	• Administer feeding at room temperature. Cold feeding increases gut peristalsis. • Consider lactose-free formula. • Consider formula with fiber. • Consider medications w/cathartic effect: antibiotics, magnesium, potassium, digoxin, theophylline, acetaminophen elixir, and others. • Administer continuous drip vs. bolus. • Consult registered dietitian regarding temporarily altering formula concentration or rate of delivery. • Rule out infection, *Clostridium difficile,* medical etiology.

(*continued*)

Tube Feedings, Nursing Management (*continued*)

Problem	Intervention
Constipation	• Consider formula with added fiber. • Monitor hydration; ensure adequate intake. • Encourage ambulation as indicated. • Assess for contributing medications (e.g., narcotics, some antacids). • Consider obstruction or medical causes.
Dehydration	• Monitor hydration: weight, intake & output, physical signs. • Ensure adequate free water intake. Need 1 mL water per 1 kcal of intake. Most formulas are 50%–75% free water (formula with >1 kcal/mL or high protein content have less free water).

Sources: Rees Parrish, C., & Falls McCray, S. (2003). Nutrition support for the mechanically ventilated patient. *Critical Care Nurse, 23,* 77–80.; Dobson, K., & Scott, A. (2007). Review of ICU nutrition support practices: Implementing the nurse-led enteral feeding algorithm. *Nursing in Critical Care, 12,* 114–123; Swanson, R. W., & Winkelman, C. (2002). Exploring the benefits and myths of enteral feeding in the critically ill. *Critical Care Nursing Quarterly, 24,* 67–75.

APPENDIXES

#1 Nursing Process: Patient Care Plan for the Postoperative Patient Following General Surgery

Assessment of Discomfort

Subjective Data:
Ask the patient to describe the pain, its location and intensity. Ask patient to rate pain from 0–10 on the pain scale.

Objective Data:
Watch for physical signs of pain including guarding, grimacing, crying, increased blood pressure (BP), heart rate (HR), and respiratory rate (RR).

Nursing Assessment and Diagnoses	Outcomes and Evaluation Parameters	Interventions with *Rationales*
Nursing Diagnosis: *Readiness for Enhanced Comfort* related to surgical incision, muscle spasm, positioning in the operating room, the presence of drains, and anxiety	**Outcome:** The patient will be comfortable and rate the pain at a 3 or less. **Evaluation Parameters:** Patient is comfortable. Patient participates in postoperative activities and exercises without discomfort.	**Interventions and Rationales:** Use pain scale (0–10) to assess pain every 2–4 hours. *Increases consistency in quantifying pain.* Watch for physical signs of pain including guarding, grimacing, crying, increased BP, HR, and RR. *Some patients are reluctant to ask for pain medication. Different cultures respond to and express pain differently.* Administer pain medication, narcotics, and anti-inflammatory agents as prescribed. *Postoperative pain is highest in the first 48 hours after surgery.* Provide teaching about patient controlled analgesia (PCA) or patient controlled epidural analgesia (PCEA) if prescribed. Elevate affected area if appropriate to *decrease tissue swelling.* Apply ice to affected area if appropriate to *decrease tissue swelling.* Teach to splint the incision. *Provides stability to injured area.* Use nonpharmacologic interventions such as massage, distraction, relaxation techniques. *These measures augment other pain control measures.*

Assessment of Nausea and Vomiting

Subjective Data:
Ask patient about feeling nauseated.

Objective Data:
Patient vomits.
Abdomen is firm, distended with hypoactive bowel sounds.

Nursing Assessment and Diagnoses	Outcomes and Evaluation Parameters	Interventions with Rationales
Nursing Diagnosis: Alteration in Nausea related to anesthesia, narcotics, antibiotics, slowed peristalsis	*Outcomes:* Patient will get relief from nausea and vomiting. Patient will have a soft abdomen and pass flatus. Patient will have adequate intake of fluids. *Evaluation Parameters:* Abdomen soft. Appetite is present. Oral fluid intake is 1,500–2,500 mL in 24 hours. Passing flatus and stool.	*Interventions and Rationales:* Assess for nausea, vomiting, abdominal distention, and flatus. *Most nausea and vomiting peaks in 24 to 36 hours after surgery.* Maintain nasogastric tube (NGT) as prescribed for comfort. *An NGT decompresses the stomach and prevents vomiting.* Maintain NPO status until nausea recedes and bowel function returns. *Flatus and passing stool are the best indicators that bowel function has returned.* Advance diet slowly from ice chips to clear liquids to full liquids and regular diet. *Vomiting can occur when the diet is advanced too rapidly.* Medicate with antinausea medication as prescribed. *Early administration of medication is more effective than waiting until the patient experiences nausea and vomiting.* Encourage patient to change positions slowly. *Movement is a trigger for nausea and vomiting.* Provide comfort measures such as rest, a cool washcloth, mouth care, and deep breathing.

(continued)

623

#1 Nursing Process: Patient Care Plan for the Postoperative Patient Following General Surgery (Continued)

Assessment of Fluid Volume

Subjective Data:
Patient reports vertigo.
Are you thirsty?

Objective Data:
Watch for signs of active bleeding including blood on dressing, hematoma, presence of blood in drainage tubes, and decreased hematocrit and hemoglobin.

Watch for signs of dehydration including heart rate (HR) >100, systolic blood pressure (BP) < 90, narrow pulse pressure, decreased urine output of < 30 mL/hour or < 0.5 mL/kg per hour.

Nursing Assessment and Diagnoses	Outcomes and Evaluation Parameters	Interventions with Rationales
Nursing Diagnosis: Deficient Fluid Volume related to hemorrhage, blood loss with surgery, fluid loss, wound drains, vomiting, or fever	*Outcome:* Patient will have adequate hemostatsis and normal intravascular volume. *Evaluation Parameters:* Normal vital signs. Urine output > 0.5 mL/kg per hour. No evidence of active bleeding.	*Interventions and Rationales:* Assess for indications of bleeding and dehydration every 1–4 hours. *There is a higher risk of bleeding if surgery is performed on tissue that is vascular. The patient is most at risk for dehydration in the first 24–48 hours postop.* Report HR > 120, systolic blood pressure (SBP) < 90, urine output < 30 mL/hour or < 0.5 mL/kg per hour, or more drainage than expected on dressing or in tubes. *Indicators of inadequate fluid volume and possible postoperative bleeding.* Check dressing and circle any new drainage with pen *to monitor for bleeding.*

Reinforce dressing as needed. *The surgeon changes the primary dressing.*
Administer IV fluids as ordered *to replace fluids lost during surgery.*
Administer normal saline fluid bolus if required. *Used to expand blood volume and increase urine output.*

Assessment of Fluid Volume

Subjective Data:
Patient reports dyspnea.

Objective Data:
Swelling in hands, feet, and eyelids, weight gain, urine output < 30 mL/hr or < 0.5 mL/kg per hour crackles in the lungs.

Nursing Assessment and Diagnoses	Outcomes and Evaluation Parameters	Interventions with *Rationales*
Nursing Diagnosis: *Risk for Excess Fluid Volume* related to response to stress hormones, excess intravenous fluids, or preexisting medical condition such as congestive heart failure	**Outcome:** Patient will have adequate fluid volume without evidence of overload. *Evaluation Parameters:* Urine output is > 30 mL/hr or > 0.5 mL/kg per hour. Intake and output (I&O) is balanced. Clear breath sounds. Normal vital signs without tachycardia or tachypnea.	**Interventions and Rationales:** Assess for swelling, weight gain, urine output < 30 mL/hr or < 0.5 mL/kg per hour, crackles in lungs, and dyspnea every 1–4 hours. *The effect of stress hormones is greatest in the first 24–48 hours.* Monitor IV fluid administration carefully. *Fluid given too rapidly can exacerbate fluid overload.*

(continued)

#1 Nursing Process: Patient Care Plan for the Postoperative Patient Following General Surgery (Continued)

Assessment of Respiratory Status

Subjective Data:

Patient states it is painful to take deep breaths.

Objective Data:

Watch for fever, diminished breath sounds, crackles in the lungs, sputum production, increased respiratory rate, and decreased oxygen saturation.

Nursing Assessment and Diagnoses	Outcomes and Evaluation Parameters	Interventions with Rationales
Nursing Diagnosis: *Ineffective Breathing Pattern* related to anesthesia, surgical pain, location of the surgery, limited mobility, a history of smoking, or preexisting medical condition	**Outcome:** Respiratory status will be stable and within normal limits. **Evaluation Parameters:** Afebrile. Clear lung sounds. Oxygen saturation > 93%. Normal respiratory rate. Denies shortness of breath and air hunger.	**Interventions and Rationales:** Monitor respiratory rate, depth, breath sounds, and oxygen saturation every 4 hours *to assess for atelectasis.* Encourage deep breathing or use of incentive spirometry 10 times every hour *to increase maximal inspiration and stimulate surfactant.* Encourage patient to cough every hour. Splint incision if appropriate. *Coughing clears mucous secretions.* Elevate head of the bed 30 degrees or higher *to lower the diaphragm and facilitate lung expansion.* Provide adequate pain relief. *Patients consistently give high pain ratings to coughing and deep breathing.*

Ambulate three times daily. *Increases RR, minute ventilation, and tidal volume.*
Titrate oxygen (O_2) to maintain the O_2 saturation at or > 93%. *Oxygen dries the airways and reduces mucociliary clearance.*

Assessment of Urine Output

Subjective Data:
Patient states he cannot void or is only able to void small amounts.

Objective Data:
Patient does not void or voids only small amounts.
Palpable fullness above symphysis pubis or a bladder scan showing a full bladder.

Nursing Assessment and Diagnoses	Outcomes and Evaluation Parameters	Interventions with Rationales
Nursing Diagnosis: Urinary Retention related to anesthesia, narcotics, anticholinergic medications, or spasm of abdominal or pelvic muscles	*Outcome:* Patient voids > 100–150 mL within 6–8 hours after surgery or after removal of Foley catheter. *Evaluation Parameters:* I&O is balanced. Voids adequate amounts without difficulty.	*Interventions and Rationales:* Monitor I&O to determine adequacy of urine output. *Inability to void may be due to dehydration.* Encourage oral fluids if appropriate. *Inability to void may be due to dehydration.* Ambulate frequently *to stimulate circulation and production of urine.* Perform measures to stimulate voiding reflex (i.e., use commode rather than bedpan; have male patients stand to use urinal; run warm water over perineum; use spirits of peppermints). If patient is unable to void 8 hours after surgery or after Foley catheter is removed, perform a bladder scan and call the surgeon for an order to perform catheterization. *The patient should feel the urge to void when the bladder has 300 mL of urine.*

(continued)

#1 Nursing Process: Patient Care Plan for the Postoperative Patient Following General Surgery (Continued)

Assessment of Activity Level

Subjective Data:
Patient states he has vertigo, fatigue, or dyspnea with activity.

Objective Data:
Positive orthostatic vital signs with activity or an increased heart rate of > 10 beats/minute, increased respiratory rate of > 10 beats/minute, decreased oxygen saturation, or labored breathing with activity.

Nursing Assessment and Diagnoses	Outcomes and Evaluation Parameters	Interventions with Rationales
Nursing Diagnosis: Activity Intolerance related to anesthesia, narcotics, surgery, and limited mobility	*Outcome:* Patient will carry out postoperative activities and activities of daily living without signs of activity intolerance. *Evaluation Parameters:* Ambulates without experiencing symptoms. Completes activities of daily living without experiencing symptoms. Postactivity vital signs and oxygen saturation are within normal limits.	*Interventions and Rationales:* Encourage muscle strengthening activities every shift *to increase circulation.* Encourage use of slow changes in position. Dangle legs at bedside before attempting to ambulate. Assist with two people during first attempt at ambulation *to provide for patient safety.* If symptomatic, take orthostatic vital signs and notify surgeon. Anticipate administering a fluid bolus. *Positive orthostatic vital signs are an indication of dehydration.* Ambulate a minimum of three times daily.

Assessment of Wound

Subjective Data:

Patient states that incision feels painful and swollen.

Objective Data:

Incision is red, painful, or swollen. Wound edges are not approximated and the wound has increased drainage.

Elevated white blood cells count (WBC) and fever.

Nursing Assessment and Diagnoses	Outcomes and Evaluation Parameters	Interventions with Rationales
Nursing Diagnosis: *Risk for Infection* related to altered skin integrity, and high-risk factors (e.g., diabetes, obesity, diminished arterial circulation, malnutrition)	**Outcomes:** The patient will be free from infection. The wound will heal within appropriately 7–10 days. **Evaluation Parameters:** The patient is afebrile. The wound edges are well approximated without drainage, redness, or swelling.	**Interventions and Rationales:** Monitor temperature, WBC count, and serum glucose. *Infection causes a fever and increased WBC and glucose.* Change dressing every shift using sterile technique and monitor for signs of infection. *The inflammatory response in an infected wound will cause redness, pain, swelling, and drainage.* Encourage adequate nutrition that is high in protein and vitamins. *Protein, calories, calcium, iron, zinc, and vitamins A, B_6, B_{12}, and C are needed for wound healing.*

Assessment of Blood Flow to the Extremities

Subjective Data:

Patient complains of pain in calf.

Objective Data:

Calf is red, painful, and swollen. Patient reports a positive Homans' sign.

(continued)

629

#1 Nursing Process: Patient Care Plan for the Postoperative Patient Following General Surgery (Continued)

Nursing Assessment and Diagnoses	Outcomes and Evaluation Parameters	Interventions with Rationales
Nursing Diagnosis: *Ineffective Tissue Perfusion, Venous Stasis* related to immobility, surgical procedure, and high-risk factors (e.g., age, use of estrogen, cancer, history of previous deep vein thrombosis [DVT])￼	**Outcome:** The patient will have adequate peripheral circulation and no evidence of DVT. **Evaluation Parameters:** Palpable dorsal pedis and posterior tibialis pulses. Calf is pain free without evidence of redness or swelling.	**Interventions and Rationales:** Assess for signs of DVT. A red, warm, swollen, or painful calf alerts the nurse to the possibility of a venous clot. *Venous thrombosis is most likely to occur 5 to 7 days after surgery.* Administer anticoagulant medication as prescribed *to prevent clot formation.* Measure the circumference of the calf and thigh of each leg and compare them prn. *The leg will increase in size with DVT formation.* Any indication of a clot is reported immediately to the health care provider. *Early treatment will decrease the risk of further clot formation.* The patient is placed on bed rest until the possibility of a clot is evaluated. *There is an increased chance of clot migration with activity.* Encourage ambulation and leg exercises three times daily *to stimulate circulation.* Apply pneumatic compression boots, antiembolism stockings or other antithrombotic devices as ordered *to increase venous return and prevent venous stasis.* Avoid pressure under the knees. *Venous compression contributes to the development of DVT.*

Assessment of Knowledge Regarding Surgery and Postoperative Care

Subjective Data:
Patient states that she needs information on how to care for herself at home.

Objective Data:
Patient is being discharged home following a recent surgery.

Nursing Assessment and Diagnoses	Outcomes and Evaluation Parameters	Interventions with Rationales
Nursing Diagnosis: Deficient Knowledge related to postoperative care	*Outcomes:* The patient will recover from surgery without complications. The patient is knowledgeable about how to care for herself at home. *Evaluation Parameters:* Demonstrates appropriate care of her wound and drains (if applicable). Verbalizes an understanding of pain management. Verbalizes an understanding of activity restrictions and other discharge instructions. Verbalizes an understanding of danger signs and what to do about them.	*Interventions and Rationales: The specific information taught depends on the surgery (refer to the appropriate disorder chapter in this text for specific information) and the preferences of the surgeon. General areas for teaching are listed below.* Teaching is done in the patient's native language, through an interpreter, if necessary. • General information about recovery • Wound care • Activity • Specific exercises to aid recovery • Diet • Medication • Symptom management: pain, constipation, fatigue • Recognition and prevention of complications • Follow-up appointments • Who to call with questions

631

#2 Nursing Process: Patient Care Plan for Postoperative Esophageal Cancer

Assessment of Airway and Gas Exchange:

Assessing level of consciousness:
  Do you know where you are? What day is it?
What is your name?
Do you know what happened to you?

Objective Data:

Lung sounds.
Oxygen saturation.
Respiratory rate and character.
Color of skin and nail beds.

Nursing Assessment and Diagnoses	Outcomes and Evaluation Parameters	Planning and Interventions with Rationales
Nursing Diagnoses: *Airway Clearance, Ineffective* related to proximity of surgery to the trachea and thoracic incision *Gas Exchange, Impaired* related to possibility of aspiration and general anesthesia	**Outcome:** Adequate oxygenation. **Evaluation Parameters:** Alert and oriented. Normal pulse oximetry and arterial blood gases. Clear lung sounds. Ability to cough to clear secretions. Unlabored respiration.	**Interventions and Rationales:** Assess level of consciousness. *Indicates possible decrease in oxygenation and brain hypoxia.* Monitor ABGs and oxygen saturation. *To evaluate gas exchange.* Assess mucous membranes and nail beds for signs of cyanosis. *Indicators of inadequate gas exchange.* Assess for diminished or adventitious breath sounds. *Indicates possible aspiration or decreased inspiratory ability related to surgical pain.* Encourage deep breathing and coughing and use of incentive spirometer at least every hour. *To promote lung expansion, mobilize secretions, and prevent atelectasis.* Assess the need for suctioning. *To maintain a patent airway.*

Monitor respiratory rate and character. *To assess for respiratory distress.*
Report respiratory distress to the health care provider. *Early intervention can prevent respiratory failure.*

Assessment of Pain

Subjective Data:
What is your level of pain on a scale of 0–10, with 10 being the worst pain?
Are you allergic to anything?
Do you have any cultural or religious practices for dealing with pain?

Objective Data:
Restlessness.
Grimacing.
Moaning or groaning.
Shallow respirations.

Nursing Assessment and Diagnoses	Outcomes and Evaluation Parameters	Planning and Interventions with *Rationales*
Nursing Diagnosis: *Pain, Acute* related to surgery	**Outcome:** Comfort level maintained. **Evaluation Parameters:** Able to communicate level of pain and relief from medications. Able to take deep breaths without pain. Appears restful without restlessness or moaning.	**Interventions and Rationales:** Assess pain using pain scale (0–10) to quantify pain level. *To increase consistency in monitoring pain.* Assess level of pain 30 minutes and 1 hour after giving pain medication. *To assess effectiveness of medications.* Explore cultural and religious practices and beliefs about pain and illness. *Different cultures and religions have varying beliefs about pain, suffering, and disease.* Teach nonpharmacologic methods of pain control, such as guided imagery, meditation, and breathing exercises. *This may augment pain relief.*

(continued)

633

#2 Nursing Process: Patient Care Plan for Postoperative Esophageal Cancer (Continued)

Assessment of Nutrition

Subjective Data:

How much weight have you lost?
How long did you have difficulty swallowing?
What had you been able to eat?

Objective Data:

Body weight.
Body mass index. Skin condition.
Wound healing.
Physical appearance.
Serum albumin.

Nursing Assessment and Diagnoses	Outcomes and Evaluation Parameters	Planning and Interventions with *Rationales*
Nursing Diagnosis: Imbalanced Nutrition: Less than Body Requirements	**Outcome:** Optimal nutrition. **Evaluation Parameters:** Maintains body weight or gains weight if underweight. Normal serum albumin. Skin is soft without evidence of dryness. Surgical incision healing. No evidence of skin breakdown.	**Interventions and Rationales:** Monitor body weight at same time every day. *Indicates a degree of adequate calorie intake and fluid balance.* Assess skin condition and healing. *Adequate dietary protein and calories are needed for wound healing and general skin condition.* Monitor laboratory values particularly serum albumin. Prepare and give parenteral or enteral nutrition as ordered. Assess for edema. *The presence of edema is one indicator of low serum proteins.* Check placement of feeding tube to prevent aspiration.

#3 Patient Care Plan for the Patient with Colon Cancer Having Surgery

Assessment of Preoperative Readiness

Subjective Data:
What did the surgeon tell you about your surgery?
Do you have any questions that you would like to ask?
Has the enterostomal therapy nurse seen the patient?
Are all preop laboratory reports in the chart?

Objective Data:
Vital signs.
Signed consent.
Character of stool post bowel prep.

Nursing Assessment and Diagnoses	Outcomes and Evaluation Parameters	Planning and Interventions with *Rationales*
Nursing Diagnosis: *Fear* related to surgical procedure and diagnosis of cancer	**Outcome:** Ready for surgery. **Evaluation Parameters:** Signed consent. Lab reports in chart. Communicates fears and anxiety. Able to verbalize the nature and extent of surgery.	**Interventions and Rationales:** Ask the patient to tell the nurse what will happen postoperatively. *This helps the nurse assess the patient's understanding of the procedure and what to expect in the postoperative period. It also assesses whether the patient understands what she signed for on the informed consent.* Administer the bowel prep as ordered and examine the stool to assess the effectiveness of the prep. Stool should be liquid and clear by the end of the prep. *The prep cleans the bowel and reduces the risk of infection postoperatively.* Contact the enterostomal therapist to arrange a preop visit with the patient *to help ease fear and anxiety about the possible colostomy.*

(continued)

#3 Patient Care Plan for the Patient with Colon Cancer Having Surgery (Continued)

Assessment of Postoperative Pain

Subjective Data:

On a scale of 1–10, with 10 being the worst pain ever, how would you rate your pain?

Are you allergic to any pain medications?

Do you have any cultural or religious beliefs that might impact your pain control?

Objective Data:

Vital signs.

Restless and irritable.

Facial grimacing when moving.

Nursing Assessment and Diagnoses	Outcomes and Evaluation Parameters	Planning and Interventions with Rationales
Nursing Diagnosis: *Pain,* Acute related to surgical incision	**Outcome:** Comfort level maintained. **Evaluation Parameters:** Communicates pain level and effectiveness of analgesia. Reports adequate pain control. No facial grimacing.	**Interventions and Rationales:** Use pain scale (1–10) to quantify level of pain *in order to be consistent from nurse to nurse, and time to time, when assessing pain.* Teach the patient to inform the nurse if the pain is not relieved. *Indicates the need to change pain management plan.* Assess cultural and religious beliefs about pain and pain relief. *Different cultures and religions may view pain as punishment or may have nontraditional ways of treating pain.* Medicate the patient prior to ambulation. *Decreased pain increases exercise tolerance, and ambulation increases intestinal motility, preventing ileus, and enhances the respiratory effort, decreasing the chance of pneumonia.*

Assessment of Skin Integrity (Postoperative)

Subjective Data:

Ask the patient whether he has feeling around the stoma.

Objective Data:

Assess stoma and skin around stoma for:

- Redness.
- Color of stoma.
- Swelling.
- Drainage.

Nursing Assessment and Diagnoses	Outcomes and Evaluation Parameters	Planning and Interventions with *Rationales*
Nursing Diagnosis: *Skin Integrity, Impaired* related to colostomy and surgical incision	**Outcome:** Good skin and stomal integrity. **Evaluation Parameters:** Stoma pink and moist. Skin surrounding stoma pink, no excoriation.	*Interventions and Rationale:* Inspect stoma and surrounding skin for color and edema. A healthy stoma is pink or beefy red and moist due to mucous production. The peristomal skin should be pink and show no signs of irritation, inflammation, excoriation, or rashes. *A bluish purple or dusky stoma indicates impaired blood flow to the stoma. Skin around the stoma can be irritated by the appliance, by a yeast infection, or from a leaking appliance.* Apply caulking agents (Stomahesive or Karaya paste) to maintain a leak-free secure ostomy appliance *to prevent leakage onto skin. Ostomy drainage is very irritating to the skin and can cause skin breakdown.* Assess surgical incision for bleeding, redness, and draining at least every 4 hours. Change dressing as ordered by surgeon to keep the incision clean and dry, *which helps prevent an infected incision.*

(continued)

#3 Patient Care Plan for the Patient with Colon Cancer Having Surgery (Continued)

Assessment of Bowel Function

Subjective Data:
Are you passing any gas through the stoma?
Do you feel any rumbling in your abdomen?
Have you been nauseated?

Objective Data:
Examination of abdomen:
- Bowel sounds.
- Palpation.
- Visual exam for contour, condition of stoma, and any drainage.

Color, consistency, and frequency of colostomy drainage.
Test stool for occult blood.

Nursing Assessment and Diagnoses	Outcomes and Evaluation Parameters
Nursing Diagnosis: Bowel Incontinence related to surgery and fecal diversion.	*Outcome:* Functioning colostomy. *Evaluation Parameters:* Stool from colostomy semiformed. Active bowel sounds.

Planning and Interventions with *Rationales*

Interventions and Rationales: Assess abdomen for bowel sounds, which indicate peristalsis has returned. *Manipulation and anesthesia have the potential for causing an ileus.* Assess for nausea and vomiting, which can also indicate an ileus. Assess the characteristics of the colostomy drainage. *Fecal-like drainage and flatulence from the stoma indicate the return of bowel function.*

#4 Patient Care Plan for Gastric Cancer and Gastric Resection

Nursing Assessment of Nutrition
What are your favorite foods?
How much did you weigh before you found out about your cancer?
Had you noticed any weight loss before that? How much?
Do you feel full after eating a small amount?
Are you nauseated?

Objective Data:
Daily weights. Intake and output (I&O). General appearance.
Laboratory studies:
- Serum albumin
- H & H
- Transferrin
- Ferritin
- TIBC
- Electrolytes

Nursing Assessment and Diagnoses	Outcomes and Evaluation Parameters	Planning and Interventions with Rationales
Nursing Diagnosis: Nutrition Imbalanced: Less than Body Requirements related to removal of part of stomach	*Outcome:* Adequate nutrition. *Evaluation Parameters:* Body weight maintained or increased. Healing incision. Normal serum albumin. Normal serum electrolytes. Normal iron studies. Normal hemoglobin and hematocrit.	*Interventions and Rationales:* See Chart 45–2 for nursing interventions for patients with feeding tubes. Weigh daily at the same time and on the same scale. *To provide an accurate assessment of fluid balance and nutritional adequacy.* Measure and record accurate intake and output. *To estimate fluid balance.* Monitor laboratory indicators of nutritional status. *These are better indicators of nutritional status than body weight alone.*

(continued)

639

#4 Patient Care Plan for Gastric Cancer and Gastric Resection (Continued)

Nursing Assessment and Diagnoses	Outcomes and Evaluation Parameters	Planning and Interventions with *Rationales*
		Assess skin for breakdown. *Can be an indicator of nutritional status, particularly protein.*
		Assess wound healing. *Decreased protein and vitamin C can hinder wound healing.*
		Medicate for nausea and pain as needed before meals. *Pain and nausea often produce anorexia and relief can increase the appetite.*
		Provide the patient with favorite foods or have family members bring home-prepared food when she is able to eat. *To increase the patient's nutritional intake.*
		Invite family or friends to visit at mealtime. Gathering for meals is a social function for many families and may improve the patient's intake.

Assessment of Emotional Status

Subjective Data:

What have the doctors told you about your cancer?

Who do you count on for support?

Do you have any religious, cultural, or spiritual beliefs that help you deal with your cancer?

Objective Data:

Family or friends visiting

Clergy visit

Initiates conversations with the nursing staff

Nursing Assessment and Diagnoses	Outcomes and Evaluation Parameters	Planning and Interventions with Rationales
Nursing Diagnosis: *Grieving, Complicated* related to diagnosis of cancer with poor prognosis	**Outcome:** Anxiety and fear controlled. **Evaluation Parameters:** Verbalizes fears about cancer and death. Communicates feelings with significant others.	**Interventions and Rationales:** Encourage family and significant others to spend as much time as possible with the patient, especially during difficult times such as visits from the health care provider, during chemo and radiation treatments. *To give purpose to the family and significant others and help them feel a part of the process.* Allow the patient to express any feelings without negating any of these feelings. *Allowing the patient to have hope may aid in coping behavior.* Inquire about the patient's cultural, religious, and spiritual beliefs about illness and death, and facilitate discussion with family and clergy where appropriate. *Spiritual and cultural beliefs can comfort the patient and family during this time.*

(continued)

#4 Patient Care Plan for Gastric Cancer and Gastric Resection (Continued)

Assessment of Pain

Subjective Data:

On a scale of 0–10, with 10 being the worst pain, how would you rate your pain?

What does your pain feel like—burning, gnawing, aching, or stabbing?

Have you felt nauseated?

Did you vomit?

Did the vomit contain blood or brown fluid?

Objective Data:

Vital signs. Abdominal examination:

- Distention?
- Pain or tenderness on palpation?
- Bowel sounds?
- Soft or rigid?

Stool for occult blood. Facial grimacing. Restless, holding abdomen.

Nursing Assessment and Diagnoses	Outcomes and Evaluation Parameters	Planning and Interventions with *Rationales*
Nursing Diagnosis: Pain, Acute related to surgical incision and metastatic cancer	*Outcome:* Pain relieved. *Evaluation Parameters:* Able to communicate level of pain and therapies that relieve it. Abdomen soft, nontender, and bowel sounds present. No restlessness or facial grimacing.	*Interventions and Rationales:* Assess pain using scale (0–10) to quantify pain. *To increase consistency in pain measurement.* Assess pain, character and location, and any related symptoms. *To give the nurse clues to the cause of the pain; i.e., incisional pain vs. infection, vs. peritonitis, vs. metastatic cancer.* Administer pain medications as ordered and assess pain level 30 minutes and 1 hour after administration. *To evaluate the effectiveness of the pain medication.*

#5 Clinical Manifestations of Cirrhosis and Physiological Causes

Clinical Manifestation	Physiological Cause
Integumentary	
• Jaundice	Blocked outflow of bile from liver due to structural change.
• Palmar erythema	Altered sex hormone metabolism (high estrogen).
• Spider angioma	High capillary pressure.
• Decreased body hair	Altered sex hormone metabolism.
• Pruritus	High levels of bilirubin cause itching.
• Ecchymosis	↓ clotting factors, ↑ platelet destruction by spleen, ↓ vitamin K.
• Caput medusae	Intrahepatic obstruction to portal blood flow.
• Edema	Low serum albumin, high hydrostatic pressure, sodium and water retention.
Gastrointestinal	
• Esophageal varices	Intrahepatic obstruction to portal blood flow.
	Stretching of Glisson's capsule or ascites.
• Abdominal pain	Increased venous pressure in GI tract.
	Hypoalbuminemia, ↑ lymph production, ↑ capillary filtration pressure, ↑ renal absorption of sodium and water.
• Anorexia	
	Intrahepatic obstruction of bile flowing into duodenum.
• Ascites	Esophageal varices bleed.
• Light-colored stools	Portal hypertension causes venous congestion.
• GI bleeding	
• Hemorrhoids	
Neurological	
• Hepatic encephalopathy	Hepatocytes unable to convert ammonia (by-product of protein metabolism) to urea to be excreted by the kidney ↑ ammonia).
• Sensory disturbances	High serum ammonia levels are neurotoxic. Caused by high serum ammonia levels.
• Asterixis (liver flap)	

(continued)

#5 Clinical Manifestations of Cirrhosis and Physiological Causes (Continued)

Cardiovascular
- Portal hypertension — Intrahepatic obstruction to portal blood flow.
- Bounding pulse — Increased fluid volume from sodium and water retention and ↑ aldosterone.
- Dysrhythmias

  Fluid and electrolyte imbalance.

Hematologic
- Decreased clotting factors — Liver unable to synthesize clotting factors and vitamin K.
- Thrombocytopenia — Enlarged spleen causes ↑ destruction of platelets.
- Anemia

  ↑ RBC destruction in spleen, bleeding.

Hepatic
- Atrophic, nodular liver — Scarring.

  Intrahepatic obstruction to portal blood flow causes engorgement
- Splenomegaly — of spleen.

Respiratory
- Dyspnea — Ascites cause pressure on diaphragm.

Reproductive
- Oligomenorrhea (female) — Altered sex hormone metabolism.
- Testicular atrophy — Altered sex hormone metabolism (high estrogen).

  Altered sex hormone metabolism (high estrogen).
- Gynecomastia (male) — Altered sex hormone metabolism.
- Loss of libido

Metabolic
- Hypoalbuminemia — Liver unable to synthesize albumin.
- Hypokalemia — Altered renal excretion.
- Hypocalcemia — Related to low serum protein levels.
- Malnutrition — Impaired metabolism of nutrients.
- Muscle wasting — Muscles are used as protein source.

#6 Nursing Process: Patient Care Plan for the Patient with Cirrhosis

Nursing Assessment and Diagnoses	Outcomes and Evaluation Parameters	Planning and Interventions with *Rationales*
Nursing Diagnosis: *Fluid Volume, Excess* related to portal hypertension and possible hepatorenal syndrome	**Outcome:** Fluid status normal.	**Interventions and Rationales:** Weigh daily at the same time of day on the same scale, and monitor I&O. *This gives an accurate assessment of fluid status because a daily change in body weight can be attributed to water retention (or loss).*
	Evaluation Parameters: Decreasing abdominal girth.	Measure abdominal girth at the same location on the abdomen at least once a day, but preferably every 8 hours to *monitor progression of ascites.*
	No peripheral edema.	Restrict dietary sodium to less than 2 grams per day and fluid as ordered. *Sodium promotes water retention, aggravating ascites and portal hypertension*
	Normal laboratory results.	Monitor lab values and report abnormalities. Low serum albumin can contribute *to ascites and edema. Hyponatremia and hematocrit may indicate hemodilu-*
	No evidence of active bleeding.	*tion. Rising BUN and creatinine can indicate impending hepatorenal syndrome.*
	No jugular venous distention.	Examine neck veins for distention and extremities for edema.
	Urine specific gravity normal.	*Distended jugular veins indicate fluid overload, and edema can result from excess fluid and low serum albumin.*
	Urine output at least 30 mL/hr.	Give prescribed diuretics to *reduce body water.*

(continued)

#6 Nursing Process: Patient Care Plan for the Patient with Cirrhosis (Continued)

Nursing Assessment and Diagnoses	Outcomes and Evaluation Parameters	Planning and Interventions with Rationales
Nursing Diagnosis: *Nutrition, Imbalanced: Less than Body Requirements* related to anorexia, impaired protein metabolism, and reduced absorption of fat soluble vitamins because of reduced liver function	**Outcome:** Adequate nutrition. **Evaluation Parameter:** No weight loss.	**Interventions and Rationales:** Provide a high-calorie, low-protein, low-sodium diet with 6 small meals per day as ordered. *Protein may be restricted if there is evidence of GI bleeding or encephalopathy in an effort to reduce nitrogenous waste products from protein metabolism.* Weekly weights after discharge. *Short-term fluctuations are usually associated with fluid balance, whereas long-term changes are a better indicator of nutritional status.* Explain the importance of avoiding substances that can be toxic to the liver, such as alcohol and acetaminophen, *in order to prevent further liver damage.* If there is no protein restriction, teach the patient to read food labels and choose foods that are high in protein and have adequate levels of vitamins and minerals, such as Instant Breakfast drink mix, *to improve nutritional status and prevent breakdown of skeletal muscle.*
Nursing Diagnosis: *Skin Integrity, Risk for Impaired* related to jaundice and resultant pruritus	**Outcome:** Skin integrity maintained. **Evaluation Parameters:** Reports diminished itching. No bruising or petechiae. No lesions from scratching.	**Interventions and Rationales:** Instruct the patient to use cool, lightweight, non-restrictive clothing and avoid woolens. *Clothing made from lightweight fabrics causes less itching.* Explain that a cool environmental temperature and cool water for bathing may increase comfort related to pruritus. Instruct the patient to keep her fingernails trimmed and well cared for to *decrease the likelihood of excoriating when scratching.*

646

Instruct the patient to take antihistamine medication as ordered to *reduce pruritus.*

Nursing Diagnosis: Fluid Volume, Deficit: Risk for related to the liver's ability to synthesize clotting factors, portal hypertension with resultant esophageal varices, and hemorrhoids

Interventions and Rationales: Give vitamin K as ordered. *Vitamin K is synthesized in the liver and may be decreased in cirrhosis.*

Teach patient to use a soft toothbrush and avoid using dental floss because *decreased clotting factors make the patient more prone to bleeding.*

Monitor for bleeding (stool, skin, urine, and mucous membranes) *because decreased clotting factors make the patient more prone to bleeding.*

Instruct patient to refrain from eating rough foods that can cause *trauma to the esophagus and cause varices to bleed.*

Outcome: No hemorrhage.

Evaluation Parameters:
Stool negative for occult blood.
No vomiting blood.
Coagulation studies normal.
Hemoglobin and hematocrit normal.
Vital signs normal.

Nursing Diagnosis: Confusion: Risk for related to hepatic encephalopathy

Interventions and Rationales: Administer Mini-Mental Status Exam (MMSE). *Hepatic encephalopathy can cause changes in mentation even in the prodromal phase.*

Provide a low-protein diet as ordered *to reduce the nitrogen metabolites of protein digestion.*

Administer medications to reduce ammonia level as ordered. *Lactulose, oral or enema, promotes diarrhea and the elimination of ammonia in the feces.*

Monitor deep tendon reflexes *as hepatic encephalopathy progresses, reflexes become exaggerated.*

Outcome: No disruption in mental status.

Evaluation Parameters:
Alert and oriented to person, place, and time.
Able to perform simple computations.
Behavior appropriate.
Normal reflexes.
MMSE score of 25 or better.

(continued)

647

#7 Nursing Process: Patient Care Plan for Pancreatitis

Nursing Assessment and Diagnoses	Outcomes and Evaluation Parameters	Planning and Interventions with Rationales
Nursing Diagnosis: Pain: Acute related to pancreatitis	*Outcome:* Comfort level maintained. *Evaluation Parameters:* Able to communicate level of pain and relief from medications. Appears restful without restlessness or moaning.	*Interventions and Rationales:* Assess pain using pain scale (0–10) to quantify pain level (restlessness, grimacing, lying in fetal position, moaning, clenched fists, periumbilical ecchymosis, abdominal tenderness) *to increase consistency in monitoring pain.* Administer pain medication, usually meperidine or morphine, and assess level of pain 30 minutes and 1 hour after giving medication. Notify health care provider if pain is unrelieved *to assess effectiveness of medications.* Explore cultural and religious practices and beliefs about pain and illness. *Different religions have varying beliefs about pain, suffering, and disease.* Teach nonpharmacologic methods of pain control, such as guided imagery, meditation, and breathing exercises. *This may augment pain relief.* Maintain a quiet, darkened, comfortable environment. *This can help decrease physical and mental stimulation,*

Nursing Diagnosis: *Nutrition, Imbalanced: Less than Body Requirements* related to nausea, vomiting, pain, and possible lack of pancreatic enzymes for digestion

Outcome: Adequate nutrition.
Evaluation Parameters: No weight loss.
Serum albumin normal.
Fasting glucose normal.
Hemoglobin and hematocrit normal.
No reported nausea.

which can lead to decreased pancreatic secretions and less pain.

Maintain bed rest and position the patient in a sitting position to *decrease the pain caused by stretched abdominal muscles that are irritated by inflammation. Close the patient's door during mealtime because the smell of food can stimulate pancreatic secretions.*

Place a nasogastric tube if ordered, and/or monitor drainage and relief of pain. *This helps to "rest" the pancreas and removes secretions that can stimulate the pancreas to produce enzymes.*

Interventions and Rationales: Weigh daily on same scale at the same time. *Fluctuations in weight from day to day are an indicator of fluid balance, but changes over a week reflect nutritional status.*

Assess laboratory results and report any abnormal values to the patient's health care provider. *The pancreas produces enzymes that aid in the digestion of protein, fat, and carbohydrates. Protein malnutrition is reflected in a low serum albumin. Transferrin is a protein that transports iron, so this level may be low. The H&H may be decreased in cases of malnutrition. Serum glucose may be elevated if the pancreatitis affects the endocrine function of the gland.*

(continued)

#7 Nursing Process: Patient Care Plan for Pancreatitis (Continued)

Nursing Assessment and Diagnoses	Outcomes and Evaluation Parameters	Planning and Interventions with Rationales
		Planning and Interventions with *Rationales*
		Monitor the frequency, color, consistency, and odor of stools. *Lack of lipase from the pancreas results in poor fat digestion and steatorrhea results. The presence of steatorrhea indicates severe pancreatitis with impaired pancreatic function.*
		Provide oral hygiene at least every 2 hours while the nasogastric tube is in place to decrease discomfort and maintain *the integrity of the oral and nasal mucosa.*
		Offer small, frequent meals, beginning with clear liquids once bowel sounds return and pain is relieved. *Smaller meals reduce the secretion of pancreatic enzymes.*
Nursing Diagnoses: *Fluid Volume Deficit* related to vascular leak syndrome resulting from inflammation, and fluid accumulation in the abdominal cavity. Potential for electrolyte	***Outcomes:*** Adequate fluid volume and electrolyte balance. ***Evaluation Parameters:*** Normal blood pressure with no orthostatic changes. Normal sinus rhythm.	***Interventions and Rationales:*** Evaluate cardiac status: heart rate and rhythm at least every 4 hours; orthostatic blood pressure, pulmonary artery pressure usually every 4 hours as indicated; peripheral pulses; capillary refill; skin color. *These assessments help establish fluid volume. The body*

imbalance related to nasogastric suction

Stable daily weight with moist mucous membranes.
Pulmonary artery pressure 8–12 mmHg.
Cardiac output at least 5 L/min.
Brisk capillary refill.
Good peripheral pulses.
Urine output 30 mL/hr.
Alert and oriented.

compensates for diminished volume by increasing the heart rate to maintain cardiac output.
Capillaries constrict to force more fluid into the general circulation and the signs are weak peripheral pulses and pale skin color. A decreased cardiac output means a decrease in the renal perfusion and decreased urine output and possibly early pre-renal renal failure.
Monitor renal function by measuring urine output every hour and notifying the health care provider if the level is less than 30 mL/hr.
Daily body weight *is an indicator of fluid status.*
Monitor neurological function by assessing level of consciousness and behavior. *Cerebral perfusion may be diminished if there is a fluid volume deficit and the cardiac output is low. Electrolytes, particularly sodium, can cause confusion when the levels are low.*
Monitor laboratory values for electrolyte status and renal function. *Electrolytes are lost in nasogastric suction or vomiting. The BUN and creatinine will rise if renal function is compromised.*

#8 Patient Care Plan for Inflammatory Bowel Disease and Ileostomy

Assessment of Bowel Elimination

Subjective Data:

How many stools do you have a day?

What is the consistency and color?

Is there any blood?

Do you have any abdominal pain or cramping?

How long have you been having this problem? When did it start?

Does stress in your life make it worse?

Does any food make the diarrhea worse?

Do you have any joint pain or fatigue?

Have you been treated before?

Do you take any home remedies, herbs, or over-the-counter medications?

Objective Data:

Vital signs. Examination of abdomen:

- Bowel sounds
- Palpation
- Visual exam for contour, scars

Visual inspection of stools. Test stool for occult blood.

Nursing Assessment and Diagnoses	Outcomes and Evaluation Parameters	Planning and Interventions with Rationales
Nursing Diagnoses: *Diarrhea* related to irritable bowel syndrome (IBS).	**Outcome:** Decreased diarrhea. **Evaluation Parameters:** Number of stools decreased by at least half.	**Interventions and Rationales:** *Take vital signs every 4 hours to assess for signs of dehydration such as tachycardia, tachypnea, or fever. Weigh daily to assess for fluid losses.*

| *Fluid Balance, Readiness for Enhanced* related to the diarrhea. | Consistency of stool: formed. Absence of blood in the stool. No abdominal cramping. | Examine skin and mucous membranes for evidence of dehydration, *such as poor turgor, dry mucous membranes, or dry, cracked tongue.* Maintain NPO if ordered *to rest the bowel, which promotes healing and improves diarrhea.* Provide good perianal care with gentle cleansing agents, and apply protective cream or ointment to the area *to prevent skin breakdown.* Administer ordered medications, assess their effectiveness, and monitor adverse effects: |

- 5-ASA compounds (sufasalazine, mesalamine, olsalazine) are anti-inflammatory drugs that decrease inflammation of the intestinal mucosa.
  1. Monitor for adverse effects, which include skin rashes, urticaria, pruritus, bleeding or easy bruising, fever, low WBC and platelet counts, low hemoglobin and hematocrit (bone marrow suppression), and decreased urine output (renal failure).
  2. Give and teach patient to take these medications after eating to avoid gastric distress.
  3. Encourage increased fluid intake (2 L/day) to prevent kidney damage.
  4. Teach patient to notify the health care provider if any of the adverse effects occur.

(continued)

#8 Patient Care Plan for Inflammatory Bowel Disease and Ileostomy (Continued)

Nursing Assessment and Diagnoses	Outcomes and Evaluation Parameters	Planning and Interventions with *Rationales*
		• Corticosteroids—adrenal hormones (prednisolone) that suppress the immune response and have anti-inflammatory properties:
		1. Monitor for side effects such as elevated blood glucose, fluid retention (edema, weight gain, hypertension, heart failure), gastric ulcers, hypokalemia (muscle weakness, nausea, dysrhythmias), and mood swings.
		2. Should be given only with meals to decrease the risk of ulcers and gastric distress.
		3. Teach the patient to increase foods high in potassium (citrus fruit, bananas, potatoes) and reduce intake of sodium (canned soup, bottled salad dressing, processed meats, cheese).
		4. Teach patient NOT TO STOP THE MEDICATION ABRUPTLY (the dose must be tapered).
		• Immunomodulators (azathioprine) suppress the immune system.
		1. Be sure to tell the patient that these drugs must be taken for 4–5 months before the full effect is seen.
		2. Monitor for adverse effects such as pancreatitis (usually within the first 2 months), and low WBC or platelet count.

654

- Infliximab (tumor necrosis factor blocker) used for refractory Crohn's disease.
  1. Given every 2–3 months and must be given intravenously.
  2. Monitor for adverse effects such as infection serum sickness–like reaction and lupus-like syndrome (Biddle, 2003).

Assessment of Body Image

Subjective Data:
How has this disease/surgery affected your life?
Are you able to continue working? Socializing with friends? Shopping?
Has this affected how you feel about your personal relationships? Sexual activity?

Objective Data:
Facial expressions.
Body language.
Attitude toward stoma.

Nursing Assessment and Diagnoses	Outcomes and Evaluation Parameters	Planning and Interventions with *Rationales*
Nursing Diagnosis: *Disturbed Body Image* related to disease process and/or surgery	**Outcome:** Normal body image. **Evaluation Parameter:** Verbalizes acceptance of body image.	**Interventions and Rationales:** Assess the patient's current perception of self and demonstrate acceptance of where the patient is now. *Acceptance of the patient's feelings can help establish a caring and trusting nurse–patient relationship.* Provide an environment in which the patient feels comfortable talking about the disease and how it has impacted his life. To build caring nurse–patient relationship.

(continued)

#8 Patient Care Plan for Inflammatory Bowel Disease and Ileostomy (Continued)

Nursing Assessment and Diagnoses	Outcomes and Evaluation Parameters	Planning and Interventions with *Rationales*
		Encourage the patient to talk about ways this disease has affected personal, work, social, and sexual relationships. *To provide understanding and demonstrate acceptance of the patient as a person.* Delineate possible treatment options, including graphic description of surgery and postop possibilities *to give the patient a sense of control.* Provide names and phone numbers of IBS support groups. If possible, arrange for the patient to meet with someone who has the disease. *This shows the patient that she is not the only person facing this problem.*

Assessment of Fecal Diversion (Ileostomy)

Subjective Data:

Are you having any cramping?

Are you passing any gas through the stoma?

Objective Data:

Vital signs. Abdominal assessment:

- Stoma color
- Stoma drainage/bleeding

Condition of skin surrounding stoma.

Condition of ostomy appliance.

Nursing Assessment and Nursing Diagnoses	Outcomes and Evaluation Parameters	Planning and Interventions with Rationales
Nursing Assessment and Nursing Diagnoses: *Bowel Incontinence* related to fecal diversion. *Skin Integrity, Impaired, Risk for* related to ostomy drainage. *Knowledge, Deficient* related to fecal diversion.	**Outcome:** Normal functioning ileostomy. **Evaluation Parameters:** Stoma color pink and moist. No bloody effluent. Effluent dark green and viscous initially, gradually turning yellow-brown. Skin around stoma free of irritation and inflammation. Ileoanal skin without irritation or inflammation. Able to communicate necessary stoma care, dietary modification, and stress reduction techniques.	**Interventions and Rationales:** Monitor stoma color. *The stoma should be pink, beefy red, and moist with no obvious cyanosis or bleeding. It should extend about 2–3 centimeters from the abdominal wall. Impaired circulation will cause the stoma to be dark, blue, or very pale.* Assess stoma function. *Immediately postop there may be small amounts of blood.* Within 1 or 2 days the drainage will be dark green and viscous, gradually turning yellow-brown and developing an odor. Empty and measure ileostomy drainage when the pouch is one-third to one-half full and explain the procedure to the patient each time. *Emptying the pouch when it is not too full eliminates the possibility of the seal in the pouch breaking and causing leaking.* Explaining the procedure to the patient each time gets the patient more comfortable with self-care. Assess the skin surrounding the stoma and around the perianal area. The skin should be pink and remain free of irritation, excoriation, or inflammation. *Ileostomy drainage is irritating to the skin because it contains bile salts and digestive enzymes that normally get reabsorbed in the large intestine.*

(continued)

#8 Patient Care Plan for Inflammatory Bowel Disease and Ileostomy (Continued)

Nursing Assessment and Diagnoses	Outcomes and Evaluation Parameters	Planning and Interventions with *Rationales*
		Apply a protecting skin barrier under the pouch *to prevent contact of drainage with skin.*
		Report abnormal assessment findings such as poor stoma color, bulging or retracted stoma, or rash around the stoma. Poor stoma color indicates poor circulation to the section of bowel that forms the stoma; bulging can indicate herniation or prolapse. Teach patient and family members to assess the stoma and to treat it gently. *Because there are no pain receptors in the stoma, it can become injured without feeling pain.*
		Teach patient to notify health care provider if there is a change in the stoma or if a rash develops in the skin surrounding the stoma. Assess the patient's ability to manage the ileostomy including knowledge of ostomy care, what medications to avoid (laxatives, enteric coated, or capsules), and signs and symptoms to report.

#9 Comparison of Female Reproductive Cancers

Etiology	Assessment	Interventions
Cervical Cancer		
Third most common reproductive cancer. 90% squamous cell. 10% adenocarcinoma. Average age 40–50. Increased risk with human papillomavirus (HPV) and herpes 2, multiple partners, and decreased socioeconomic status. Increased in African American and Hispanic women.	Preinvasion is often asymptomatic. Invasive shows postcoital bleeding and abnormal bleeding. Late symptoms include rectal bleeding, hematuria, back and leg pain, and anemia. Pap smear is the single most reliable diagnostic test (it will show 90% of early cervical cancers). Other diagnostic tests include colposcopy, biopsy, and conization.	Preinvasive lesions often entail cryosurgery, laser surgery, or loop electrosurgical excision procedure (LEEP: an electrically charged thin wire is used to remove a thin layer of cells from the cervix). Typically done as an outpatient procedure. Invasive treatment is hysterectomy with internal or external radiation.
Vulvar Cancer		
Fourth most common gynecologic cancer. Average age 60–70. Those under 35 are linked to condolymata. 90% squamous cell. Slow growing.	Lesion usually asymptomatic until 1–2 centimeters. Symptoms include vulvar pruritus and burning pain.	Local, wide excision, or vulvectomy. External radiation.

(continued)

659

#9 Comparison of Female Reproductive Cancers (Continued)

Etiology

90% survival even with late diagnosis if nodes are negative.

Less than 50% survival with node involvement.

Diagnosed by biopsy with histologic evaluation using toluidine blue.

Endometrial Cancer

Most common gynecologic malignancy. Average age 50–65.

Risk factors include obesity, nullipara, infertility, diabetes mellitus, hypertension, family history, Caucasian, and hormone imbalance, which is the most significant risk factor.

Symptoms include abnormal uterine bleeding, lower back pain, lower pelvic pain, uterine enlargement, and positive Pap smear.

Diagnosis by fractional curettage or endometrial biopsy.

Total abdominal hysterectomy with bilateral salpingectomy and oophorectomy.

Radiation (internal or external) before or after surgery.

Chemotherapy with advanced stage or recurrent.

Ovarian Cancer

Second most frequent gynecologic cancer. Causes more deaths than any other reproductive cancer.

Risks include nullipara, infertility, and family history.

Affects all ages but increased in the 50s.

No definitive tests.

Often diagnosed in late stage.

Symptoms include lower abdominal discomfort and digestive complaints.

Increased pain, weakness, and malnutrition are late signs.

Treatment varies from removal of the ovary to total hysterectomy.

Chemotherapy.

Antineoplastic drugs. Radiation is controversial.

Vaginal Cancer

Rare.

Two types: squamous cell (increased in ages 60–80) and adenocarcinoma (increased in ages 12–30).

Risks include young women of mothers who received diethylstilbestrol (DES) in 1945–1970 as a treatment for miscarriage.

Bleeding or discharge not related to menstruation.

Pain during intercourse (dyspareunia). Pelvic pain.

Treatment depends on the stage of the cancer and may include:

- Surgery (to remove the cancer)
- Radiation (to kill cancer cells and/or shrink tumors)
- Chemotherapy (to kill the cancer cells).

#10 Nursing Process: Patient Care Plan for SIRS, Sepsis, Shock

Nursing Assessment and Diagnoses	Outcomes and Evaluation Parameters	Planning and Interventions with *Rationales*
Nursing Diagnoses: *Tissue Perfusion Ineffective* related to alterations in circulating volume and organ dysfunction. *Fluid Volume Deficient* related to alterations in circulating volume *Cardiac Output, Decreased* related to alterations in circulating volume and cardiac pump function	**Outcome:** Improved tissue perfusion. ***Evaluation Parameters:*** Presence of peripheral pulses by palpation or Doppler. Capillary refill < 2 seconds. Maintenance of a perfusing blood pressure. Improved mental status. Glascow Coma Scale (GCS) 15. Follows commands. No restlessness/fatigue. Oxygen saturation within normal limits.	**Interventions and *Rationales*:** Assess peripheral pulses and compare to central pulses. *Decrease in or loss of peripheral pulses indicates decreased tissue perfusion.* Assess skin color, temperature. *Capillary refill indicates body's attempt to compensate for decreased perfusion by diverting blood flow from the periphery to the central circulation.* Assess patient's GCS and ability to follow commands. Monitor restlessness and confusion *as an indication of decreased cerebral perfusion and worsening shock state.* Assess for obvious signs of bleeding, *which will cause blood loss and alter circulating volume.* Apply direct pressure and pressure dressings, assist with clamping of bleeding vessels, and prepare patient for operative intervention *to prevent blood and volume loss.* Apply PASG to manage large-volume loss from such injuries as a pelvic fracture *to prevent blood and volume loss.* Initiate large-bore IV catheters.

Control of blood and fluid loss.	Assist with insertion of central venous access *to replace volume and blood loss to maintain adequate circulation and improve perfusion.*
Adequate hydration.	Administer appropriate isotonic solution at 20 mL/kg and increase as indicated by patient's urinary output of 0.5 mL/kg/hr *to maintain adequate circulation and improve perfusion.*
Corrected acid–base balance.	Prepare for administration of blood and blood products *to replace lost blood and increase oxygen to the tissues.*
Improved core body temperature.	Administer O-negative blood if needed immediately.
Adequate cardiac output and blood pressure.	Administer blood components such as fresh frozen plasma and platelets *to maintain adequate circulation and improve perfusion.*
	Place warm blankets on the patient.
	Use a commercial warming device.
	Warm fluids and blood *to prevent hypothermia and maintain adequate circulation and improve perfusion.*
	Turn and position patient frequently *to prevent skin breakdown and development of DVT.*
	Obtain 12-lead ECG to assess the status of the myocardium.
	Increase cardiac contractility by administering a fluid bolus.

(continued)

663

Nursing Assessment and Diagnoses	Outcomes and Evaluation Parameters	Planning and Interventions with *Rationales*
		Initiate medications to improve contractility:
		• Dopamine hydrochloride
		• Dobutamine hydrochloride
		• Amrinone lactate.
		Initiate medications to decrease afterload:
		• Nitroprusside sodium
		• Nitrates.
		Initiate medications to increase afterload:
		• Norepinephrine bitartrate
		• Epinephrine.
		To improve cardiac output.
		Prepare the patient for interventions that may increase reperfusion to an injured myocardium, e.g., percutaneous transluminal coronary angioplasty (PCTA) or insertion of an intraaortic balloon pump *to improve cardiac output.*

Nursing Diagnoses/Outcome/Evaluation Parameters	Interventions and Rationales
Nursing Diagnoses: *Gas Exchange, Impaired* related to inadequate tissue perfusion *Airway Clearance, Ineffective* related to altered mental status from inadequate tissue perfusion **Outcome:** Patient will maintain a patent airway. Normal arterial blood gases. Decreased respiratory rate because of a decreased need to compensate for metabolic acidosis; 12–20 breaths per minute. Adequate perfusion for the patient to become alert and oriented. Clear breath sounds. **Evaluation Parameters:** Regular rate, depth, and pattern of breathing. Bilateral chest expansion. Effective cough and gag reflex.	**Interventions and Rationales:** Assess for symptoms of increased work of breathing, which indicate inadequate tissue perfusion: oxygen saturation, length of capillary refill, skin temperature, and color *to assess tissue perfusion.* Monitor ABGs and oxygen saturation to assess adequacy of gas exchange and level of shock state. *When the body responds to shock, it will divert blood from the periphery and direct it to the brain, lungs, and kidneys.* Monitor for changes in mental status such as restlessness and confusion. *Indicators of inadequate gas exchange with resultant cerebral hypoxia.* Observe for pallor and cyanosis, especially in the mucous membranes. *Indicators of inadequate gas exchange with resultant tissue hypoxia.* Administer 100% oxygen by nonrebreather mask. *To increase available oxygen and decrease tissue hypoxia.* Report respiratory distress and hypoxia to the health care provider. *Intubation and mechanical ventilation may be needed to deliver greater amounts of oxygen and maintain adequate tissue perfusion* Open and clear airway. *Patient may have secretions in mouth.* Insert oro- or nasopharyngeal airway. *Patient may have adequate respiratory drive but needs support to keep airway open.* Prepare to assist with endotracheal intubation. *Level of consciousness too low to protect and maintain airway.*

(continued)

#10 Nursing Process: Patient Care Plan for SIRS, Sepsis, Shock (Continued)

Nursing Assessment and Diagnoses	Outcomes and Evaluation Parameters	Planning and Interventions with Rationales
Nursing Diagnoses: Infection related to a focus of infection	*Outcomes:* Identification of focus of infection. Infection resolved. *Evaluation Parameters:* Decrease or absence of fever. Removal of source of the infection, for example, draining of an abscess or removal of an invasive catheter. Normal white blood cell count and differential.	*Interventions and Rationales:* Measure and monitor the patient's body temperature using the most appropriate method. For example, rectal, esophageal or bladder so the most accurate temperature is measured. *Effects of treatment can also be monitored.*
		Perform measures to decrease the patient's fever such as administration of an antipyretic or application of a cooling blanket. *To prevent side effects of fever such as dehydration.*
		Note the presence of a source of an infection, for example, urinary catheter, draining wound, rigid abdomen, and colored sputum. *To determine cause and infection site.*
		Obtain blood cultures by drawing blood from two sites. At least one should be drawn percutaneously and one drawn through each vascular access device unless the device was recently inserted to identify infectious agent. *To diagnose the presence of sepsis.*
		Obtain cultures from other sites such as urine, CSF, or other body fluids to identify source and infectious agents. *To identify source of infection.*

Nursing Diagnosis:	Outcome: Patient will ingest daily nutritional requirements for activity level and metabolic needs.	Use aseptic technique when changing dressings or drawing blood from invasive lines *to prevent introduction of further sources of infection.*
Imbalanced Nutrition Risk for: Less than Body Requirements related to decreased appetite secondary to treatments, fatigue, environment, and increased protein and vitamin requirements for healing		Perform hand hygiene frequently and use infection control measures when indicated *to prevent introduction of further sources of infection.*
		Instruct the patient's family about hand hygiene *to prevent further introduction of infection.*
		Report to the health care provider changes in temperature as prescribed *so appropriate interventions and medications can be given to manage a fever.*
		Administer antibiotics per health care provider's orders.
		Interventions and Rationales: Communicate the need for adequate caloric intake of carbohydrates, fats, protein, vitamins, minerals, and fluids. *Adequate nutrition can reduce the risk of complications and promote healing.*
	Evaluation Parameters: Patient maintains adequate weight.	Consult with the nutritionist to establish appropriate daily caloric requirements. *Consultation helps to ensure optimal intake.*
	Patient maintains adequate caloric intake.	Offer small frequent meals *to help prevent gastric distention.*
		Determine the patient's food preferences and arrange to have those foods provided.
		Encourage family to bring allowed foods from home.
		Eliminate any offensive odors.
		Control pain and nausea.
		Provide a relaxed atmosphere during meals.
		These interventions can improve appetite and lead to increased intake.

(continued)

667

#10 Nursing Process: Patient Care Plan for SIRS, Sepsis, Shock (Continued)

Nursing Assessment and Diagnoses	Outcomes and Evaluation Parameters	Planning and Interventions with Rationales
Nursing Diagnosis: *Coping, readiness for enhanced grieving*	**Outcome:** Patient and/or family are able to make decisions about care. **Evaluation Parameters:** Patient and family verbalize realistic perception of the patient's condition and chances of survival. Spiritual care is provided as identified by the patient and family. End-of-life decisions are made by the patient and/or family to ensure a painless and dignified death.	***Interventions and Rationales:*** Provide the patient and the family with information about their illness or injury especially related to outcomes *to assist the patient and family with grieving.* Allow the family to see the patient as soon as possible, especially if the patient is near death. Explain to the family what the patient looks like and how comfort has been provided for the patient *to assist the patient and family with grieving.* Provide requested spiritual care by contacting appropriate personnel. Respect cultural rituals related to the patient and family beliefs. Consult with personnel such as the ethics committee when problems arise with end-of-life decisions *to assist the patient and family with grieving.* Help the staff to recognize signs and symptoms of their own grief and provide them with resources *to assist them with the grieving process.* Prepare patient and family for end-of-life decisions. *To prepare the family for possible death.*

#11 Diagnostics Cardiac Valvular Disorders

Test and *Normal Value*	Expected Abnormality	Rationale for Abnormality
Echocardiogram and transesophageal echocardiography (TEE) Echocardiogram (ultrasound): *Normal chamber size and normal cardiac structures*	Abnormal structure and function of heart valves, able to identify thickened valve leaflets, vegetative growths, myocardial function, and chamber size. TEE is particularly useful not only for diagnosing but also for tracking the progression of the disease.	Vegetative growths and infection cause a thinning of valve leaflets leading to abnormal function.
Chest x-ray: *Clear lungs and normal heart size*	Pulmonary congestion, cardiac hypertrophy, chamber and great vessel enlargement, and calcification of the valves.	Abnormal valve function causes a change in blood flow leading to changes in chamber size and valve structure.
Cardiac catheterization: *Normal coronary artery blood flow, chamber size, and valve function*	The size of the valve opening and pressure gradients across valve surfaces is abnormal. Pressure in the heart chambers and pulmonary system is increased. Cardiac output typically is decreased.	Abnormal valve structure causes changes in openings leading to increased pressures in the cardiac chambers and decreased cardiac output.

(continued)

669

#11 Diagnostics Cardiac Valvular Disorders (Continued)

Test and *Normal Value*	Expected Abnormality	Rationale for Abnormality
Electrocardiogram (ECG): *Normal conduction time intervals*	Conduction delays, atrial and ventricular dysrhythmias, and the presence of cardiac ischemia. Is useful in detecting increased ischemia and the presence of life-threatening dysrhythmias.	Changes occur due to diminished blood flow to the myocardium due to decreased cardiac output caused by abnormal valvular function.
Cardiac MRI (CMR): *Normal heart valve function*	Valve size and competence.	Abnormal valve structure causes changes in openings, leading to increased pressures in the cardiac chambers and decreased cardiac output.

#12 Summary of Medications for Cardiac Valvular Disorders

Cardiac Valve Disease

Cardiac medications:		
Digoxin	Increases force and velocity of myocardial systolic contraction. Decreases conduction through AV node.	Convert and then control atrial fibrillation.	Digoxin requires periodic laboratory testing to ensure therapeutic drug level. Assess pulse prior to administration of digoxin. The pulse rate needs to be > 60 beats/min.
Calcium channel blockers:			
Cardizem		Control atrial fibrillation.	Never given if heart block, sick sinus syndrome, severe hypotension, and shock are present.
Calan		Manage heart failure if present.	Assess heart rate, blood pressure, lung sounds, and ECG monitor regularly.
ACE inhibitors	See above.		Monitor for hypotension especially when being given intravenously.
Antiarrhythmic agents	Reduces automaticity in the SA node and slows impulse conduction through the AV node. Used for supraventricular dysrhythmias.	To manage the dysrhythmias that are common with valve disease.	
	See above.		
Diuretics	See above.	To manage heart failure if present.	
Antibiotics	See above.	Prophylactically for dental work and invasive diagnostic studies as well as for the treatment of acute endocarditis episodes.	

(continued)

671

#12 Summary of Medications for Cardiac Valvular Disorders (Continued)

Anticoagulant therapy: Coumadin Heparin	See above.	Prevent strokes, pulmonary emboli, and deep venous thrombosis, especially if atrial fibrillation is occurring.	See above.
Nitrates (nitroglycerin)	Relaxes both atrial and venous smooth muscle, causing decreased preload and afterload.	Used with aortic valve disease to increase peripheral dilation and decrease preload, thereby allowing the heart to pump more effectively, hence decreasing myocardial oxygen demand. Dilate the coronary arteries to increase perfusion to the myocardium.	Assess blood pressure above and during therapy. Hypotension could result. Should be given with other vasodilators. Patient education includes: No alcohol use. Rotate patches. Keep medication with you at all times and away from excessive heat and light. Report blurred vision, dry mouth, and severe headache.

Sources: Adams, M. P., Josephen, D. L., & Holland, L. N. (Eds.). (2005). *Pharmacology for nurses: A pathophysiologic approach.* Upper Saddle River, NJ: Pearson Prentice Hall; American Heart Association. (2005). *Handbook of emergency cardiovascular care for health providers.* Dallas, TX: Author; Wilson, B., Shannon, M., & Stang, C. (Eds.). (2005). *Nurses drug guide.* Upper Saddle River, NJ: Pearson Prentice Hall.

#13 Patient Teaching & Discharge Priorities for Use of Anticoagulant Medications

Medication Need	Teaching
All anticoagulant/ antiplatelet agents	Take as directed by the health care provider. Do not skip doses. Consider an alert bracelet/necklace. Avoid activities that can cause injury or falling. Early warning signs of bleeding include bruising, nosebleeds, or bleeding gums. Serious bleeding can occur and includes: • Pink or brown urine • Red or black stool • Spitting up or coughing up bloody secretions or secretions that look like coffee grounds • Severe headache • Dizziness, fatigue, or weakness. Report any excessive bruising or bleeding to the health care provider.
Heparin	Patients need to be taught subcutaneous injection techniques.
Low molecular weight heparin	Patients need to be taught subcutaneous injection techniques. Frequent monitoring of lab work is generally not required for patients on low molecular weight heparin.
Warfarin/Coumadin	Patients need to take the exact dose as prescribed by their health care provider or pharmacist. They may need to take different doses of warfarin/Coumadin on different days of the week. Many patients taking warfarin are monitored by an interdisciplinary anticoagulation clinic rather than their health care provider. Instruct patients to know who is monitoring their warfarin/Coumadin.

(continued)

#13 Patient Teaching & Discharge Priorities for Use of Anticoagulant Medications (Continued)

Medication Need	Teaching
	If patients miss two or more doses in a row, they should call whoever is managing their medication for further instructions.
	Regular blood testing of the INR level is required. Instruct patients to know their optimal INR range. For many cardiovascular patients, it is between 2 and 3.
	Drug interactions can occur. Patients should use care when taking many over-the-counter drug preparations.
	The most likely drugs to affect the INR include aspirin, ibuprofen, cold remedies, antacids, and vitamin supplements. Herbal supplements can impact the INR, especially dan shen, garlic, *Ginkgo biloba,* ginseng, green tea, or kava.
	Food interactions can occur. Because the drug reduces the liver's ability to use vitamin K, any foods that change the amount of vitamin K in the body can affect the INR. These foods include brussels sprouts, kale, green tea, asparagus, avocado, broccoli, cabbage, cauliflower, collard greens, liver, soybean oil, soybeans, certain beans, mustard greens, peas (black-eyed peas, split peas, chick peas), turnip greens, parsley, green onions, spinach, and lettuce.
	Patients may be advised to limit their alcohol intake.
	Warfarin/Coumadin can cause birth defects; it should NOT be taken by patients planning to become pregnant.

#14 Diagnostic Tests for Cardiac Inflammatory Disorders

Test and *Normal Values*	Expected Abnormality	Rationale for Abnormality
White blood cells (WBC): *5,000–10,000/mm³*	Elevated with rheumatic fever, pericarditis, and myocarditis. Mild elevation with infective endocarditis (IE).	Elevated levels are associated with inflammation and infection.
Red blood cells (RBC): *Male: 4.7–6.1 mm³ Female: 4.2–5.4 mm³*	Mild to moderate decrease with rheumatic fever.	Occurs due to the inflammatory inhibition of erythropoiesis.
Erythrocyte sedimentation rate: *Male: up to 15 mm/hour Female: up to 20 mm/hour*	Elevated rheumatic fever, pericarditis, IE, and myocarditis.	The test measures inflammation. Chronic inflammation and infection cause an elevation.
C-reactive protein: *< 10 mg/L*	Elevated rheumatic fever, pericarditis, IE, and myocarditis.	Acute-phase reactant protein used to indicate an inflammatory illness.
Antistreptolysin O titer (ASO): *1:85 international unit/mL*	> 250 international unit/mL with rheumatic fever.	Streptococcal antibody test used to determine whether a previous streptococcal infection has caused a poststreptococcal infection such as rheumatic fever.

(continued)

#14 Diagnostic Tests for Cardiac Inflammatory Disorders (Continued)

Test and *Normal Values*	Expected Abnormality	Rationale for Abnormality
Cardiac marker: creatinine kinase MB (CK-MB), troponin T, and troponin I *Troponin T: < 3% or 0–7.5 ng/mL Troponin T: < 0.2 ng/mL Troponin I: < 0.35 ng/mL*	Elevated if carditis is present with all of the inflammatory disorders.	May be transiently elevated during the acute stages of myocardial cell damage.
BNP: *< 100 pg/mL or < 100 ng/L*	Elevated with ventricular hypertrophy, severe hypertension, and heart failure.	Marker of ventricular systolic and diastolic dysfunction. Useful to determine presence of heart failure.
Throat culture: *Negative or normal flora*	Positive for A beta-hemolytic streptococci with rheumatic fever.	Quantifies and differentiates bacterial from viral throat infections.
ECG: *Normal conduction time intervals (see Chapter 38)*	Prolonged PR interval with rheumatic fever. Diffuse ST segment abnormalities, T wave changes, dysrhythmias and heart block with myocarditis. ST segment changes associated with myocardial ischemia and the conduction delays typical of IE.	Conduction delays may be present with inflammation. ST segment changes may be present when myocardial ischemia is occurring.

Chest x-ray: *Clear lungs and normal heart size*	Enlarged heart and lung congestion with pancarditis and heart failure. May show cardiac enlargement if a pericardial effusion is present. Diagnoses of heart failure and in right-sided IE may show evidence of septic pulmonary emboli.	Cardiac enlargement occurs with inflammation, heart failure, and pericardial effusion. Congestion occurs with heart failure.
Echocardiogram (ultrasound): *Normal chamber size and normal cardiac structures*	Valve damage and dilated chamber size, abnormal pressure gradients, decreased ventricular function, and/or pericardial effusion with structurally abnormal valves. Depressed systolic function, dilated chambers, and mild to no pericardial effusion may occur with myocarditis. Determines the presence of pericardial fluid, motion of the heart walls, and the presence of restriction with pericarditis. Presence of thickening and calcification of the pericardium for IE.	The inflammation causes structural changes in cardiac chambers and function.

(continued)

#14 Diagnostic Tests for Cardiac Inflammatory Disorders (Continued)

Test and *Normal Values*	Expected Abnormality	Rationale for Abnormality
Cardiac catheterization: *Normal coronary arteries, chambers, and valve pressures*	Valve damage, enlarged chamber size, decreased ventricular and/or function with rheumatic fever. Valvular and ventricular function abnormalities, and assists in evaluating need for valve replacement surgery.	Inflammation causes changes in chamber size and valve function. Valve stenosis disrupts blood flow causing enlarged chamber size. Valve regurgitation causes a backflow of blood into the previous chamber.
Blood cultures: *Negative for organisms*	Positive and organism specific in 90–95% of cases with IE and therefore guide antibiotic therapy.	Organisms enter the bloodstream, adhere to the valve surface, and multiply.
Viral titers: *Negative*	Elevated.	Viral titers are present for 8 to 10 days after onset of illness.
Endomyocardial biopsy: *Normal tissue*	Presence of patchy cell necrosis and inflammatory changes confirm the diagnosis.	Often done within 6 weeks of acute illness while lymphocytic infiltration and myocyte damage is present.
Autoimmune serum markers: *Negative*	Presence of intracellular adhesion molecules on cardiac myocytes.	Intracellular adhesion molecules on cardiac myocytes is specific to autoimmune myocarditis.

Source: From *Laboratory Tests and Diagnostic Procedures with Nursing Diagnosis*, 6th edition, by J. V. Corbett, 2004, Upper Saddle River, NJ: Pearson Prentice Hall.

#15 Pharmacology Summary of Medications to Treat Inflammatory Heart Disease

Medication Category	Action	Application/Indication	Nursing Responsibility
Inflammatory Heart Disease Antibiotics Erythromycin Penicillin Specific type depends on the organism	Inhibits protein synthesis of microorganisms by binding reversibly to a ribosome, thus interfering with transmission of genetic information.	*Rheumatic fever:* treats Lancefield group A beta-hemolytic streptococcus. *Pericarditis and myocarditis:* indicated if it is a bacterial infection. *Endocarditis:* indicated if infecting organism is bacterial and prophylactic for invasive procedures and dental work.	Assessment of history of drug allergies prior to administration. Assessment of clinical manifestations of allergic reaction. Assessment of relief of clinical manifestations to determine drug effectiveness. Patient education regarding need to complete the entire regimen and report any clinical manifestations of drug allergy.
Nonsteroidal Anti-Inflammatory Agents (NSAIDs) Indomethacin (Indocin) Ibuprofen Aspirin	Inhibits cyclooxgenase, an enzyme responsible for the formation of prostaglandins. When cyclooxygenase is inhibited, inflammation and pain are reduced.	*Rheumatic fever:* joint pain and fever. *Pericarditis:* chest pain and swelling. *Myocarditis:* pain. *Endocarditis:* fever.	Assess pain before and after administration to determine effectiveness. Medications should not be taken on an empty stomach. Monitor renal and liver function tests for abnormalities related to drug side effects. Assessment of bleeding and gastric ulcer development.

(continued)

#15 Pharmacology Summary of Medications to Treat Inflammatory Heart Disease (Continued)

Medication Category	Action	Application/Indication	Nursing Responsibility
Steroids Solu-Cortef Cortisone Solu-Medrol	Stabilizes leukocyte lysosomal membrane; inhibits phagocytosis and release of allergic substances; reduces capillary dilation and permeability. Modifies immune response to various stimuli.	*Myocarditis*: to prevent cardiac damage when the cause is autoimmune.	Careful assessment of relief of clinical manifestations. Assessment of side effects: Infection due to depressed immune response. Blood glucose monitoring. Gastric bleeding. Emotional lability. Lack of wound healing. Patient education regarding need to eventually reduce dosage.
Cardiac Medications ACE inhibitors: Lisinopril Enalapril Ramipril Captopril	ACE inhibitor: Lowers peripheral resistance and reduces blood volume by enhancing the excretion of sodium by inhibition of angiotensin-converting enzyme.	*Myocarditis*: heart failure. *Rheumatic fever, pericarditis, and myocarditis*: to control atrial and ventricular dysrhythmias caused by inflammation and stretching of myocardium.	Monitor blood pressure carefully after first dose for hypotension. Educate patient that it takes 2 weeks for therapeutic effect. May experience dizziness.

Antiarrhythmic Agents Adenosine Amiodarone Atropine sulfate Sotalol	Alters the electrophysiological properties of the heart by either blocking flow through the channels or altering autonomic activity.	To control dysrhythmias.	There is a narrow margin between therapeutic effect and toxicity; therefore, careful and ongoing cardiac monitoring is essential. Patient teaching includes avoiding the use of alcohol, drugs, and tobacco.
Diuretics Furosemide Torsemide	Blocks reabsorption of sodium and chloride in the loop of Henle. Reduces edema associated with heart failure.	*Myocarditis:* heart failure.	Potassium levels also need monitoring because low levels are a side effect of certain diuretics, especially furosemide. May need potassium replacement. Measure urine output prior to administration to gauge the response to the medication.
Anticoagulant Therapy Coumadin Heparin Aspirin	Can either inhibit specific clotting factors in coagulation cascade or diminish the clotting action of platelets.	*Myocarditis:* to prevent thromboembolism from mural wall blood clots.	Ongoing assessment of therapeutic blood level per health care provider orders. Assess for bleeding including nosebleeds, bruising, "coffee-grounds" emesis, tarry stools, fatigue, and pale skin. Assess for decreases in hemoglobin, hematocrit, RBCs, and platelets.

(continued)

#15 Pharmacology Summary of Medications to Treat Inflammatory Heart Disease (Continued)

Medication Category	Action	Application/Indication	Nursing Responsibility
Antianxiety Agents Valium Versed Xanax	Acts by binding with the gamma-aminobutyric acid (GABA) receptor-chloride channel molecule. This intensifies the effect of GABA, which is a natural inhibitory neurotransmitter.	*Rheumatic fever, pericarditis, myocarditis, and endocarditis:* may be necessary for anxiety-onset heart disease and its impact on the quality of life.	Assess patient's anxiety levels and ability to sleep. Assess for excessive sleepiness and respiratory depression as side effects.

Sources: Adams, M. P., Josephen, D. L., & Holland, L. N. (Eds.). (2005). *Pharmacology for nurses: A pathophysiologic approach.* Upper Saddle River, NJ: Pearson Prentice Hall; American Heart Association. (2005). *Handbook of emergency cardiovascular care for health providers.* Dallas, TX: Author; Wilson, B., Shannon, M., & Stang, C. (Eds.). (2005). *Nurses drug guide.* Upper Saddle River, NJ: Pearson Prentice Hall.

#16 Nursing Process: Patient Care Plan for Inflammatory Heart Disease

Assessment of Respiratory Status

Subjective Data:

Do you feel short of breath?

When does it occur?

How far can you walk before you have to rest due to shortness of breath?

Do you have a cough and, if so, do you cough anything up?

Do you become more short of breath when lying down?

Objective Data:

Acid–base balance.

Lung sounds.

Respiratory rate.

Assess for adventitious or diminished breath sounds.

Note presence of cough, and amount and color of sputum.

Monitor ABGs and oxygen saturation.

Monitor respiratory rate and depth.

Monitor restlessness and confusion.

Observe for cyanosis, especially in the mucous membranes.

Nursing Assessment and Diagnoses	Outcomes and Evaluation Parameters	Planning and Interventions with *Rationales*
Nursing Diagnosis: *Impaired Gas Exchange* related to heart failure	**Outcome:** Adequate gas exchange achieved. **Evaluation Parameters:** Normal arterial blood gases.	**Interventions and *Rationales*:** Monitor: Turn, cough, deep breathe, elevate head of bed. instruct on use of incentive spirometry. *Measures to promote gas exchange.*

(continued)

#16 Nursing Process: Patient Care Plan for Inflammatory Heart Disease (Continued)

Nursing Assessment and Diagnoses	Outcomes and Evaluation Parameters	Planning and Interventions with *Rationales*
	No dyspnea: unlabored respirations < 24/minute.	Administer humidified oxygen as prescribed by the health care provider. *Medical intervention may be indicated to prevent respiratory failure.*
	No ischemic ECG changes such as ST segment changes and dysrhythmias.	Report respiratory distress to the health care provider. *Medical intervention may be indicated to prevent respiratory failure.*
	Alert and oriented.	Assess need for suctioning and/or endotracheal intubation *to maintain adequate gas exchange.*
	Clear breath sounds.	
	No restlessness, cyanosis, or fatigue.	Monitor fluid status *to assess heart failure.*
	Oxygen saturation is within normal limits.	
Assessment of Pain Subjective Data:	**Objective Data:**	
Do you have problems with pain?	Use pain scale (0–10) to quantify pain level.	
Where is the pain (joints, chest)?	Assess cultural and religious impact on patient's responses.	
What brings the pain on; what makes it go away?	Assess the onset of increased pain to evaluate the presence of disease.	
What do you use to relieve it and is it effective?	progression and/or an embolic event.	
Is the pain getting worse?		

| Nursing Diagnosis: *Pain, acute* related to fluid build up and inflammatory response | Outcome: Comfort level maintained. Evaluation Parameters: Patient able to communicate pain level and therapies that help alleviate it. Pain reduced and/or absent as evidenced by patient report and no pain behaviors: grimacing. Nonpharmacologic method of control is effective as evidenced by patient report and no pain behaviors. Patient reports satisfaction with pain management program. Patient is compliant with both antibiotics and pain medication schedule. Reports understanding of need to report a change in pain level to health care provider. | Interventions and Rationales: Instruct patient to inform nurse if pain is not relieved. *Indicates need to change pain management plan.* Obtain a clear description of source of discomfort. *This will assist in developing a pain management plan.* Correct misconceptions about risk of addiction and overdose *to decrease anxiety related to medication addiction.* Provide a supportive environment where patient is able to express pain level. *Opens communication and facilitates pain management.* Use pain control measures before pain becomes severe. *This increases comfort and decreases need for medication.* |

(continued)

#16 Nursing Process: Patient Care Plan for Inflammatory Heart Disease (Continued)

Nursing Assessment and Diagnoses	Outcomes and Evaluation Parameters	Planning and Interventions with *Rationales*
		Teach nonpharmacologic method of control, i.e., guided imagery and massage, and breathing exercises. *These measures augment pain relief.* Teach the patient/family the correct dosage and time intervals for medication administration *to increase compliance and prevent complications.*

Assessment of Anxiety Related to Inflammatory Heart Disease

Subjective Data:
Has anyone explained your health problems to you?
Would you tell me what you know about your disease?
How does this disease affect your daily life?
Do you feel anxious about your health problems?
Do you have family members or close friends who provide emotional support?

Objective Data:
Observe for manifestations of anxiety: restlessness, apprehension, withdrawal.

Nursing Diagnosis: *Fear and Anxiety* related to inflammatory heart disease

Outcomes: Anxiety level minimized and manageable.
Evaluation Parameters: Verbalizes anxious feelings.
Verbalizes what relieves anxiety.

Interventions and Rationales: Provide factual information concerning diagnosis, treatment, disfigurement, disabilities, and prognosis. *Truthful explanations increase trust and potentially decrease anxiety.*

Verbalizes absence of sensory perceptual disorders.
Verbalizes absence of physical manifestations of anxiety.
Behavioral manifestations of anxiety absent.

Explain all procedures and allow time for mental preparation. *This decreases fear and anxiety of the unknown.*

Allow time and encourage verbalization of fears related to illness *to assist in relieving anxiety.*

Explore with the patient/family techniques to reduce anxiety. *This gives the patient a sense of control and opens communication about the subject.*

Explore with patient effective ways to minimize anxiety. *This gives the patient a sense of control.* Instruct patient on use of relaxation techniques *to relieve anxiety.*

Assess need for and administer antianxiety and pain medication. *If alternative measures are not effective, may need antianxiety agents.*

(continued)

#16 Nursing Process: Patient Care Plan for Inflammatory Heart Disease (Continued)

Nursing Assessment and Diagnoses	Outcomes and Evaluation Parameters	Planning and Interventions with *Rationales*
Assessment of Cardiac Output **Subjective Data:** Do you become short of breath at rest or with activity? Has your shortness of breath become worse? Do your legs become swollen at any time during the day? Have you noticed a blue tinge in your nail beds?		**Objective Data:** Determine heart rate and rhythm. Assess: Blood pressure Lung sounds Urine output Capillary refill Right-sided heart failure (JVD, hepatomegaly, peripheral edema).
Nursing Diagnoses: Decreased Cardiac Output and *Ineffective Tissue Perfusion* related to infection, incompetent valves, and heart failure	*Outcome:* Sufficient cardiac output to perfuse organs. *Evaluation Parameter:* Minimal valve damage that decreases cardiac output.	*Interventions and Rationales:* Auscultate heart sounds for murmur and S_3, S_4 *to evaluate valve function and onset of heart failure.* Provide oxygen per order *to increase oxygen to the heart and peripheral tissues.* Administer diuretics, inotropics, and a low sodium diet *to treat heart failure.* Plan rest period *to reduce cardiac workload.*

Assessment of Tissue Perfusion

Subjective Data:

Do you have any pain in either leg?

Have you noticed any swelling or hard reddened areas?

Have you had any sudden chest pain that becomes worse when you take a deep breath?

Have you had any headaches, loss of consciousness, or dizzy spells?

Nursing Diagnosis: *Ineffective Tissue Perfusion* related to dislodging of vegetative growths and immobility-related thrombophlebitis

Outcome: Occurrence of emboli diagnosed early and treatment instituted.

Evaluation Parameter: Effective prevention of DVT.

Objective Data:

Assess:

Lung congestion. Urine output and color. Abdominal pain. Neurological function.

Skin and eyes.

Nail beds.

Calf deep vein thrombosis (DVT).

Glasgow Coma Scale.

Interventions and Rationales: Apply elastic compression stocking *to provide venous support.*

Teach leg exercises *to promote venous return and decrease risk of DVT.*

Report any new abnormal clinical manifestations to the health care provider.

Monitor for therapeutic levels of anticoagulant therapy.

Monitor for bleeding.

(continued)

#16 Nursing Process: Patient Care Plan for Inflammatory Heart Disease (Continued)

Nursing Assessment and Diagnoses	Outcomes and Evaluation Parameters	Planning and Interventions with *Rationales*

Assessment of Knowledge of Health Problems

Subjective Data:

What have you been told about your health problems?

Tell me what you know about your health problems.

What do you do when symptoms occur?

Do you see your health care provider on a regular basis?

Do you know what symptoms are important to report to your health care provider immediately?

Nursing Diagnosis: Deficient Knowledge related to disease process and prognosis

Outcome: Verbalizes understanding of prevention. **Evaluation Parameter:** Reports regular dental appointments and follow-up visits. Verbalizes adherence and compliance to therapy.

Objective Data:

Assess knowledge of need to rest the heart and decrease the oxygen needs Explore patient's understanding of purpose of preventive antibiotic therapy.

Interventions and Rationales: See Chart 41-8 for home care and remainder of teaching needs.

Assessment of Activity Tolerance

Subjective Data:

What type of activity fatigues you?

Has it been getting progressively worse?

Does activity increase joint tenderness and swelling?

Are you able to complete your ADLs without fatigue or shortness of breath?

Objective Data:

Assess for joint tenderness, swelling, and decreased range of motion. Monitor vital signs during activity.

Nursing Assessment and Diagnoses	Outcomes and Evaluation Parameters	Planning and Interventions with *Rationales*
Nursing Diagnosis: Activity Intolerance related to decreased cardiac output, fatigue, and inflammation	*Outcome:* Able to complete ADLs without fatigue. *Evaluation Parameter:* Able to increase activity level with resolution of clinical manifestations.	*Interventions and Rationales:* Take 30- to 60-minute rest periods between all activities *to decrease cardiac workload.* Perform only essential activities until endurance improves *to decrease cardiac workload during the healing process.*

Assessment of Fever

Subjective Data:
Do you feel hotter than normal?
If so, how long have you been feeling that way?
Have you had the chills?

Objective Data:
Monitor temperature and WBC count.

Nursing Assessment and Diagnoses	Outcomes and Evaluation Parameters	Planning and Interventions with *Rationales*
Nursing Diagnosis: Hyperthermia related to the infection	*Outcomes:* Normal temperature. Absence of chills. *Evaluation Parameters:* Effective antibiotic treatment. Resolution of infection.	*Interventions and Rationales:* Administer antipyretics *to decrease temperature.* Administer antibiotics *to treat causative organism.* Cover patient *to prevent shivering and subsequent temperature elevation.*

#17 Patient Teaching & Discharge Priorities for Inflammatory Heart Disease

Need	Teaching
Knowledge of disease process and prognosis	Home care needs include verbal and written instructions for:
Understanding of medications	• Treatment plan
Oral hygiene	• Follow-up care
Disease prevention	• Activity restriction
Safety	These instructions will reinforce need to comply with therapy.
Reportable clinical manifestations	The patient/family are
Family/Support system	taught to administer the antibiotics and to care for the infusion site
Emotional adjustment of patient/family due to the chronic nature of the disease.	using aseptic technique.
	Teach the purpose, dose, and possible side effects of all medications to increase compliance and prevent over/underdosing.
	Emphasize the importance of good dental hygiene and regular checkups to decrease the risk of pathogen entry via the mouth.
	Explain the need for antibiotic prophylaxis before invasive procedures to prevent reoccurrence.
	Encourage avoidance of people with upper respiratory infections to prevent an increased risk of infection.
	Avoid IV drug use.
	Stress the importance of a medic alert bracelet to identify a heart problem to health care workers.

Instruct patient/family to report:

- Change of exercise tolerance
- New onset chest pain and fever
- Clinical manifestations of heart failure

Assess availability, knowledge and compliance with treatment regimen.

Assess respite needs and resources. Assess discharge placement needs:

- Home
- Rehabilitation facility
- Extended care facility

Assess home environment for need for assistive devices.

Assess for need for professional home health needs.

Assess need for follow-up appointments.

Answer questions honestly.

Encourage verbalization of frustrations and anger.

Encourage positive reinforcement from the family.

Stress that it is not uncommon to feel a let down or depressed after discharge.

#18 Nursing Process: Patient Care Plan for Cardiomyopathy

Assessment of Knowledge of Disease

Subjective Data:

What have you been told about your health?

What is your understanding of the treatments you are on?

Do you drink alcohol or use any recreational drugs?

Do you take rest periods during the day?

What is your level of activity?

Do you feel any change in your ability to perform your activities of daily living (ADLs)?

How much activity can you do before you become short of breath?

What symptoms need to be reported to your health care provider?

Objective Data:

Assess:

Level of understanding of disease and treatment.

Compliance with therapy.

High-risk behaviors.

Lung sounds.

Vital signs.

Peripheral edema.

Shortness of breath.

Cough—type of sputum.

Nursing Assessment and Diagnoses	Outcomes and Evaluation Parameters	Planning and Interventions with *Rationales*
Nursing Diagnosis: Deficient Knowledge related to disease process, care needs, and complications	*Outcomes:* Understanding of disease process, care needs, and importance of compliance with treatment.	*Interventions and Rationales:* Avoid high-risk behaviors (alcohol, cocaine).
	Evaluation Parameters: Compliance with treatment plan. Activity level appropriate for cardiac workload.	Report any increases in clinical manifestations to your health care provider. *To retard the progression of the disease.*
		Comply with therapy *to prevent progression of the disease.*
		Activity restriction *to decrease cardiac workload.*

Assessment of Heart Failure

Subjective Data:
How much activity are you able to do before becoming short of breath? Do you have a cough? If so, is it productive?
Do your feet swell?

Objective Data:
Assess:
Vital signs.
Lung sounds.
Jugular venous distention.
Dyspnea.
Confusion.
Decreased urine output.
Orthopnea.
Pink frothy sputum.
Skin temperature.
Peripheral edema.

Nursing Assessment and Diagnoses	Outcomes and Evaluation Parameters	Planning and Interventions with Rationales
Nursing Diagnosis: *Tissue perfusion ineffective* related to hypercontractility and aortic outflow obstruction	**Outcome:** Prevention of heart failure. **Evaluation Parameters:** Lungs clear. Patient denies shortness of breath. Patient verbalizes understanding and willingness of treatment plan.	**Interventions and Rationales:** Monitor BUN, creatinine, liver enzymes, bilirubin *to assess blood supply to liver and kidneys.* Monitor fluid balance and record as prescribed *to assess fluid retention that would exacerbate the symptoms of heart failure.* Report significant imbalances to the health care provider *to obtain the necessary intervention(s) to correct the imbalance.*

(continued)

695

#18 Nursing Process: Patient Care Plan for Cardiomyopathy (Continued)

Assessment of Anxiety

Subjective Data:

What do you know about your disease process?

How do your health-related issues impact your daily life?

Do you feel anxious about your health?

Do you have family members or close friends who provide emotional support?

Objective Data:

Observe for manifestations of anxiety: restlessness, apprehension, withdrawal.

Nursing Assessment and Diagnoses	Outcomes and Evaluation Parameters	Planning and Interventions with Rationales
Nursing Diagnosis: Fear and Anxiety related to disease process and sudden cardiac death	**Outcome:** Anxiety level minimized and manageable. **Evaluation Parameters:** Verbalizes anxious feelings. Verbalizes what relieves anxiety. Demonstrates anxiety-relief by consistently controlling aggression, impulsiveness, and self-mutilation, and by improving coping and social interaction skills.	**Interventions and Rationales:** Allow time and encourage verbalization of fears related to illness *to assist in relieving anxiety.* Explore with the patient/family techniques to reduce anxiety. *This gives the patient a sense of control and opens communication about the subject.* Provide factual information concerning diagnosis, treatment, disfigurement, disabilities, and prognosis. *Truthful explanations increase trust and potentially decrease anxiety.* Explain all procedures and allow time for mental preparation. *This decreases fear and anxiety of the unknown.* Explore effective ways to minimize anxiety. *This gives the patient a sense of control.*

Instruct patient on use of relaxation techniques to relieve anxiety.
Assess need for and administer antianxiety and pain medication. *If alternative measures are not effective, may need antianxiety agents.*

Verbalizes absence of sensory perceptual disorders. Verbalizes absence of physical manifestations of anxiety. Behavioral manifestations of anxiety absent.

Assessment of Ability to Function in Usual Role

Subjective Data:
What is your role in your family?
Are you able to perform that role?
Who takes over your role function when you are not able to?
How do you feel about your inability to function in your role?

Objective Data:
Determine knowledge of health status (see *Deficient Knowledge* nursing diagnosis).
Assess level of functioning.
Assess alternatives or alterations in role function.

Nursing Assessment and Diagnoses	Outcomes and Evaluation Parameters	Planning and Interventions with Rationales
Nursing Diagnosis: Powerlessness over altered role function due to chronic progressive illness	**Outcomes:** Verbalizes a realistic perception of control. Verbalizes realistic perception of abilities to perform. **Evaluation Parameters:** Identifies health outcome priorities. Verbalizes powerlessness. Identifies actions that are within his/her control and demon-	**Interventions and Rationales:** Discuss realistic options for self-care. *Gives patient hope and realistic view of limitations.* Reinforce personal strengths. *Decreases sense of powerlessness.* Encourage verbalization of feeling of powerlessness. *Opens communication.* Assist patient to increase independence when realistic. *Decreases powerlessness.*

(continued)

#18 Nursing Process: Patient Care Plan for Cardiomyopathy (Continued)

strates ability to perform those actions. Reports adequate support from staff and family.	Allow control over surroundings and schedule when possible. *Decreases powerlessness.* Keep items within reach. *Decreases powerlessness.* Set short-term realistic goals. *Decreases powerlessness.* Explore patient's support mechanisms: family, church, and friends. *Needed as a source of support.*

Assessment of Compliance with Treatment Regimen

Subjective Data:

What do you understand about your treatment plan?

Are you able to comply with the restrictions necessary to prevent further progression of your disease?

What can the health care team do to help you with treatment compliance?

Objective Data:

Assess motivation and willingness to comply with therapy.

Assess where health care team can assist with barriers to compliance.

Nursing Assessment and Diagnoses	Outcomes and Evaluation Parameters	Planning and Interventions with *Rationales*
Nursing Diagnosis: *Noncompliance* with medication and activity restrictions	**Outcomes:** Shows willingness to comply with therapy.	**Interventions and *Rationales*:** Suggest alternative solutions to barriers *to determine interventions that will increase compliance.* Monitor and

Evaluation Parameters: Accepts imposed restrictions and complies with treatment plan.

Evaluation Parameters: Accepts imposed restrictions and complies with treatment plan.

evaluate compliance with therapy *to determine patient's ability to sustain treatment.*

Assessment of Fatigue

Subjective Data:

What level of activity fatigues you?

Have you been becoming more fatigued with less activity recently?

Are you able to complete your ADLs without fatigue?

Objective Data:

Monitor tolerance to activities while on bed rest in order to obtain a baseline to plan activities. Monitor for changes in symptoms and vital signs (VS) during activity.

Determine if pulse, respirations, and BP return to normal within 3 minutes after stopping activity.

Nursing Assessment and Diagnoses	Outcomes and Evaluation Parameters	Planning and Interventions with *Rationales*
Nursing Diagnosis: Fatigue and *Activity Intolerance* related to decreased cardiac output	*Outcomes:* No increase in fatigue or decrease in activity levels. *Evaluation Parameters:* Absence of or no progression of peripheral edema, congested lungs, decreased CO, dyspnea, pink frothy sputum, diaphoresis, and decreased renal and liver perfusion.	*Interventions and Rationales:* Identify activities that increase fatigue *to avoid increasing cardiac workload.* Discontinue activity if chest pain, dyspnea, cyanosis, dizziness, hypotension, sustained tachycardia, or dysrhythmias develop *to aid in evaluating tolerance of activities.* Explore sedentary activities the patient may enjoy *to provide diversion that does not place a demand.*

(continued)

#18 Nursing Process: Patient Care Plan for Cardiomyopathy (Continued)

Assessment of Tissue Perfusion

Subjective Data:

Do you become short of breath? If so, what causes it to occur?

How far can you walk before becoming short of breath?

Do you experience leg pain? If so, what brings it on and is it getting worse?

Do your hands and feet feel cold on a warm day?

Objective Data:

Assess:

Acid–base balance.

Lung sounds.

Respiratory rate.

Nursing Assessment and Diagnoses	Outcomes and Evaluation Parameters	Planning and Interventions with *Rationales*
Nursing Diagnosis: *Ineffective Tissue Perfusion* related to decreased cardiac output	**Outcome:** Adequate gas exchange. **Evaluation Parameters:** Normal ABGs. No dyspnea: unlabored respirations < 24/minute. Alert and oriented. Clear breath sounds. No restlessness, cyanosis, or fatigue. Oxygen saturation is within normal limits.	**Interventions and Rationales:** Assess for adventitious or diminished breath sounds. *Indicates decreased gas exchange and heart failure.* Note presence of cough, and amount and color of sputum. *Assessing for heart failure.* Monitor ABGs and oxygen saturation *to assess adequacy of gas exchange.* Monitor respiratory rate and depth *to assess for respiratory distress.* Monitor fluid status *to assess heart failure.* Monitor restlessness and confusion. *Indicators of inadequate gas exchange with resultant brain hypoxia.*

Assess need for suctioning and/or endotracheal intubation to *maintain adequate gas exchange.*

Observe for cyanosis, especially in the mucous membranes. *Indicators of inadequate gas exchange with resultant tissue hypoxia.*

Turn, cough, deep breathe, elevate head of bed, instruct on use of incentive spirometry. *Measures to promote gas exchange.*

Administer humidified oxygen as prescribed *to increase oxygen levels.*

Report respiratory distress to the health care provider. *Medical intervention may be indicated to prevent respiratory failure.*

Assessment of Cardiac Output

Subjective Data:

Do you feel weak or light-headed with activity?
Do you become short of breath? If so, what causes it to occur?
Is the shortness of breath getting worse?

Objective Data:

Assess:
Vital signs.
Lung sounds.
Weight.
Cardiac output.
Fluid intake and output.

(continued)

#18 Nursing Process: Patient Care Plan for Cardiomyopathy (Continued)

Nursing Assessment and Diagnoses	Outcomes and Evaluation Parameters	Planning and Interventions with Rationales
Nursing Diagnosis: Decreased Cardiac Output related to hypercontractility and obstruction to outflow	*Outcomes:* Patient able to tolerate decreased cardiac output. Stabilization of cardiac output. *Evaluation Parameters:* Clear lung sounds. No dyspnea. Normal vital signs. Skin warm and dry. Normal heart rate and rhythm. No abnormal heart sounds (S_3 and S_4). No jugular venous distention, peripheral edema, and ascites. Normal urine output.	*Interventions and Rationales:* Monitor vital signs, lung sounds, skin, heart rate and rhythm, edema, JVD, and ascites *in order to monitor response and tolerance of altered cardiac output (CO).* Administer negative inotropic medications as ordered *to decrease the hypercontractility.* Avoid a valsalva maneuver *because it impedes venous return (preload).*

#19 Patient Teaching for Cardiomyopathies

Need	Teaching
Prevention of disease progression	Teach the importance of following a treatment plan that includes medications (that slow disease progression) and lifestyle changes. Teaching includes: • Timed rest periods between activities. • Space activities to prevent dyspnea. • Avoid alcohol and drug use (cocaine). • Restrict sodium and fluid intake to prevent fluid overload.
Compliance with therapy	Teach the importance of complying with the treatment plan in order to slow the progress of the disease and prevent sudden death. Determine motivation factors for individual patients and create a plan that utilizes these factors. Comply with follow-up health care provider visits.
Prevent exacerbation of heart failure	Explain to patient/family what clinical manifestations to monitor and report to the health care worker: • Sudden increase in weight in a short period of time; i.e., greater than 2–3 lb in a few days • Shortness of breath at rest, possibly with chest pressure • Increased shortness of breath with activities • Persistent productive cough • Swelling ankles, feet, or abdomen • Waking breathless at night Diet therapy: limit sodium to 2–3 g and 2 liters of fluid daily. Eat small, frequent meals Plan rest periods between activities
Reportable clinical manifestations	Clinical manifestations of heart failure Clinical manifestations of infective endocarditis New onset chest pain

#20 Postoperative Nursing Care of the Valve Surgery Patient

- Following valve surgery patients will be admitted to the critical care area (24 to 43 hours) where the ECG, hemodynamic status, cardiac output, and pulmonary artery pressures can be monitored and ventilatory support provided.
- Vasoactive agents optimize cardiac output. Inotropic agents improve cardiac contractility, and vasodilators decrease afterload.
- Monitor for the usual complications such as hemorrhage, wound infection, and pulmonary complications.
- ECG monitoring
  - Dysrhythmias may occur because the mitral and aortic valves lie close to the conduction pathway.
  - Transient or permanent heart blocks may occur due to edema, ischemia, or damage to the conduction pathway, pacemaker may be required.
  - Atrial dysrhythmias are a common symptom.
- Anticoagulant therapy is started within 48 hours of valve surgery.

#21 Indications for Prophylactic Antibiotic Therapy with Infective Endocarditis

Medical Indications	Procedural Indications
Prosthetic heart valve	A dental procedure in which bleeding is likely, including cleaning and extractions
Previous episodes of IE	
Rheumatic heart disease	
Hypertrophic cardiomyopathy	Periodontal procedures/dental implants
Mitral valve prolapse with regurgitation and murmur	Bronchoscopy and/or pulmonary biopsy
Sclerotic aortic valve	Cystoscopy/colonoscopy
Most congenital heart malformations	Urinary catheterization when infection is present
Surgically constructed systemic-pulmonary shunts or conduits	Incision and drainage of infective tissue, especially soft tissue
	Vaginal delivery if infection is present
	Most surgeries

Source: Eble, B.E., Reyeds, G., and Wiewall-Winkellmann, J. eMedicine—Endocarditis, Bacterial.
http://intranet.santa.lt/thesaurus/REZIDENTUI/Valvular/endocarditis%20bacterial%20child.htm

#22 Summary of Medications to Treat Heart Failure

Medication Category	Action	Application/Indication	Nursing Responsibility
Angiotensin-converting enzyme (ACE) inhibitors: Benazepril Captopril Enalapril Lisinopril Quinapril Ramipril	Works within the renin-angiotensin-aldosterone system (RAAS) to inhibit the vasoconstricting action of angiotensin II and the angiotensin-mediated secretion of aldosterone, thus causing blood vessels to dilate, and systemic vascular resistance is decreased. Results in decreased afterload, decreased sodium resorption, and increased contractility.	Use in all patients with reduced ventricular function; left ventricular ejection fraction (LVEF) < 40%. HF patients on ACE inhibitors have improved survival and delayed progression of heart failure due to the favorable blockade of the RAAS.	Monitor for ACE inhibitor-induced cough, dizziness, hypotension, hyperkalemia, and worsening renal insufficiency. Angioedema may also occur in rare settings.
Angiotensin II receptor blockers (ARBs): Candesartan cilexetil Eprosartan mesylate Irbesartan	Causes inhibition by blocking RAAS activation at the angiotensin II receptor site. Angiotensin receptor blockers have been found to have similar clinical effects as	Use in heart failure (HF) patients who are intolerant to ACE inhibitors with an LVEF < 40%. HF patients on ARBs have improved	Monitor for dizziness, hypotension, hyperkalemia, and worsening renal insufficiency.

(continued)

#22 Summary of Medications to Treat Heart Failure (Continued)

Losartan potassium Telmisartan Valsartan	ACE inhibitors with regard to the interference with the RAAS. They decrease afterload, decrease sodium resorption, and increase contractility.	survival and delayed progression of heart failure due to the favorable blockade of the RAAS.
Beta-adrenergic blockers: Carvedilol Metoprolol succinate	Acts primarily by blocking the sympathetic nervous system (SNS) in patients with heart failure. By blocking these effects, there is an improvement in coronary blood flow and less ischemia. There also is a decreased workload on the heart and less myocyte hypertrophy resulting in decreased myocardial ischemia and hypertrophy.	Use in HF patients with LVEF < 40% or postmyocardial infarction. HF patients on beta-blockers have been found to have improved survival, improvement in symptoms, a decrease in the risk of sudden death, and improved overall exercise tolerance.	Observe for signs of hypotension or bradycardia, as either condition may require adjustment to the beta-adrenergic-blocker dose or other background medications. Patient education is imperative about the initial response or up-titration of this drug, which can cause fatigue, dizziness, fluid retention, and worsening heart failure. It is also imperative

Drug	Mechanism of Action	Uses	Nursing Implications
			that nurses instruct patients on how to monitor their pulse and blood pressure and to help them recognize when they should notify their provider if these parameters become too low. Beta-adrenergic blockers can worsen bronchospasm in patients with reactive airway disease and therefore should be monitored.
Diuretics: Bumetanide Furosemide Metolazone Torsemide	Interferes with the sodium retention of HF by inhibiting the reabsorption of sodium or chloride at specific sites in the renal tubules.	Use in HF patients exhibiting signs and symptoms of fluid overload. Diuretic drugs increase urinary sodium excretion and decrease physical signs of fluid retention in patients with HF.	Nursing assessment for patients on diuretics includes monitoring for signs of hypokalemia, hypotension, and dehydration. It is also imperative that nurses provide patient self-management instruction, including daily

(continued)

#22 Summary of Medications to Treat Heart Failure (Continued)

Medication Category	Action	Application/Indication	Nursing Responsibility
			weights, sodium and fluid restrictions, and instruction on when to notify their health care provider about worsening symptoms.
Digitalis Digoxin	A weak, positive inotrope that increases the contractility of the weakened heart muscle thus, improving the volume of cardiac output. It has also been found to have an impact on enzyme inhibition in noncardiac tissues, thus, eventually leading to a suppression of renin secretion from the RAAS.	Use in HF patients with New York Heart Association (NYHA) class III or IV symptoms. This medication has been found to decrease hospitalizations and to improve symptoms, quality of life, and exercise tolerance.	Nursing assessment for patients on digitalis includes monitoring for toxic drug levels that can cause cardiac dysrhythmias and conduction disturbances, gastrointestinal symptoms, and neurological complaints.
Aldosterone antagonists: Spironolactone	Blocks the release of aldosterone hormone secreted by the adrenal glands that, when activated in heart failure, causes sodium and fluid retention.	Use in HF patients with continued symptoms, despite therapies listed above. Found to have a favorable mortality	Monitor for signs of hyperkalemia and renal dysfunction. Should not be used in combination with ACE inhibitors and ARBs. Side effect

benefit and has shown to decrease hospitalizations. These benefits are greatest in those patients with NYHA class IV symptoms.

of some aldosterone antagonists is gynecomastia, which may require a change in antagonist used. Nursing instruction should include a discussion with the health care provider regarding the reduction or discontinuation of potassium supplements and also the avoidance of high-potassium-containing foods. Nonsteroidal anti-inflammatory drugs and cyclooxygenase-2 inhibitors should be avoided, which can worsen hyperkalemia and renal dysfunction.

(continued)

#22 Summary of Medications to Treat Heart Failure (Continued)

Hydralazine and isosorbide dinitrate	This combination of vasodilators acts on both arteries and veins. Theoretically, it may act as an antioxidant on nitric oxide.	African American HF patients on standard therapy (i.e., ACE inhibitors or ARBs) and beta-blockers may benefit when this combination is added. Patients unable to tolerate ACE inhibitor or ARB therapy may consider this alternative combination. This combination has shown improved survival, reduced hospitalizations, and improved quality of life.	Monitor for headache, hypotension, and gastrointestinal complaints. Should not be used in patients that have not had a trial of ACE inhibitor or ARBs. Compliance must be reinforced due to the multidose schedule required.

| Antiarrhythmic: Amiodarone Bretylium Dofetilide Ibutilide Sotalol | This class III antiarrhythmic agent has sympatholytic (or antiadrenergic) effects on the heart and AV nodal blocking properties. | May be used for rate and rhythm control for patients in atrial fibrillation, and to suppress significant ventricular dysrhythmias, or may suppress implantable cardioverter defibrillator (ICD) shocks. | Possible side effects include pulmonary toxicities, skin discoloration, hepatic and/or thyroid derangements, corneal deposits, optic neuropathy, and interactions with warfarin and digoxin. May be proarrhythmic; monitor cardiac rhythm. |

Sources: Adams, K. F., Lindenfeld, J., Arnold, J. M., et al. (2006). Executive summary: HFSA 2006 comprehensive heart failure practice guideline. *Journal of Cardiac Failure, 12*(1), 10–38; Crawford, P. A., & Lin, T. L. (2004). *The Washington manual cardiology subspecialty consult* (pp. 122–126). Philadelphia: Lippincott Williams & Wilkins; and Hunt, S. A., Abraham, W. T., Chin, M. H., Feldman, A. M., Francis, G. S., Ganiats, T. G., et al. (2005). ACC/AHA 2005 guideline update for the diagnosis and management of chronic heart failure in the adult: Summary article: A report of the American College of Cardiology/American Heart Association Task Force on Practice Guidelines (Writing Committee to Update the 2001 Guidelines for the Evaluation and Management of Heart Failure). *Journal of the American College of Cardiology, 46,*1116–1143.

#23A Nursing Process: Patient Care Plan for Heart Failure

Assessment of Hypervolemia

Subjective Data:

Are you having difficulties breathing at rest or with activity?

How long have you had shortness of breath (SOB)?

Do you need to sleep with your head propped up, or do you awaken short of breath in the middle of the night?

Do you have a cough?

Do you have abdominal bloating or lower extremity swelling?

Have you had recent weight increase over a short period of time (2–3 days)?

Objective Data:

Vital signs: weight blood pressure, heart rate (HR).

Oxygen saturation.

Dyspnea with exertion.

Lethargy.

Anxiety.

Lung sounds: crackles/wheezes.

Restlessness.

Elevated neck veins.

Ascites and/or lower extremity edema.

Daily weight.

Hemodynamic parameters:

1. Right atrial pressure (RAP) or central venous pressure (CVP)
2. Pulmonary artery pressure (PAP mean)
3. Pulmonary artery occlusion pressure (PAOP)
4. Cardiac output (CO) or cardiac index (CI)

Peripheral circulation:

1. Peripheral pulses
2. Presence of edema using the edema scale

3. Color and temperature
4. Capillary refill time

Intake and output:

1. Assess volume of fluid intake by any route (e.g., oral, intravenous).
2. Assess volume of fluid expelled by any route (e.g., urinary, nasogastric (NG), drainage, blood)

Evaluate laboratory/diagnostic findings associated with hypervolemia:

1. Serum sodium (may be decreased, normal, or elevated based on cause of hypervolemia)
2. BUN (may be normal to decreased)
3. Urine specific gravity (may be decreased)
4. Hematocrit (may be decreased)
5. Chest x-ray (may show pulmonary congestion or cardiomegaly)
6. Right heart catheterization (may indicate elevated filling pressures)

(continued)

713

#23A Nursing Process: Patient Care Plan for Heart Failure (Continued)

Nursing Assessment and Diagnosis	Outcomes and Evaluation Parameters	Planning and Interventions with *Rationales*
Nursing Diagnosis: Fluid volume excess related to ventricular dysfunction and sodium/water retention	*Outcomes:* Diuresis: improved volume status (i.e., euvolemia) and improved symptoms. *Evaluation Parameters:* Blood pressure target: 120/80 mmHg. Heart rate target: 60–100 beats/min. Improved New York Heart Association (NYHA) class. No signs of pulmonary congestion: airway patent; respiratory rate < 20 breaths/min; pattern regular and unlabored; lungs clear to auscultation all lobes bilaterally. Oxygen saturation > 90% in patients breathing room air.	*Interventions and Rationales:* Insert intravenous catheter. *To facilitate intravenous medication administration.* Administer and titrate intravenous (IV) medications. *To facilitate diuresis.* Record amount of Intravenous (IV) fluid infused. *To monitor fluid intake.* Assess vital signs and urine output regularly (every hour or less). *To assess adequacy of diuresis.* Monitor central venous pressure and pulmonary artery occlusion pressure (PAOP), if possible. *To assess response to diuresis.* Obtain and track daily morning weight. *To monitor adequacy of diuresis.* Monitor serum electrolytes, hematocrit, serum creatinine, and report critical abnormalities to the provider. *To monitor hematological changes associated with hypervolemia, possibly*

Hemodynamic parameters (normals):

1. RAP 1–7 mmHg or CVP 2–8 cm H_2O
2. PAP 10–20 mmHg
3. PCWP 6–12 mmHg
4. CO 3.5–5.5 L/min or CI 2.0–3.2 L/min/m²

Peripheral circulation:

1. Pulse 2–3 + on pulse grading scale
2. No edema
3. Skin warm, natural color
4. Capillary refill time less than 3 seconds

Intake and output:

1. Intake/output difference greater than 1,000 mL/24 hours or as defined for diuresis per provider
2. Urinary output average of greater than or equal to 30mL/hr

hypovolemia, electrolyte changes, and diuresis. Instruct patient on fluid and sodium restrictions. To prevent excess oral intake, which negates the effect of diuresis.

(continued)

#23A Nursing Process: Patient Care Plan for Heart Failure (Continued)

Daily morning weight less than the day prior. Abdomen soft, nondistended; no ascites.

Laboratory/diagnostic workup indicates:

1. Serum sodium 135–140 mEq/L
2. Blood urea nitrogen (BUN) 10–20 mg/dL
3. Urine specific gravity 1.005–1.030
4. Hematocrit, male: 42–52%, female: 37–47%

Assessment of Cardiac Output

Subjective Data:

How is your energy level?

Are symptoms limiting your level of activity?

Are you light-headed?

Are you having memory problems or troubles concentrating?

Are you making the same amount of urine as usual?

Objective Data:

Cardiovascular system:

1. Heart rate
2. Heart rhythm
3. Blood pressure
4. Peripheral pulses
5. Presence of edema using the edema scale

6. Color and temperature
7. Capillary refill time.

Heart sounds: murmurs, clicks, rubs, splitting.

Pulmonary status.

Oxygen saturation.

Hemodynamic parameters (as applicable):

1. Right atrial pressure (RAP) or central venous pressure (CVP)
2. Pulmonary artery pressure (PAP mean)
3. Pulmonary artery occlusion pressure (PAOP)
4. Cardiac output (CO) or cardiac index (CI).

Intake and output:

1. Assess volume of fluid intake by any route (e.g., oral, intravenous).
2. Assess volume of fluid expelled by any route (e.g., urinary, NG, drainage, blood).

ECG waveform (rhythm and intervals) as ordered (including cardiac rhythm, PR interval, QRS interval, QT/QTc interval, dysrhythmias). Obtain weight.

(continued)

#23A Nursing Process: Patient Care Plan for Heart Failure (Continued)

Evaluate laboratory/diagnostic findings associated with decreased cardiac output:

1. Serum BUN and creatinine (may be elevated)
2. Serum hematocrit, hemoglobin (may be decreased)
3. Echocardiogram (may show depressed ventricular function, pericardial effusion)
4. 12-lead ECG (may show dysrhythmias, myocardial infarction, heart block, tachycrdia, or bradycardia)
5. Blood gases (may show acidosis, hypoxemia)
6. Arterial–mixed venous blood gases may show an increased SaO_2/SvO_2 ratio.

Nursing Assessment and Diagnosis	Outcomes and Evaluation Parameters	Planning and Interventions with *Rationales*
Nursing Diagnosis: Decreased Cardiac Output related to ventricular dysfunction	*Outcome:* Adequate cardiac output as seen by improved organ, tissue, and cerebral perfusion related to *Evaluation Parameters:* Cardiovascular system: 1. Heart rate: 60–100 beats/min 2. Regular rhythm or patient's normal asymptomatic rhythm 3. BP: 120/80 mmHg	*Interventions and Rationales:* Insert intravenous catheter *to facilitate intravenous medication administration.* Administer and titrate IV medications *to facilitate diuresis and inotropic support.* Record amount of IV fluid infused *to monitor intake.* Assess vital signs and urine output regularly (every hour or less) *to assess adequacy of diuresis and inotropic support.* Monitor hourly urine output *to assess adequacy of diuresis.*

4. Pulses 2–3 + on pulse grading scale
5. No edema
6. Skin warm and natural color
7. Capillary refill time less than or equal to 3 seconds. Heart sounds: normal S_1 and S_2

Airway patent; respiratory rate < 20 per minute, pattern regular and unlabored; lungs clear to auscultation all lobes bilaterally. Oxygen saturation > 90% in patients breathing room air. Hemodynamic parameters:

1. RAP 1–7 mmHg or CVP 2–8 cm H_2O
2. PAP 10–20 mmHg
3. PCWP 6–12 mmHg

Monitor central venous pressure and pulmonary artery occlusion pressures (PAOP, CO/CI), if possible *to assess adequacy of diuresis and inotropic support of cardiac output.*

Monitor integument and neurological status *to assess for adequacy of tissue and cerebral perfusion.*

Administer oxygen *to ensure proper oxygenation and tissue perfusion.*

Administration of medications *to improve cardiac output, tissue perfusion, and diuresis.*

(continued)

#23A Nursing Process: Patient Care Plan for Heart Failure (Continued)

4. CO 3.5–5.5 L/min or CI 2.0–3.2 L/min/m^2

Intake and output:

1. Intake/output difference greater than 1,000 mL/24 hours or as defined for diuresis per provider.

2. Urinary output average of greater than or equal to 30 mL/hr.

ECG is stable, with regular rhythm or patient's normal asymptomatic rhythm, without evidence of ischemia, myocardial infarction, tachycardia/bradycardia, or heart block.

Cardiac intervals are within normal limits:

- PR interval: 0.12–0.20 second
- QRS interval: < 0.10 second
- QTc interval: 0.37–.047 second.

Daily morning weight less than the day prior. Laboratory/diagnostic findings:

1. BUN 10–20 mg/dL
2. Creatinine 0.8–1.3 mg/dL
3. Hematocrit, male: 42–52%, female 37–47%; hemoglobin, male: 14–18 g/dL, female 12–16 g/dL
4. May show depressed ventricular function
5. Sinus rhythm, sinus dysrhythmia, or patient's normal asymptomatic rhythm
6. pH 7.35–7.45, PCO_2 35–45 mmHg, HCO_3 21–28 mEq/L, PO_2 80–100 mmHg, O_2 saturation 95–100%
7. Normal SaO_2/SvO_2 ratio

(continued)

#23A Nursing Process: Patient Care Plan for Heart Failure (Continued)

Assessment of Activity Tolerance

Subjective Data:

How much activity are you able to do (i.e., walk for 5, 10, 30 + minutes, or not at all)?

Are you more or less active now than 1, 3, and 6 months ago?

Are you able to walk up 1 or 2 flights of stairs without stopping?

Do you have symptoms during exercise (chest pain, shortness of breath, palpitations, and light-headedness)?

Objective Data:

Vital signs: blood pressure (BP) and heart rate (HR).

Oxygen saturation.

NYHA classification for heart failure assessment.

Pain scale.

6-minute walk.

Nursing Assessment and Diagnosis	Outcomes and Evaluation Parameters	Planning and Interventions with *Rationales*
Nursing Diagnosis: Risk for Activity Intolerance related to impaired cardiac function secondary to chronic heart failure	*Outcomes:* Activity tolerance stabilizes or improves as seen by improved NYHA classification for heart failure, and decreased symptoms. *Evaluation Parameters:* Normal vital signs.	*Interventions and Rationales:* Monitor vital signs at rest and with activity and 3 minutes after activity (heart rate, BP, respiratory rate) *to obtain a baseline for comparison.* Monitor oxygenation before, during, and after activity *to obtain a baseline for comparison.* Assess baseline activity level (including strength and balance) and tolerance to activity *to use as basis for individualized plan.*

Oxygen levels are within normal range: oxygen saturation $> = 90\%$.	Assess symptoms at rest and with activity *to use as a baseline for comparison.*
Patients have clear plan for activity, with reasonable goals.	Monitor level of pain.
Patients have access to activity.	Assess degree of symptoms (NYHA class) *to use as a baseline for comparison.*
Patients understand what symptoms to monitor during activity: increased shortness of breath, chest pain, palpitations, lightheadedness.	Assess quality of life (QOL) *to use as a baseline for comparison.*
	Promote activity: Start with reasonable daily plan, increasing slowly, set reachable goal, plan around periods of rest, and reassure that small improvements will lead to physical, emotional, and psychosocial benefits. *An individualized plan of care will promote change.*
Symptoms during activity are minimal.	Promote exercise prescription: type, activity, duration, intensity. Monitor level of strength *to individualize each patient's plan.*
Patients have action plan for symptoms that occur.	
NYHA classification for heart failure has improved.	Teach appropriate diet to accompany activity plan. Assess current level of body mass index (BMI). Monitor current level of

(continued)

#23A Nursing Process: Patient Care Plan for Heart Failure (Continued)

Indexes of quality of life are improved.
Pain scale improves.
Strength and balance improve.
Nutrition improves.
Weight reduction occurs (if needed).
Stress is reduced.
Smoking cessation is successful.

nutrition and calorie content *to enhance balance nutrition and promote weight loss as needed.*
Teach strengthening exercises *to promote muscular strength to improve balance.*
Discuss level of stress and anxiety. Teach stress reduction techniques *to facilitate well-being and foster activity plan.*
Stress smoking cessation. *Smoking decreases oxygenation to muscles during activity.*
Teach heart failure symptoms to monitor: shortness of breath, chest pain, light-headedness, and passing out, palpitation *to obtain a baseline for comparison.*

Assessment of Dysrhythmias

Subjective Data:
Do you experience palpitations or feel that your heart races?
Do you become light-headed or pass out?
Do palpitations or light-headedness occur at the same time?

Objective Data:
Vital signs: BP and HR.
Oxygen saturation.
Level of consciousness.
ECG.

Lab values: electrolytes and Lung/cardiac.
Abdomen.
Integument.
Urine output.
Cardiac devices (if present).

Nursing Assessment and Diagnosis	Outcomes and Evaluation Parameters	Planning and Interventions with *Rationales*
Nursing Diagnosis: Cardiac output decreased due to dysrhythmias related to impaired cardiac function related to secondary to ischemia, acidosis, hypoxemia, electrolyte abnormalities, structural/conduction abnormalities, or device implantation.	*Outcome:* Absence of hemodynamically significant dysrhythmias. *Evaluation Parameters:* Heart rate is within normal range (60–80, or not > 100 beats per minute). Breath sounds are normal and clear, without respiratory distress. Oxygen levels are within normal range: SaO_2 > = 90%.	*Interventions and Rationales:* Assess cardiovascular status: heart rate, regularity of rhythm (pattern), and blood pressure. *To assess baseline, monitor for changes and response to therapy.* Assess lung sounds. *To assess for presence of lung fluid from increased dysrhythmias.* Assess oxygenation (SaO_2 and absence of acidosis). *To monitor baseline, for changes with dysrhythmias and response to therapy.* Assess level of consciousness (LOC). *To assess for changes/increases in dysrhythmias.*

(continued)

#23A Nursing Process: Patient Care Plan for Heart Failure (Continued)

Patient has no altered level of consciousness (LOC) or anxiety.

ECG is stable, with regular rhythm or patient's normal asymptomatic rhythm, without evidence of ischemia, myocardial infarction, tachycardia/bradycardia, or heart block.

Cardiac intervals are within normal limits:

- PR interval: 0.12–0.20 second
- QRS interval: <0.10 second
- QTc interval: 0.33–0.47 second

Lab values are within normal limits:

1. Potassium 3.5–5.1 mEq/L
2. Magnesium 1.3–2.1 mEq/L
3. Digoxin level, optimal = <1.1 ng/mL, toxic: >2.0 ng/mL
4. pH 7.35–7.45

Assess ECG and waveforms (rhythm, PR, QRS, and QTc intervals, dysrhythmias) *to establish a baseline, determine degree of abnormality and response to therapies.*

Assess lab and blood gas values (potassium, magnesium, calcium, digoxin level, presence of acidosis) *to establish a baseline, determine degree of abnormality and response to therapies.*

Assess abdomen to assess for ascites, abdominal pain, *presence of bowel sounds, organomegaly.*

Assess urine output to assess for decreases that may occur with dysrhythmias.

Assess integument to assess for cyanosis, pallor, or diaphoresis.

Assess cardiac device if present (i.e., pacemaker, cardiac defibrillator) *to assess proper position of leads and for appropriate device function.*

5. $PaCO_2$ 35–45 mmHg
6. HCO_3 21–27 mEq/L
7. Base excess +/− 2 mEq/L

Abdomen is soft, without pain, ascites, organomegaly. Urine output remains normal. Integument is dry, warm, well perfused. Cardiac device interrogation: shows properly functioning device with settings optimized and optimal battery life with leads intact.

Assessment of Knowledge Deficit

Subjective Data:

Patient/family express concerns about the diagnosis of heart failure, in terms of prognosis, changes in lifestyle, and progression of disease.

Patient/family express lack of understanding of therapies to treat heart failure.

Patient/family express concerns about how to take medications and their potential side effects.

Objective Data:

Patients may be anxious, confused, and may need repeated information.

(continued)

#23A Nursing Process: Patient Care Plan for Heart Failure (Continued)

Patient/family express concerns about what symptoms they might have and how to monitor them at home.
Patient/family express concerns about continuing a sexual relationship.
Patient/family express concerns about treatment options if medicines fail.
Patient/family express concerns about the mode of death.

Nursing Assessment and Diagnosis	Outcomes and Evaluation Parameters	Planning and Interventions with Rationales
Nursing Diagnosis: *Deficient Knowledge* related to the diagnosis of heart failure.	**Outcomes:** Patient/family understand: The diagnosis of heart failure. Their prognosis. Treatments for heart failure. Lifestyle changes. Progression of the disease. Symptoms to monitor. Sexuality. End-stage treatment options. Mode of death.	**Interventions and Rationales:** Discuss with patient/family the course of heart failure, using the diagram. *This will enhance their understanding of the chronic and progressive nature of the disease, which usually presents with periods of exacerbation and stabilization.* Discuss how heart failure is treated with the patient and family. *This will provide the fundamental treatment strategies for heart failure including medications, surgical strategies, and devices.* Discuss with patients/family the MAWDS-based curriculum of self-management support (see Figure 42–9). *This will teach the basic concepts that will help them to*

(continued)

understand their medications, about their activity, the importance of daily weights, their diet, and what to do when their symptoms worsen.

Discuss the common symptoms of heart failure with the patient and family, describing shortness of breath, cough, fatigue, activity intolerance, weight gain/edema, palpitations, chest tightness, and poor concentration. *This will enable the patient to recognize her symptoms and reinforce calling early when her symptoms worsen, so she can be seen and have adjustments made in her medications, preempting an urgent hospitalization.*

Discuss ways for the patient and significant other to maintain a sexual relationship. *Patients will understand that having sexual intercourse is about the amount of effort in climbing 2 flights of stairs. If they are able to complete this activity without significant symptoms, then sexual intercourse will likely be safe. Patients will understand other means of sexual intimacy and will understand what to do if symptoms worsen during sexual activities.*

Evaluation Parameters:
Patient/family will:

- Ask appropriate questions about the course of heart failure.
- Follow appropriate medication adjustments, and consider recommendations for surgical procedures and devices.
- Come in with a completed self-care diary, following instructions between visits.
- Call when their symptoms worsen for urgent evaluation when needed.
- Express attempts at maintaining a sexual relationship.
- Understand which end-stage therapies are available and for which they qualify.

#23A Nursing Process: Patient Care Plan for Heart Failure (Continued)

- Understand the usual mode of death of heart failure and have made appropriate plans with their health care team and family regarding their wishes. Advanced directives and power of attorney will have been filled out.

Describe end-stage treatment options to the patient and family. Those who fail standard therapy might be considered for cardiac transplantation, mechanical assist devices, and heart failure research studies or for hospice care. *The patient and family will understand which of the preceding end-stage therapies they might be considered for and why they might not be a candidate for others.*

Describe the mode of death for patients with heart failure. *Most patients with heart failure die either by a sudden dysrhythmia (caused by ventricular tachycardia or fibrillation) or by progressive deterioration of the cardiac muscle and its function. Dying suddenly will be a fast, typically painless, way to die. Dying of progressive disease is typically associated with more symptoms that will require an individualized plan for symptom relief by medicines such as narcotics, anxiolytics, nitrates, diuretics, and oxygen.*

#23B Patient Teaching & Discharge Priorities for Heart Failure

Patients discharged from the hospital have multiple needs. Teaching strategies should be based on these needs, with the goal to prevent readmissions, decrease disease progression, and improve quality of life.

Need	Teaching
Patient/family • Prevent recurrent symptoms of congestion. • Optimize medical therapy for heart failure and comorbid conditions. • Increase activity tolerance. • Minimize risk factors. • Provide palliative care.	MAWDS self-management instruction (medications, activity, weights, diet, symptoms). Provide list of current medications to patients with dose and schedule, with clear instructions on changes from prehospitalization. Instruct purpose of medications; refill prescriptions before running out; do not double up for missed doses; call with adverse effects. Increase activity as tolerated, monitoring for symptoms; become active most days; call with new or worsened symptoms. Review health maintenance strategies: smoking cessation, limited ethyl alcohol (ETOH), regular exercise, stress reduction, eating balanced diet, and optimally treating comorbid conditions. Discuss chronic nature of disease; encourage multidisciplinary team meeting regarding overall plans for care.
Family/support system • Assess resources to assist with chronic illness in the home setting.	Provide resources based on individual's needs: home health; hospice; family/friends/neighbors to help with home care; meals; transportation.
Setting • Assess home needs.	Assess safety from falls for those who are weak and at risk for falling; use occupational therapy to assess home safety and for home aids for debilitated patients.

#24 Differential Diagnosis of Chest Pain

Pain Description	Associated Findings	History
Angina/Myocardial Infarction	• Tachycardia	• Cardiac risk factors
• Usually retrosternal	• Tachypnea, dyspnea	• Smoking
• Can originate or radiate at the back, anterior chest, epigastric area, jaw, shoulder, elbow, forearm, wrist	• Weak heart sounds	• Male gender
	• Rales	• African American
	• Diaphoresis	• Sedentary lifestyle
• May be relieved with rest, lasts < 30 minutes	• Abnormal precordial impulses	• Social stressors
	• Evidence of dysrhythmias	• High-fat diet
• Heaviness, burning, tight pressure, aching, indigestion	• Fever, elevated white blood count (WBC) count, elevated sedimentation rate	• Cardiovascular disease
		• Heart failure
• Is not relieved with position change		• Dysrhythmias
• May increase while supine	• Anxiety, sense of impending doom	• PVD
• Is not aggravated by deep breathing	• Nausea/vomiting	• Heart valve disease
		• Angina, unstable angina, myocardial infarction (MI) cardiac interventions
		• Cardiac surgery
		• Catheter-based interventions

Pulmonary Embolism

- Sudden onset
- Sharp
- Pleuritic
- Lateral chest
- Increases on deep inspiration

- Shock
- Syncope
- Dyspnea, shortness of breath (SOB), cyanosis
- Tachycardia
- Hemoptysis
- Pleural friction rub
- Expiratory wheeze
- Fever

- Hypercoaguable state
- Immobility
- Surgery
- Trauma
- DVT

Gastrointestinal Disorders

- Burning, squeezing, gripping
- Retrosternal without radiation
- Lasts many hours or days, constant in nature
- Precipitated by bending over, drinking very hot/cold liquids, meals
- Relieved w/food or beverage

- Reflux
- Dysphagia
- Dyspepsia

- GERD
- Esophageal motility disorders
- Esophageal malignancy

(continued)

#24 Differential Diagnosis of Chest Pain (Continued)

Costochondritis
- Usually superficial and localized
- Described as tender, ache, sharp
- Can be in any location
- Duration variable
- Aggravated/provoked by movement or touch

- Sudden movement	- Falls or trauma
- Tachypnea, shallow breathing	- Immobility
- Tachycardia	- Chest tubes newly removed
- Elevated blood pressure	

Acute Anxiety
- Dull, stabbing

- Breathlessness, hyperventilation	- Acute stress, phobia
	- Inability to cope

Pain Description	Associated Findings	History
Pericarditis		
- Sudden, sharp	- Pulsus paradoxsus	- AMI
- Dull, aching	- Dyspnea	- Dressler's syndrome
- Stabbing, knife-like	- Low-grade erratic fever	- Tamponade
- Retrosternum or precordial	- Pericardial friction rub	- Pericardial effusion
- Can radiate to neck, left shoulder and arm,	- Elevated neck veins	- Constrictive pericarditis
back, epigastrium	- Tachycardia	- Myocardial/pericardial injury
	- Hiccups	- Connective tissue disease
	- Nausea/vomiting	- Infection

- Aggravated by deep inspiration, cough, rotation of the chest
- Alleviated by sitting up and forward

- Dizziness
- Generalized malaise
- Hoarseness
- Abdominal pain

- Radiation therapy
- Neoplasm

Dissecting Aortic Aneurysm
- Acute sharp onset w/o warning
- Tearing, ripping
- In synch w/heartbeat
- Lasts for hours or days
- Upper back, anterior chest, epigastric, shoulders, retrosternal
- Radiates to hips, groin, lower extremity, neck, shoulders, costovertebral area, epigastric area, jaw
- Settles in lower back

- Syncope
- Diaphoresis
- Tachycardia
- Hyper/hypotension
- Confusion
- Fever
- Blood pressure different in each arm
- Absent or diminished pulses uni/bilateral
- Decreased LOC
- Melena, hematemesis, nausea, vomiting

- Hypertension
- Congenital heart defects
- Syphilitic aortitis
- Blunt trauma
- Males > 50–70 years
- Third trimester of pregnancy

Spontaneous Pneumothorax
- Sudden
- Severe
- Over lateral thorax

- Dyspnea
- Tachycardia
- Blood pressure difference in each arm
- Hyperresonance and decreased breath sounds

- Severe underlying lung disease
- Necrotizing pneumonia
- ARDS
- High airway pressures while on mechanical ventilation

(continued)

735

#24 Differential Diagnosis of Chest Pain (Continued)

• Tracheal deviation toward affected side • Decreased respiratory excursion • Bulging intercostal muscles	• Common ages 16–25 years • COPD • Cystic fibrosis • Blebs
Cholecystitis • Severe abdominal pain • Epigastric area • Tenderness in abdomen, right upper quadrant • May radiate to back and scapula	• Nausea/vomiting • Fever • Jaundice • Changes in bowel habit • Intolerance to fatty foods
Pancreatitis • Extreme epigastric pain, alternating with dull aching sensation • Radiates to back, flank	• Hypotension • Fever • Change in bowel habit • Weight loss, malnutrition

Sources: Williams, J. L. (2003). Gastroesophageal reflux disease: Clinical manifestations. *Gastroenterology Nursing, 26*(5), 195–200; Zoorob, R. J., & Campbell, J. S. (2003). Acute dyspnea in the office. *American Family Physician, 68*,1803–1810; Lissin, L. W., & Vagelos, R. (2002). Acute aortic syndrome: A case presentation and review of the literature. *Vascular Medicine, 7*(4), 281–287; Pope, J. H., & Selker, H. P. (2002). Diagnosis of acute cardiac ischemia. *Emergency Medical Clinics of North America, 21*(1), 27–59; and Kontos, M. C. (2001). Evaluation of the emergency department chest pain patient. *Cardiology Review, 9*(5), 266–275.

#25 Risk Stratification for Unstable Angina

	High Risk (Any of the Following)	Intermediate Risk (Absence of High Risk Features and Presence of Any of the Following)	Low Risk (Absence of High or Intermediate Risk Features but May Have the Following)
History	Prior cardiovascular disease history, including myocardial infarction	Prior cardiovascular disease history; male sex; history of diabetes mellitus; age > 70	No prior cardiovascular disease history; recent cocaine use
Symptoms	Pain at rest or with increased tempo, persistent, or recurrent	Prolonged pain now resolved	New and/or progressive angina past 2 weeks
Physical exam	Adverse clinical presentation: presence of shock (pallor, diaphoresis, tachycardia, hypotension)	Presence of extracardiac vascular disease	Chest discomfort reproduced by palpation
	Left ventricular dysfunction including S_3, S_4, pulmonary edema		

(continued)

#25 Risk Stratification for Unstable Angina (Continued)

	Right ventricular dysfunction including jugular venous distention (JVD), hepatomegaly, BP sensitivity to nitrates New or worsening mitral regurgitation		
ECG	New left bundle branch block (LBBB); new, transient ST segment deviation (>0.05 millivolt) or T wave inversion (>0.2 millivolt) with symptoms; new SVT	Abnormal ST segments of T waves not documented to be new; presence of fixed pathologic Q waves	Normal or unchanged ECG during chest pain; T wave flattening or inversion in leads with dominant R waves
Cardiac markers	Elevated markers	Normal	Normal levels of markers
Diagnostic tests	Presence of left ventricular dysfunction on echocardiography	Angiography may be performed	

Treatment setting	Admit to telemetry or critical care area such as a coronary care unit, depending on intensity of monitoring and nursing care required	Admit to 24-hour observation unit or telemetry	Outpatient; return to clinic in 72 hours

Source: Braunwald, E., Antman, E. M., Beasley, J. W., et al. (2002). ACC/AHA 2002 guideline update for the management of patients with unstable angina and non-ST-segment elevation myocardial infarction: A report of the American College of Cardiology/American Heart Association Task Force on Practice Guidelines (Committee on the Management of Patient with Unstable Angina). *Journal of the American College of Cardiology, 40,* 10. Retrieved on July 23, 2008, from http://www.acc.org/qualityandscience/clinical/guidelines/unstable/update_index.htm

#26 ECG Changes During an MI, Correlated with Coronary Anatomy

	Areas and Structures Supplied	Type of MI and Leads Involved	Associated Symptoms and Complications
Right Coronary Artery (RCA)	SA node (55%), AV node (90%) Bundle of His Right atrium and ventricle Inferior surface of left ventricle Posterior 1/3 of septum Left bundle branch Posterior/inferior division of right bundle branch	**INFERIOR MI (RCA)** II, III, aVF Reciprocal changes in I, aVL	Vagal symptoms: nausea and bradycardia AV blocks: most common = 1st degree and 2nd degree type I (Wenckebach); 3rd degree possible Usually transient; treat only if symptomatic
Left Anterior Descending (LAD)	Anterior wall of left ventricle Anterior 2/3 of septum Right bundle branch Anterior/superior division of left bundle branch	**ANTERIOR MI (LAD)** $V_1 - V_4$ Reciprocal changes in II, III, aVF	Often associated with loss of large muscle mass. If large myocardial infarction (MI), prone to develop diminished left ventricular branch function, signs and symptoms of heart failure (HF), cardiogenic shock. Rhythm disturbances: atrial and ventricular dysrhythmias,

Left Circumflex Artery (CIRC, CX)	SA node (45%), AV node (10%) Inferior surface of left ventricle Lateral wall of left ventricle Left atrium Posterior/inferior division of left bundle branch		bundle branch blocks, AV blocks with 2nd degree type II most common; may progress to 3rd-degree block (complete heart block).
		ANTEROLATERAL (LAD/CIRC) I, aVL, V$_5$, V$_6$ Reciprocal changes in II, III, aVF	Frequently seen with large anterior MIs. Occasionally seen with inferior MIs. Least likely to alter hemodynamics or cause dysrhythmias.
		LATERAL MI (CIRC/LAD) I, aVL, V$_5$, V$_6$ Reciprocal changes in V$_1$, V$_3$	
		ANTEROLATERAL MI (LAD/CX) V$_1$ – V$_4$ Reciprocal changes in II, III, aVF	Uncommon; involves both right coronary artery (RCA) and circumflex (CIRC). Hard to diagnose on traditional 12-lead; researchers developing 18-lead EKG.
		POSTERIOR MI (RCA, CIRC) Reciprocal changes only in V$_1$, V$_2$ unless 18-lead EKG is done	Bradycardia with possible AV block; usually transient.

#27 Summary of Medications to Treat Coronary Artery Disease

Medication Category	Action	Application/Indication	Nursing Responsibility
Medical Management of Acute Coronary Syndrome (ACS)			
Calcium channel blockers: Diltiazem (Cardizem) Amlodipine (Norvasc)	Inhibits calcium ion movement across the cell membrane in cardiac and vascular muscle, thereby relaxing the smooth muscle and dilating coronary and peripheral arteries.	Chronic stable angina. Vasospastic angina. Unstable angina. Hypertension. Postcoronary intervention. Dysrhythmias.	Monitor blood pressure, heart rate, and rhythm. Monitor electrocardiogram (EKG) intervals. Monitor for response; i.e., decrease in angina, blood pressure, and dysrhythmias. Assess for increase in heart failure (HF), as edema may increase.
Nitrates: Nitroglycerin (NTG) Nitro–Bid Nitro–Dur Tridil	Dilates coronary and systemic arteries, thereby decreasing preload and afterload.	Angina: chronic, unstable, or vasospastic.	Monitor blood pressure. Monitor for response; i.e., decrease in anginal pain, decrease in blood pressure. Assess patient for headache (known to cause headaches in some patients).

Drug	Action	Uses	Nursing Considerations
Beta-adrenegic blockers: Metoprolol (Lopressor) Atenolol	Selective: completely blocks beta-1 receptor stimulation in cardiac smooth muscle. Nonselective: causes a decrease in blood pressure through a mixture of beta-blocking effects but does not cause reflex tachycardia or decreased heart rate.	Hypertension. Ventricular dysrhythmias.	Store drug in dark container, as it is sensitive to light. Do not administer within 24 hours of Viagra, Cialis, or Levitra. Closely monitor blood pressure and heart rate. Monitor for response; i.e., decreased blood pressure, heart rate decreased, ventricular dysrhythmias. Monitor blood chemistries, especially those related to renal function. Use with caution in patients with chronic obstructive pulmonary disease (COPD), asthma, renal disease, or diabetes mellitus.

(continued)

#27 Summary of Medications to Treat Coronary Artery Disease (Continued)

Angiotensin-converting enzyme inhibitors (ACE inhibitors): Benazepril (Lotensin) Captopril (Capoten) Enalapril (Vasotec)	Inhibits the conversion of angiotensin I to angiotensin II; suppresses renin-angiotensin-aldosterone system.	Hypertension. Congestive heart failure.	Monitor blood chemistries, specifically renal function and electrolytes. Monitor lower extremity edema. Monitor signs and symptoms of heart failure. Monitor response; i.e., decreased blood pressure, decreased shortness of breath (SOB), decreased rales. Weigh patient every day.
Angiotensin II receptor blockers (ARBs): Candesartan (Atacand) Eprosartan (Teveten) Irbesartan (Avapro)	Blocks the vasoconstrictor and aldosterone-secreting effects of angiotensin.	Hypertension.	Monitor for response; i.e., decrease in blood pressure (BP). Monitor blood chemistries.

Lipid Lowering Therapy	Inhibits HMG-CoA reductase enzyme, thereby preventing the formation of cholesterol in the liver. Statins lower total cholesterol, low density lipoproteins-cholesterol (LDL-C), and triglycerides while increasing high density lipoprotein-cholesterol (HDL-C). Statins have also been connected with stabilizing *rupture-prone* atherosclerotic plaque, improving vasomotor tone, decreasing levels of proinflammatory proteins, decreasing factors that contribute to thrombosis, and improving myocardial perfusion.	Hypercholesterolemia.	Monitor liver function studies. Monitor lipid panel. Monitor patient for myalgias. Administer medication in the evening to take advantage of the fact that the liver produces more cholesterol at nighttime than during the day. Patients may experience abdominal discomfort from gas or constipation, which usually subsides with continued therapy. Rarely causes elevated liver enzymes and muscle soreness, pain, and weakness, which may require changes in dose or discontinuance of statin therapy. Monitor liver function tests (LFT).
HMG-CoA reductase inhibitors (statins): Atorvastatin (Lipitor) Lovastatin (Mevacor) Simvastatin (Zocor) Pravastatin (Pravachol) Fluvastatin (Lescol) Crestor (Rosuvastatin)			

(continued)

#27 Summary of Medications to Treat Coronary Artery Disease (Continued)

Medication Category	Action	Application/Indication	Nursing Responsibility
Resins, or bile acid sequestrants: Cholestyramine (Questran) Colestipol (Colestid) Colesevelam (WelChol)	Binds with cholesterol-containing bile acids in the intestines and are then eliminated via stool.	Hypercholesterolemia.	Monitor lipid panel. Administered orally as powders or tablets and taken with water or fruit juice once, twice, or three times a day. May interfere with the absorption of other medications and, like statins, can cause constipation, bloating, nausea, and gas.
Fibrates: Gemfibrozil (Lopid) Fenofibrate (Tricor)	Fibrates lower triglycerides and can increase HDL-C levels.	Hypercholesterolemia.	Monitor serum LDL, very low density lipoprotein (VLDL), total cholesterol, and triglycerides. Monitor for gastrointestinal upset and bleeding. Assess for bloody stools, nosebleeds, cloudy or bloody urine, bleeding gums, and ecchymoses.

| Antihyperlipidemics:
Ezetimibe (Zetia)
Ezetimibe/Simvastatin (Zetia and Zocor)
Combination drugs:
Ezetimibe and Simvastatin (Vytorin) Work best when given with statin. | Ezetimibe: reduces blood cholesterol by inhibiting the absorption of cholesterol at the small intestine. This will decrease the level of cholesterol delivered to the liver.
Simvastatin: inhibits HMG-CoA reductase enzyme, thereby decreasing cholesterol production; increases HDL-C and decreases VLDL and triglycerides. | Hypercholesterolemia. | Monitor liver function studies.
Monitor lipid panel.
Monitor patient for myalgias and headaches.
Administer medication in the evening. |
| Niacin B vitamin | In high doses lowers triglycerides and LDL-C levels, and increases HDL-C. | Hypercholesterolemia.
Increased triglycerides. | Patients should be advised not to start taking megadoses without being under the care of a clinician.
Dose levels need to be gradually increased over time.
Flushing or hot flashes (due to vasodilation) may occur, often requiring changes in antihypertensive medication dosage. |

(continued)

#27 Summary of Medications to Treat Coronary Artery Disease (Continued)

Gastrointestinal symptoms of nausea, indigestion, gas, vomiting, diarrhea, and aggravation of peptic ulcers, liver problems, gout, and elevated blood sugar.

Aspirin can be prescribed 30 minutes prior to the dose to decrease flushing.

Fibrinolytic (thrombolytic therapy)

TNK — Modified human tissue plasminogen activator that binds to fibrin and converts plasminogen to plasmin. It is fibrin specific, thus decreasing the systemic activation of plasminogen.

Acute myocardial infarction.

Do not administer if the patient has active internal bleeding; history of cerebrovascular accident; intracranial or intraspinal surgery or trauma within 2 months; intracranial neoplasm, arteriovenous malformation, or aneurysm; known bleeding diathesis; or severe uncontrolled hypertension.

Medication Category	Action	Application/Indication	Nursing Responsibility
RPA	Nonglycosylated deletionmutein of tissue plasminogen activator, made by recombinant DNA technology.	Same as above.	Monitor for bleeding postdrug infusion. Administered as single bolus. Same as above. Administered as double bolus.
Antiplatelet Agents Acetylsalicylic acid aspirin (ASA)	Powerfully inhibits platelet aggregation by impairing hepatic synthesis of blood coagulation factors VII, IX, and X and possible inhibiting action of vitamin K.	Acute myocardial infarction and prevention of recurrence.	Monitor for gastrointestinal upset and bleeding. Assess for bloody stools, nosebleeds, cloudy or bloody urine, bleeding gums, and ecchymoses. Administer with food. Do not administer if the patient has active internal bleeding. Discontinued use if ringing in ears. Maintain adequate fluid intake. Avoid medications with aspirin in them.

(continued)

#27 Summary of Medications to Treat Coronary Artery Disease (Continued)

ADP receptor blockers: Clopidrogrel (Plavix) Ticlopidine (Ticlid)	Inhibits platelet aggregation by selectively preventing the binding of adenosine diphosphate to its platelet receptor.	Secondary prevention of myocardial infarction. Reduction in restenosis after stent placement.	Monitor for gastrointestinal upset and bleeding. Assess for bloody stools, nosebleeds, cloudy or bloody urine, bleeding gums, and ecchymoses. Do not take other drugs that inhibit platelet aggregation.
Glycoprotein IIb/IIIa blockers: Eptifibatide (Integrilin) Abciximab (ReoPro) Tirofiban (Aggrastat)	Binds the IIb/IIIa receptor sites on platelets, preventing fibrinogen and von Willebrand factor from adhering to the platelet.	Treatment of acute coronary syndrome.	Monitor for bleeding. Stop infusion if bleeding occurs. Avoid invasive procedures including needle sticks.

Sources: Adams, M. P., Josephen, D. L., & Holland, L. N. (Eds.). (2005). *Pharmacology for nurses: A pathophysiologic approach.* Upper Saddle River, NJ: Prentice Hall Health; and Wilson, B. A., Shannon, M. T., & Stang, C. L. (2005). *Nurse's drug guide.* Upper Saddle River, NJ: Prentice Hall Health.

#28 Cardiac Laboratory Markers' Pattern Consistent with Acute Myocardial Infarction

Laboratory Test	Time to Elevation	Mean Time to Peak Elevation	Time to Return to Normal
Myoglobin	1–3 hours	6–7 hours	24 hours
Troponin I	3–12 hours	24 hours	5–10 days
Troponin T	3–12 hours	12 hours–2 days	5–14 days
CK-MB	3–12 hours	24 hours	48–72 hours
C-reactive protein	24 hours	2–3 days	2 weeks

Source: Antman, E. M., & Braunwald, E. (1997). In E. Braunwald (Ed.), *Heart disease: A textbook in cardiovascular medicine* (5th ed., p. 1202). Philadelphia: W. B. Saunders.

#29 Nursing Process: Patient Care Plan for Acute Coronary Syndrome

Nursing Assessment and Diagnoses	Outcome and Evaluation Parameters	Planning and Interventions with *Rationales*
Nursing Diagnosis: Activity Intolerance related to insufficient oxygenation secondary to decreased cardiac output	*Outcomes:* Patient enrolls in cardiac rehabilitation program and attends post-MI lectures. *Evaluation Parameters:* Patient uses exercise log to record distances walked and symptoms experienced. Patient is able to monitor vital signs and adjust activity accordingly.	*Interventions and Rationale:* Encourage participation in cardiac rehabilitation program. Teach patient to use exercise log to monitor distances walked and symptoms. Teach patient how to monitor heart rate, blood pressure, and respirations as response to activity. *To increase endurance and strength and prevent weight gain.*

Assessment of Cardiac Output

Subjective Data:

Do you ever feel your heart beat fast, beat irregularly, or skip beats?

Do you ever feel light-headed?

Do you get short of breath when you walk distances?

Objective Data:

Assess heart rate and rhythm for abnormalities.

Monitor medications given and evaluate their response, especially those given for tachy/brady dysrhythmias.

Monitor blood pressure and respirations.

Nursing Assessment and Diagnoses	Outcome and Evaluation Parameters	Planning and Interventions with Rationales
Nursing Diagnosis: Decreased Cardiac Output related to dysrhythmias secondary to acute myocardial ischemia and infarction	*Outcomes:* Patient maintains normal and regular heart rate and rhythm. Patient verbalizes less fear and anxiety. *Evaluation Parameters:* Vital signs within normal limits. Exercise endurance increases. No anginal-type chest pain. Cardiac output within normal limits. No clinical manifestations of heart failure. Alert and oriented. Lungs clear.	*Interventions and Rationales:* Administer and teach antiarrhythmic medications, as ordered by health care provider *to ensure proper dosages and time intervals.* Provide comfort measures to patient and assurance *to decrease fear and anxiety.*

Assessment of Patient Ability to Cope

Subjective Data:

How are you feeling about your heart attack?

What are your thoughts about your future health?

Objective Data:

Evaluate patient response to written and verbal teaching materials about the patient's heart attack.

Evaluate patient response to discussion about current and future health concerns.

(continued)

#29 Nursing Process: Patient Care Plan for Acute Coronary Syndrome (Continued)

Nursing Assessment and Diagnoses	Outcome and Evaluation Parameters	Planning and Interventions with *Rationales*
Nursing Diagnosis: Ineffective Coping secondary to denial related to decreased physical status after myocardial infarction	*Outcome:* Patient verbalizes a decrease in problems and concerns. *Evaluation Parameters:* Vital signs within normal limits. Denies apprehension. Able to state an understanding of disease process.	*Interventions and Rationale:* Determine degree of denial; do not directly confront patient's denial; support patient's behavior. Provide active listening *to ensure patient you are working with her, not against her.*

Assessment of Pain

Subjective Data:

Do you have chest pain? Does your jaw hurt or throat hurt?

Does it radiate anywhere on your body?

Does it go away with a deep breath?

What makes the pain better or worse?

Objective Data:

Use pain scale (0–10) to quantify pain level.

Assess cultural or religious impact on the patient's response.

Assess location, duration, and onset of pain.

Nursing Assessment and Diagnoses	Outcome and Evaluation Parameters	Planning and Interventions with *Rationales*
Nursing Diagnosis: *Acute Pain* related to cardiac ischemia	**Outcome:** Pain free or controlled with medication. **Evaluation Parameters:** Patient notifies nurse immediately on experiencing pain. Patient's ECG is normal and pain is relieved with sublingual NTG. Patient is able to verbalize how to take sublingual NTG and its side effects.	**Interventions and Rationale:** Instruct patient to notify nurse immediately of chest pain. Implement health care provider's orders; i.e., ECG, sublingual NTG, morphine, oxygen. Teach patient about how to take sublingual nitroglycerin and its side effects. *This encourages the patient to participate in his own care and teaches one of the most important interventions for patients with CAD.*

Assessment of Fluid Status
Subjective Data:
Are you short of breath?
Do you monitor your weight?
Do you eat a lot of salt?

Objective Data:
Assess lung sounds for rales or crackles.
Monitor blood pressure, jugular venous distension (JVD), vital signs, urine output, daily weight, and peripheral edema.

(continued)

#29 Nursing Process: Patient Care Plan for Acute Coronary Syndrome (Continued)

Nursing Assessment and Diagnoses	Outcome and Evaluation Parameters	Planning and Interventions with *Rationales*
Nursing Diagnosis: Excess Fluid Volume related to fluid retention secondary to impaired myocardial contractility	*Outcomes:* Patient's body weight is within normal range; electrolytes will be maintained in normal range. *Evaluation Parameters:* Weight. Electrolyte values daily until stable. Lungs clear. No peripheral edema. Neck vein distention not present. Cardiac index and ejection fraction with normal limits.	*Interventions and Rationales:* Administer diuretics as ordered and teach patient rationale and side effects of medication. Weigh patient daily and stress to patient the importance of daily weights. Instruct patient to notify health care provider with greater than 2–3 pound gain. *This will allow the patient to identify weight gain from fluid.* Fluid restriction and low-sodium diet as ordered *in order to decrease excess fluid accumulation.*

Assess Patient/Family Knowledge of Disease and Treatment

Subjective Data:

Tell me what you know about your problems with your heart.

Tell me what you are doing about your risk factors.

Tell me about your dietary intake and your exercise program.

When do you develop chest pain and what makes it go away?

Objective Data:

Patient/family may be anxious, confused, and need repeated information. Mistakes being made with treatment plan. Self-care deficit.

What medications are you on, when are you supposed to take them, and
what are the side effects you should watch for?
When are you supposed to see your doctor?
Are you participating in a cardiac rehabilitation program?

Nursing Assessment and Diagnoses	Outcome and Evaluation Parameters	Planning and Interventions with *Rationales*
Nursing Diagnosis: *Deficient Knowledge* related to disease and treatment plan	**Outcome:** Patient/family have an understanding of and comply with treatment plan. **Evaluation Parameters:** Patient and family understand treatment plan and safely become compliant. Patient and family understand the importance of risk factor control in preventing a progression of the disease. Patient and family participate in a cardiac rehabilitation program.	**Interventions and Rationales:** Describe the required diet, medications, activity, and limitations *to increase knowledge of disease and treatment.* Describe what clinical manifestations need to be reported to the health care provider and when to access the emergency medical system *to ensure immediate care when necessary.* Have patient/family repeat instructions *to assess understanding.* Provide information about the type, setting, and cost of a cardiac rehabilitation program, and assist with contacting the program *to decrease anxiety about the process.*

Sources: Wilkinson, J. M., & Ahearn, N. R. (2009). *Prentice Hall Nursing Diagnosis Handbook.9/E.* Upper Saddle River, NJ: Prentice Hall.

#30 Pharmacology Summary of Medications to Treat Lower Airway Disorders

Medication Category	Action	Application/Indication	Nursing Responsibility
Mucolytics • Dornase alpha (Pulmozyme) • Acetylcysteine* (Mucomyst) • Amiloride**	Liquefies bronchial secretions by altering the structure of mucous molecule.	Cystic fibrosis, acute and chronic bronchitis, pneumonia, TB.	Monitor for adverse effects: nausea, vomiting. Observe for possible bronchospasm. Establish a routine for elimination of secretions post-treatment. Use with caution in patients with compromised ability to cough.
Decongestants • Sympathomimetics • Ephedrine (Efedron) • Oxymetazoline (Afrin 12 hour, Neo-Synephrine 12 hour) • Phenylephrine (Afrin 4–6 hour, Neo-Synephrine 4–6 hour) • Pseudoephedrine (Chlor-Trimeton, Drixoral, Sudafed) **Anticholinergic** • Intranasal ipratropium (Atrovent, Combivent)	Decreases nasal membrane edema by constricting nasal arterioles. Decreases rhinorrhea by blocking muscarinic receptors in nasal passages.	Common cold, sinusitis, allergic rhinitis, nasal congestion.	Monitor for adverse effects: insomnia, tremors, weakness, anxiety, hypertension, tachycardia, palpitations, arrhythmias. Observe for rebound nasal congestion with intranasal administration, CNS stimulation with oral administration. Monitor for severe reactions: hallucinations, convulsions. Be aware of drug interactions (MAOIs, methyldopa, tricyclic antidepressants and others).

Drug	Action	Use	Nursing Considerations
Antitussives • Nonopioid dextromethorphan* (Benylin, Robitussin, Delsym)	Suppresses cough by direct action on the cough center in the medulla.	Nonproductive or hyperactive cough.	Monitor for adverse effects: drowsiness, sedation (especially patients on CNS depressants), nausea, vomiting, constipation, dizziness, **pruritus. *Be aware of drug interaction with MAOIs. Monitor for CNS stimulation, hypotension, hyperpyrexia.
Opioid • Codeine** • Hydrocodone bitartrate (Hycodan, Mycodone)			Monitor for adverse effects: tightness of chest, drowsiness, excitability, stomach pain or upset, constipation, diarrhea
Antibiotics • Fluoroquinolones/quinolones • Ciprofloxacin (Cipro) • Ofloxacin (Floxin) • Levofloxacin (Levaquin) • Moxifloxacin (Avelox)	Exerts bacteriocidal effect by disrupting synthesis of gram-negative and gram-positive bacterial DNA.	Acute exacerbation of chronic bronchitis, community-acquired pneumonia, sinusitis.	Monitor for adverse effects: nausea, headache, diarrhea, some may cause dysrhythmias or liver failure. Monitor WBC count, liver and renal function. Monitor for signs of CNS toxicity especially if given in presence of epilepsy, cerebral artery disease,

(continued)

#30 Pharmacology Summary of Medications to Treat Lower Airway Disorders (Continued)

		alcoholism. Be aware of drug interactions (warfarin, NSAIDs, theophylline, antacids, caffeine). Monitor for altered efficacy or toxicity. Do not give with antacids or vitamins containing calcium, magnesium, iron, or zinc.
Tetracyclines • Doxycycline (Vibramycin) • Tetracycline (Sumycin)	Exerts bacteriostatic effect by inhibiting bacterial protein synthesis in gram-positive and gram-negative bacteria. May be bactericidal at higher doses.	Respiratory tract infections, *Chlamydia*, gonorrhea, tetanus, *Helicobacter pylori*, Lyme disease.	Monitor for adverse effects: nausea, vomiting, diarrhea, signs of superinfection. Be aware of drug interactions (iron, calcium, magnesium, antacids, lipid lowering drugs, oral anticoagulants, oral contraceptives). Observe for decreased drug efficacy or toxicity. Do not give with milk products, iron, magnesium laxatives, or antacids. Warn patient of photosensitivity and need for sun block.

Medication Category	Action	Application/Indication	Nursing Responsibility
Macrolides • Clarithromycin* (Biaxin) • Erythromycin (Erythrocin) • Azithromycin (Zithromax)	Exerts bacteriostatic effect by inhibiting bacterial protein synthesis in gram-positive and gram-negative organisms. May be bactericidal at higher doses.	Legionnaire disease, *Mycoplasma pneumoniae* pneumonia, diphtheria, chlamydial infections.	Monitor for adverse effects: urticaria, nausea, vomiting, diarrhea, abdominal cramping, *Clostridium* overgrowth. Observe for exacerbation of existing heart disease or, if given IV, torsades de pointes. Monitor hepatic function. Be aware of multiple drug interactions (warfarin, anticonvulsants, theophylline, and others). Monitor for toxicity or altered drug efficacy. Warn patient not to take OTC drugs without contacting health care provider. Do not give with fruit juice
Aminoglycosides • Tobramycin (Nebcin) • Amikacin (Amikin) • Gentamicin (Garamycin)	Exerts bacteriocidal effect on gram-negative organisms and staphylococcus by altering bacterial protein synthesis.	TB, serious respiratory infections, sepsis, meningitis, osteomyelitis.	Monitor for adverse effects: signs of ototoxicity (dizziness, loss of balance, tinnitus, headache), superinfection. *Note:* Hearing loss is usually irreversible.

(continued)

761

#30 Pharmacology Summary of Medications to Treat Lower Airway Disorders (Continued)

			Be aware of increased risk of nephrotoxicity and/or ototoxicity if given concurrently with amphotericin B, furosemide, acetylsalicylic, and others. Monitor renal function for signs of nephrotoxicity.
Sulfonamides • Trimethoprim-sulfamethoxazole (SMZ-TMP) (Bactrim, Septra)	Exerts bacteriostatic activity by inhibiting bacterial folic acid synthesis needed for cell growth.	Exacerbation of chronic bronchitis, pneumonia, traveler's diarrhea, urinary tract infections, otitis media.	Monitor for adverse effects: nausea, vomiting, urticaria. Be aware of drug interactions (warfarin, digoxin, phenytoin and others). Observe for drug toxicity. Monitor CBC, renal function, urinalysis (crystalluria can occur). Increase fluid intake unless contraindicated.

Medication Category	Action	Application/Indication	Nursing Responsibility
Miscellaneous antibiotics • Chloramphenicol (Chloromycetin)	Exerts broad-spectrum bacteriostatic activity by interfering with bacterial protein synthesis. May be bacteriocidal in some organisms.	Serious infections, cystic fibrosis regimes, bacteremia, meningitis, typhoid fever.	Monitor for adverse effects: nausea, vomiting, headache, fungal overgrowth. Monitor blood studies regularly. May cause blood dyscrasias and irreversible bone marrow depression. Increase monitoring of blood glucose in patients on oral antidiabetic agents. Monitor serum drug levels, especially in the presence of renal or hepatic impairment.
Antifungals • Polyene • Amphotericin B (Fungizone)	Causes fungal cell death by altering fungal cell membrane.	Progressive or potentially fatal systemic fungal or protozoal infections.	Monitor for anorexia, nausea, vomiting. May require premedication with antiemetic. During IV infusion, monitor vital signs, observe for infusion reaction: headache, fever, chills, nausea, vomiting, hypotension,

(continued)

763

#30 Pharmacology Summary of Medications to Treat Lower Airway Disorders (Continued)

			bronchospasm (premedication with diphenhydramine and acetaminophen may reduce infusion reactions). Monitor I&O, renal function, appearance of urine, CBC, electrolytes, hepatic function. Monitor IV site for extravasation, thrombophlebitis. Be aware of multiple drug incompatibilities when given IV.
Azoles • Fluconazole (Diflucan) • Itraconazole (Sporanox)	Exerts fungistatic effect by interrupting fungal cell membrane function. May be fungicidal at higher concentrations.	Systemic candidiasis, pneumonia, esophageal candidiasis.	Monitor for adverse effects: headache, nausea, abdominal pain, diarrhea. Monitor liver function. Be aware of multiple drug interactions (oral hypoglycemics, Coumadin, phenytoin, theophylline, and others).

		Monitor for decreased drug efficacy or toxicity. Monitor for hypoglycemia in diabetic patients. Be aware of multiple drug incompatibilities when given IV.
Echocardins • Anidulafungin (Eraxis)	Exerts antifungal effect by inhibiting synthesis of major component of fungal cell wall.	Esophageal candidiasis, candidemia.	Monitor for adverse effects: nausea, vomiting, diarrhea, hypokalemia, rash. Monitor liver function.
Antiviral • Amantadine (Symmetrel) Rimantadine (Flumadine) • Oseltamivir* (Tamiflu) • Zanamivir* (Relenza)	Thought to exert antiviral effect by inhibiting early viral replication.	Prevention and treatment of influenza A. *Treatment of influenza A and B.	Monitor for adverse effects: dizziness, light-headedness, insomnia, nausea. Observe for increased seizure activity in presence of seizure disorder.

(continued)

765

#30 Pharmacology Summary of Medications to Treat Lower Airway Disorders (Continued)

Medication Category	Action	Application/Indication	Nursing Responsibility
Anti-TB • Isoniazid* (INH, Nydrazid, Laniazid) • Rifapentine** (Priftin) • Rifampin** (Rifadin)	Exerts bacteriostatic or bacteriocidal effects by disrupting synthesis of bacterial cell wall or impairing cell metabolism.	Prevention and treatment of pulmonary TB.	Monitor for adverse effects: visual disturbances, orthostatic hypotension*, signs of hepatotoxicity (anorexia, fatigue, nausea, malaise), signs of peripheral neuropathy (burning, tingling, pain, numbness). Monitor hepatic function, CBC. Monitor for hyperglycemia in presence of diabetes. **Be aware of multiple drug interactions (phenytoin, warfarin, diazepam, theophylline and others). Monitor for altered drug efficacy. **Warn patient on oral

Drug	Action	Use/Indication	Nursing Considerations
			contraceptives to use alternate birth control method. Instruct patient to restrict alcohol and intake of foods rich in tyramine (dairy, beef, chicken, bananas, caffeine, and others) and histamine (tuna, yeast extract, brine).
Digestive Enzyme • Pancrelipase (Viokase)	Breaks down fats, proteins, and starches in the final stage of digestion for easier absorption.	Steatorrhea from malabsorption syndrome in cystic fibrosis.	Monitor for adverse effects: nausea, abdominal cramps, diarrhea. Assess for improved nutritional status and decreased steatorrhea. Be aware of religious considerations; drug is pork based.
Bronchodilators • Corticosteroids (see the Pharmacology Summary in textbook Chapter 36)			

*Acetaminophen toxicity, prevention of contrast-induced renal complications.

**A diuretic that reduces mucous viscosity by altering sputum electrolytes.

*Binds with hepatotoxic metabolite of acetaminophen, protects liver and renal cells from damage.

#31 Comparative Effects of Common Insulin Preparations

Type/Generic Name	Brand Name(s)	Onset (hours)	Peak (hours)	Duration (hours)
Rapid Acting				
Insulin lispro (analog)	Humalog	<0.25	1–2	3–4
Insulin aspart	NovoLog			
Insulin glulisine	Apidra			
Short Acting				
Regular	Humulin R	0.5–1.0	2–3	3–6
	Novolin R			
	Humulin R (U-500)*			
Intermediate Acting				
NPH (isophane)	Humulin N	2–4	4–10	12–18
	Novolin N			
Long Acting				
Insulin glargine	Lantus	2–4	Peakless	20–24
Insulin detemir	Levemir	0.8–2	Relatively flat	~24

Combinations

50% lispro protamine/50% insulin lispro	Humalog Mix 50/50	0.5–1	Dual	~18–24
70% NPH/30% regular	Humulin 70/30 Novolin 70/30	0.5–1	Dual	~18–24
50% NPH/50% regular	Humulin 50/50	0.5–1	Dual	~18–24
75% aspart protamine/25% aspart	NovoLog Mix 75/25	<0.25	Dual	~18–24
75% lispro protamine/25% lispro	Humalog Mix 75/25	<0.25	Dual	~18–24

Note: The concentration of commercial insulin in the United States is 100 units/mL (U-100); however, regular insulin is also available as 500 units/mL (U-500). This concentration is usually used only in patients who are extremely insulin resistant.

#32 Summary of Medications to Treat Type 2 Diabetes

Medication/ Category	Action	Application/ Indication	Nursing Responsibility
Chlorpropamide (First-generation sulfonylurea)	**General Mechanism:** Sulfonylureas stimulate insulin secretion from the pancreatic beta cells. **Mechanism of Action (MOA):** These medications bind with a cell surface protein on the pancreatic beta cell. The binding of the sulfonylurea with the sulfonylurea receptor (SUR) results in the closure of potassium channels and depolarizes the cell membrane, opening calcium channels and stimulating insulin release. **Primary Mechanism of Clearance:** Renal chlorpropamide has the longest duration of action of any of the sulfonylureas (>48 hours). This enhanced activity may place selected groups (e.g., elderly, renal disease) at risk for hypoglycemia.	Used to lower blood glucose in patients with type 2 diabetes.	Assess patient for allergy to other sulfonylureas or sulfa medications. Assess patient for renal or liver disease. Assess patients who are at high risk for injury from hypoglycemia (e.g., elderly). Assess patient for signs and symptoms of hyponatremia (chlorpropamide specific effect). Assess patient for weight gain. Instruct patient on the signs and symptoms of hypoglycemia. Instruct patient on the treatment of hypoglycemia. Instruct patient to avoid ingesting alcohol with medication to prevent a disulfiram reaction.

Tolbutamide (First-generation oral sulfonylurea)	**General Mechanism:** Sulfonylureas stimulate insulin secretion from the pancreatic beta cells. **MOA:** See above **Primary Mechanism of Clearance:** Hepatic	Lowers blood glucose in patients with type 2 diabetes.	As above
Tolazamide (First-generation sulfonylurea)	**General Mechanism:** Sulfonylureas stimulate insulin secretion from the pancreatic beta cells. **MOA:** See above **Primary Mechanism of Clearance:** Hepatic and renal	Lowers blood glucose in patients with type 2 diabetes.	As above
Glyburide (Second-generation sulfonylurea)	**General Mechanism:** Sulfonylureas stimulate insulin secretion from the pancreatic beta cells. **MOA:** See above **Primary Mechanism of Clearance:** Hepatic and renal	Lowers blood glucose in patients with type 2 diabetes.	As above

(continued)

#32 Summary of Medications to Treat Type 2 Diabetes (Continued)

Glipizide (Second-generation sulfonylurea; available in extended-release formulations)	**General Mechanism:** Sulfonylureas stimulate insulin secretion from the pancreatic beta cells. **MOA:** See above **Primary Mechanism of Clearance:** Hepatic	Lowers blood glucose in patients with type 2 diabetes.	As above *In addition:* Instruct patient to take glipizide with meals.
Glimepiride (Second-generation sulfonylurea)	**General Mechanism:** Sulfonylureas stimulate insulin secretion from the pancreatic beta cells. **MOA:** See above **Primary Mechanism of Clearance:** Hepatic and renal	Lowers blood glucose in patients with type 2 diabetes.	As above
Metformin (Biguanide) (available in extended-release formulations)	**General Mechanism:** Metformin reduces hepatic glucose production and improves insulin sensitivity. **MOA:** Metformin reduces hepatic glucose production through decreased hepatic glycogenolysis and decreased hepatic	Lowers blood glucose in patients with type 2 diabetes.	Assess patient for allergy to metformin. Assess patient for contraindications to metformin (renal, cardiorespiratory, hepatic dysfunction, and alcohol abuse). Assess patient for the development of gastrointestinal symptoms, such as diarrhea, nausea,

772

gluconeogenesis. It also improves insulin sensitivity through mechanisms that are not entirely clear.

Primary Method of Clearance: Metformin is not metabolized but is cleared rapidly from the kidney. Metformin is contraindicated in patients with renal, cardiorespiratory, hepatic dysfunction, and alcohol abuse. These conditions may precipitate lactic acidosis, which is a rare, but life-threatening, complication.

Renal dysfunction is defined as:
Serum creatinine: ≤ 1.4 mg/dL in females; ≤ 1.5 mg/dL in males; or abnormal creatinine clearance. Elderly patients need a 24-hour urine for creatinine clearance prior to starting on metformin.

vomiting, flatulence, abdominal discomfort, and indigestion.

Encourage patients to report continued gastrointestinal symptoms to their health care provider, because the symptoms may resolve with slower titration of the metformin dose. Discuss with patient the risk of lactic acidosis.

Instruct patient on the signs and symptoms of hypoglycemia.

In general, metformin does not cause hypoglycemia as monotherapy. However, hypoglycemia may occur when metformin is combined with other medications.

Discuss with patients the need to discontinue metformin prior to any procedure using a radio contrast dye, and to resume the medication only when normal renal function has been assessed.

(continued)

#32 Summary of Medications to Treat Type 2 Diabetes (Continued)

Acarbose (Alpha-glucosidase inhibitor)	**General Mechanism:** Alpha-glucosidase inhibitors reduce postprandial hyperglycemia. **MOA:** The actions of the alpha-glucosidase inhibitors occur in the intestinal lumen where they competitively inhibit enzymes that convert polysaccharides into simple sugars. The alpha-glucosidase inhibitors delay the absorption of dietary carbohydrates until they reach the distal bowel. As a result, these inhibitors reduce postprandial hyperglycemia. **Primary Method of Clearance:** Renal and feces	Lowers postprandial hyperglycemia in patients with type 2 diabetes.	Assess patient for allergy to alpha-glucosidase inhibitors. Assess patient for any gastrointestinal conditions (e.g., inflammatory bowel disease, colonic ulceration, partial intestinal obstruction) that may deteriorate as a result of increased intestinal gas formation. Instruct patient to contact her health care provider for continued bloating and flatulence, because the symptoms may resolve with slower titration of the alpha-glucosidase dose. Instruct patient to take the medication with the first bite of each meal. Instruct patient to recognize the signs and symptoms of hypoglycemia. In general, alpha-glucosidase inhibitors do not cause hypoglycemia when used as monotherapy.

	General Mechanism: Alpha-glucosidase inhibitors reduce postprandial hyperglycemia.	Lowers postprandial hyperglycemia in patients with type 2 diabetes.	Hypoglycemia can occur when used in combination with other hypoglycemic medications.
Miglitol (Alpha-glucosidase inhibitor)	MOA: See above		Instruct patient on the treatment of hypoglycemia. Patients using alpha-glucosidase inhibitors need to treat their reactions with pure glucose, such as glucose gels, glucose tablets, or fruit juice, because the absorption of other carbohydrates may be delayed.
	Primary Method of Clearance: Renal		
	General Mechanism: Meglitinides cause a rapid increase in insulin secretion.	Lowers postprandial hyperglycemia in patients with type 2 diabetes.	As above
Repaglinide (Meglitinide)	MOA: Meglitinides are nonsulfonylureas medications that act through the SUR on the		Assess patient for any allergies to meglitinide. Instruct patient to take the medication at the start of the meal and to withhold the dose if no meal is eaten. Instruct patient on the signs and symptoms of hypoglycemia.

(continued)

#32 Summary of Medications to Treat Type 2 Diabetes (Continued)

			Instruct patient on the treatment of hypoglycemia.
	pancreatic beta cells. The meglitinides bind with the SUR at a site distinct for the traditional sulfonylureas (see above). The binding of the sulfonylurea with the SUR results in the closure of potassium channels and depolarizes the cell membrane, opening calcium channels and stimulating insulin release. The meglitinides differ from the sulfonylureas in that the insulin response is rapid and exerts it major effect on postprandial hyperglycemia. **Primary Method of Clearance:** Hepatic		
Nateglinide (Meglitinide)	**General Mechanism:** Meglitinides cause a rapid increase in insulin secretion. **MOA:** See above **Primary Method of Clearance:** Hepatic and renal	Lowers postprandial hyperglycemia in patients with type 2 diabetes.	As above

| Sitagliptin (Dipeptidyl peptidase-4 [DPP-4] inhibitor) | **General Mechanism:** DPP-4 inhibitors lower postprandial hyperglycemia. **MOA:** Glucagon-like peptide 1 (GLP-1) is a hormone that is secreted by the intestinal L-cell, which suppresses elevated glucagon levels, promotes satiety, decreases food intake, and slows gastric emptying. DPP-4 is an enzyme that inactivates the GLP-1 peptide. DPP-4 inhibitors slow the breakdown of GLP-1 and thereby extend the effects of the hormone. **Primary Method of Clearance:** Hepatic and renal | Lowers postprandial hyperglycemia in patients with type 2 diabetes. | Assess patient for allergies to DPP-4 inhibitors. Instruct patient to notify health care provider if a skin rash develops. |
| Pioglitazone (Thiazolidinedione) | **General Mechanism:** Thiazolidinediones improve insulin sensitivity. **MOA:** The actions of thiazolidinediones occur through the actions of a group of nuclear regulatory proteins, peroxisome-proliferator-activated (PPAR) receptors, which are important in fat and carbohydrate metabolism. Thiazolidinediones | Lowers postprandial hyperglycemia in patients with type 2 diabetes. | Assess patient for the presence of liver disease. Monitor patient for weight gain and fluid retention. Instruct patient to contact his health care provider if shortness of breath, edema, and fatigue develop. Instruct patient to contact her health care provider if signs and symptoms develop of liver disease: nausea, vomiting, fatigue, jaundice, and dark urine. |

(continued)

#32 Summary of Medications to Treat Type 2 Diabetes (Continued)

	bind and activate the PPARγ isoform and improve insulin sensitivity. **Primary Method of Clearance:** Hepatic	Instruct anovulatory premenopausal women (e.g., polycystic ovarian syndrome) that these medications may cause ovulation to resume and pregnancy to occur.
Rosiglitazone (Thiazolidine-dione)	**General Mechanism:** Thiazolidinediones improve insulin sensitivity. **MOA:** See above **Primary Method of Clearance:** Hepatic	As above
Exenatide (Incretin mimetics)	**General Mechanism:** Exenatide reduces postprandial hyperglycemia. **MOA:** Exenatide is an analog of GLP-1 (see DPP-4 inhibitors) that suppresses elevated glucagon levels, promotes satiety, decreases food intake, and slows gastric emptying. The medication is injected prior to meals to reduce postprandial hyperglycemia. **Primary Method of Clearance:** Renal	Lowers postprandial hyperglycemia in patients with type 2 diabetes. Assess patient for any allergies to incretin mimetics. Instruct patient on proper injection techniques. Instruct patient to check the injection site for swelling and irritation. Instruct patient to inject medication prior to meals. Instruct patient on the signs and symptoms of hypoglycemia. Instruct patient on the treatment of hypoglycemia. Instruct patient to call his health care provider with continued gastrointestinal symptoms, because slower titration of the dose may alleviate this problem.

| Pramlintide (Amylin analog) | **General Mechanism:** Pramlintide reduces postprandial hyperglycemia.

MOA: Amylin is a neuroendocrine hormone that is secreted with insulin from the pancreatic beta cells. This hormone can reduce postprandial blood glucose control through slowing gastric emptying, suppressing glucagon secretion, and promoting satiety. Pramlintide is an amylin analog that is injected prior to meals to reduce postprandial hyperglycemia.
Primary Method of Clearance: Renal | Pramlintide is used in patients with type 1 diabetes and insulin-treated type 2 diabetes. Patients with type 1 diabetes are amylin deficient. Patients with type 2 diabetes have a poor amylin response to meal. Treatment with pramlintide can address each of these problems. | Assess patient for any allergies to pramlintide. Assess patient for gastroparesis and hypoglycemic unawareness because these conditions may predispose the patient to severe hypoglycemia. Instruct patient on proper injection techniques. Instruct patient to check the injection site for swelling and irritation. Instruct patient to inject medication prior to meals. Instruct patient on the signs and symptoms of hypoglycemia. Instruct patient on the treatment of hypoglycemia. |

Sources: American Diabetes Association. (2008a). *Diabetes forecast resource guide 2008.* Alexandria, VA: Author; Burant, C. F., & American Diabetes Association. (2008). *Medical management of type 2 diabetes* (6th ed.). Alexandria, VA: American Diabetes Association; Campbell, R. K., & White, J. R., Jr. (2000). *Medications for the treatment of diabetes.* Alexandria, VA: American Diabetes Association; Gutierrez, K. (2008). *Pharmacotherapeutics: Clinical reasoning in primary care* (2nd ed.). St. Louis: W. B. Saunders; Kaufman, F., & American Diabetes Association. (2008). *Medical management of type 1 diabetes* (5th ed.). Alexandria, VA: American Diabetes Association; Youngkin, E. Q., Sawin, K. J., Kissinger, J. F., & Isreal, D. S. (Eds.). (2005). *Pharmacotherapeutics* (2nd ed.). Upper Saddle, NJ: Pearson Prentice Hall.

#33 Transfusion Reactions

Class	Cause	Clinical Manifestations	Nursing Care
Allergic reaction	Recipient's sensitivity to foreign plasma proteins. Common in patients with allergies.	Itching, hives, flushing, and chills.	Slow the transfusion. Take vital signs. Notify the health care provider. May be necessary to medicate with antipyretic and/or antihistamine. Then resume the transfusion.
Febrile nonhemolytic reaction	Due to leukocyte or thrombocyte incompatibility (donor's WBCs or platelets react with recipient's antibodies). Usually occurs after multiple transfusions. Accounts for 90% of transfusion reactions. Fever begins about 2 hours after the transfusion. WBC reduced blood helps prevent these reactions.	Increased pulse rate, temperature > 1°C, chills, headache, nausea and vomiting, anxiety, flushing, back pain, muscle aches.	Stop transfusion, but maintain IV site. Give antipyretics as prescribed. Take vital signs. Notify health care provider. Obtain urine and blood sample. Send blood bag, normal saline, and IV tubing to the laboratory. Consider using leukocyte-poor blood.

Delayed hemolytic reaction	May occur up to 14 days after a transfusion when the level of the antibodies has increased to the extent that a reaction occurs.	Fever, anemia, increased bilirubin level, decreased or absent haptoglobin, and jaundice.	Generally not dangerous, but it is important to recognize the reaction because subsequent transfusions may cause a more severe hemolytic reaction. Typically not recognized or treated due to the mild nature of the reaction.
Acute hemolytic reaction	ABO incompatibility of the blood and recipient. May be due to a mistake in labeling by laboratory or blood bank or nursing error. Causes agglutination of cells, which causes obstruction of the capillaries and blockage of blood flow.	Bloody urine and decreased urine output. Petechiae, jaundice, decreased BP, chest tightness, low back pain, nausea, anxiety, and dyspnea. Hypotension, bronchospasm, and vascular collapse may occur. Hemoglobinemia, acute renal failure, shock, cardiac arrest, death. Symptoms	Emergent life-threatening situation. Stop transfusion, but maintain IV site and infuse IV colloid solutions to maintain BP. Give diuretics as prescribed to maintain urine flow. Insert urinary catheter to assess output and color. Obtain vital signs. Treat shock. Start CPR if necessary. Give epinephrine. Notify health care provider.

(continued)

#33 Transfusion Reactions (Continued)

Class	Cause	Clinical Manifestations	Nursing Care
		typically occur within the first 15 minutes of the transfusion.	Obtain urine and blood sample. Send blood bag, normal saline, and IV tubing to the laboratory.
Hemolytic or anaphylactic reaction	Reaction to donor plasma proteins. Specifically, infusion of IgA proteins to an IgA-deficient recipient who has an IgA antibody.	Wheezing, restlessness, anxiety; progressing to cyanosis, shock, and possibly cardiac arrest.	Stop infusion, but maintain IV site. Give epinephrine per doctor's order. Initiate CPR if necessary. Notify health care provider. Obtain urine and blood sample. Send blood bag, normal saline, and IV tubing to the laboratory.

Sources: Josephson, D. (2004). *Intravenous infusion therapy for nurses* (2nd ed.). Clifton Park, NY: Thompson Delmar Learning; Porth, C. M. (2005). *Pathophysiology: Concepts of altered health status* (7th ed.). Philadelphia: Lippincott Williams & Wilkins.

#34 Diagnostic Tests for Burns

Test	Initial Expected Abnormality	Later Expected Abnormality	Rationale for Abnormality
Potassium level	Increased.	Decreased after burn shock; fluid shifts back to intracellular and intravascular spaces.	Increased due to cell lysis and fluid shifts to extracellular spaces. Decreases with fluid resuscitation.
Sodium level	Increased.	Normalizes with fluid replacement. Will decrease with repeated Hubbard tank treatments.	Due to dehydration and then decreased with fluid shifts.
Hematocrit (HCT)	For the first 12–48 hours after the burn injury, there is an increase in the hematocrit due to hemoconcentration related to intravascular fluid volume loss.	Decreased with adequate hydration due to cell destruction from injury. Once fluid balance has been reestablished, a lower and more accurate hematocrit reading occurs.	Red blood cells are lost both directly in the burn and as a result of increased fragility. Circulating red blood cell mass becomes trapped and destroyed within the burn wound at the time of injury. Erythrocyte losses continue to occur for several days after the injury.

(continued)

#34 Diagnostic Tests for Burns (Continued)

Test	Initial Expected Abnormality	Later Expected Abnormality	Rationale for Abnormality
Hemoglobin (Hgb)	Increased due to hemoconcentration.	Decreased with adequate hydration due to cell destruction from injury.	Red blood cells are lost both directly in the burn and as a result of increased fragility. Circulating red blood cell mass becomes trapped and destroyed within the burn wound at the time of injury. Erythrocyte losses continue to occur for several days after the injury.
Platelets	Decreased due to dilution and consumption.	Normal if bone marrow manufactures enough. May be increased in the presence of infection.	Dilution and consumption immediately after a burn injury cause an abnormal decrease both in the platelet count and in clotting factors. It is believed that a large number of platelets are utilized to stabilize the vasculature in and around the burned area.
White blood cells (WBC)	Granulocytes continue to increase for the first 24 hours after the injury, and then the count begins to fall.	Increased with infection and decreased in immunodeficient states.	This increase is due to mobilization of preexisting stores. The decrease in the granulocyte level is due in part to the dilutional effects of fluid replacement therapy, and due to concentration in the injured areas.

Creatinine/blood urea nitrogen (BUN)	Normal to increased depending on fluid replacement.	Low if malnourished. Increased in presence of renal insufficiency.	Increases seen with electrical burns where extensive tissue damage is suspected.
Blood glucose; nondiabetic	Increased.	Increased or decreased depending on nutritional replacement.	Due to stress response and changes that occur with fluid resuscitation and type of nutritional replacement.
Total protein	Decreased.	Increased or decreased depending on nutritional status.	Fluid shifts cause a decrease, and nutritional replacement will increase it.
Prealbumin	Decreased.	Increased or decreased depending on nutritional status.	Massive inflammation causes a decrease, and nutritional replacement will increase it.
Creatine kinase (CK) level	Elevated.	Returns to normal after 48 hours.	Electrical burns due to extensive tissue damage.
Urine specific gravity	Elevated.	Decreased to normal levels with rehydration.	Dehydration.

#35 Nursing Process: Patient Care Plan for Thrombocytopenia and Bleeding Disorders

Nursing Assessment and Diagnoses	Outcomes and Evaluation Parameters	Planning and Interventions with Rationales
Nursing Diagnoses: *Risk for Injury* related to increased intracranial pressure, abdominal bleeding, pericardial bleeding, and/or bleeding into pleural space	**Outcome:** Free of injury due to bleeding. **Evaluation Parameters:** Laboratory: Hemoglobin values remain within normal limits. Laboratory: Platelet, APTT, PT, and INR values remain within normal limits. Vital signs: Vital signs remain within baseline normal limits for patient. Cerebral: Patient remains alert and well oriented. Cerebral: Pupils remain equal, round, and reactive to light. Cerebral: Gross reflex assessment remains unchanged from baseline.	*Interventions and Rationales:* Frequently monitor laboratory values for signs of precipitous decrease in hemoglobin *to detect changes in level of circulating red blood cells.* Frequently monitor laboratory values for signs of increased bleeding times *to detect tendencies to bleed.* Assess vital signs especially blood pressure *as indicators of vascular space volume. In the event of bleeding, blood volume leaves vascular space.* Report critical values immediately *because health care provider may wish to initiate blood product transfusion.* Frequently monitor neurological signs including level of Glasgow Coma Scale, papillary changes, and cranial nerves *to detect changes in level of consciousness and nerve damage.* Monitor restlessness, and confusion *as indicators of increased intracranial pressure and/or decreased oxygenation due to bleeding.*

Abdominal: Patient denies abdominal pain.

Abdominal: Bowel sounds at baseline or present in all four quadrants.

Patient denies chest pain, shortness of breath.

Frequently assess (inspection, auscultation, palpation, percussion) abdominal status and seek patient report of abdominal pain to detect signs of bleeding into abdominal cavity and hypoxia in abdominal structures due to blood loss.

Assess abdomen for pain, tenderness, distention as indicators of internal abdominal bleeding.

Assess for adventitious or diminished breath sounds. Indicates decreased gas exchange and hypoxia.

Monitor respiratory rate and depth to assess for respiratory distress.

Urine color clear. Free of blood in stool.

Frequently assess urine and stool color. Possible early indicator of systemic internal bleeding. Detection of early signs allows for timely administration of platelet transfusion.

Outcome:

Free of serious injury due to internal bleeding.

Evaluation Parameters: Alert and oriented. Clear breath sounds and absence of respiratory distress.

Free of reports of abdominal pain.

Interventions and Rationales:

Frequently assess skin, mucosa membrane for evidence of color change, tenderness, and bleeding. For clinical manifestations of bleeding.

Frequently assess urine and stool color. Possible early indicator of systemic internal bleeding. Detection of early signs allows for timely administration of platelet transfusion.

Monitor respiratory rate and depth to assess for respiratory distress.

Impaired Skin Integrity related to abnormal bleeding into cutaneous areas and mucosal surfaces

(continued)

#35 Nursing Process: Patient Care Plan for Thrombocytopenia and Bleeding Disorders (Continued)

Nursing Assessment and Diagnoses	Outcomes and Evaluation Parameters	Planning and Interventions with Rationales
	Lab values (platelet/Hct/Hgb) within normal limits for patient. Free of petechiae, ecchymosis, hematuria. Blood pressure within normal limits. **Outcome:** Minimal or no bleeding observed. *Evaluation Parameters:* Free of petechiae, ecchymosis. Free of bleeding from gums, mucosa, and catheter sites. Urine color clear. Free of blood in stool.	Assess abdomen for pain, tenderness, distention *as indicators of internal abdominal bleeding.* Assess vital signs, especially blood pressure *as indicators of vascular space volume. In the event of bleeding, blood volume leaves vascular space.*

Nursing Diagnosis: Deficient Knowledge related to management of thrombocytopenia	Outcome: Patient and family verbalize understanding of required skills and knowledge required in the management of thrombocytopenia.	Interventions and Rationales: Frequently reinforce patient education regarding bleeding precautions *to minimize risk of injury.* Educate patient and family about tests and procedures *to increase understanding of disease process.*
	Evaluation Parameters: Patient verbalizes understanding of bleeding precautions including avoidance of contact sports, use of razors, oral care. Patient reports signs and symptoms that warrant immediate attention by health care provider. Patient reports understanding of medications that should be avoided including aspirin and other drugs specific to patient's history.	Educate patient and family concerning the disease, treatment, and potential complications *to increase understanding of disease process.* Collaborate with multidisciplinary team to *reinforce pharmaceutical, nutritional, and rehabilitation/educational interventions.*

#36 Nursing Process: Patient Care Plan for Cancer

Nursing Assessment and Diagnoses	Outcomes and Evaluation Parameters	Planning and Interventions with *Rationales*
Nursing Diagnosis: *Risk for Infection* related to skin reactions, skin breakdown, multiple invasive lines, and myelosuppression	**Outcome:** No evidence of infection. **Evaluation Parameters:** Skin integrity is maintained. Urine appearance is clear, yellow, and possesses no foul odor. Invasive lines are free from signs of infection. Patient demonstrates appropriate self-care behaviors.	***Interventions and Rationales:*** Perform hand hygiene before and after working with patient. *Prevents spread of infection.* Monitor and record vital signs. *Elevated temperature and heart rate may indicate infection.* Assess for signs of infection and notify health care provider immediately: • Increased WBCs • Changes in temperature; >101°F (38.3°C) • Presence of chills, diaphoresis • Presence of myalgias • Cough, with or without sputum • Purulent drainage from site of skin reactions, intravenous site, or invasive line sites • Pain with urination, frequency with urination, foul-smelling urine • Mental status changes • Diarrhea

Identifies need for prompt treatment.

Obtain cultures and sensitivities prior to administering antibiotic therapy. *Identifies organism responsible for infection, which directs appropriate treatment.*

Administer antibiotics, antifungals, and antivirals as prescribed. Note presence of drug allergy. *Treatment of infection and prevention of drug reaction.*

Initiate measures to reduce infection:

- Private room if absolute neutrophil count (ANC) < $1,000/mm^3$
- Avoid contact with those who have known or recent infection or recent vaccination.
- Hand hygiene
- Avoid rectal or vaginal procedures (temperatures, examinations, medications).
- Administer stool softeners to prevent straining
- Meticulous hygiene
- Avoid use of straight-edge razor.
- Avoid raw meat and fish, fresh fruit and vegetables, fresh flowers and plants.

(continued)

#36 Nursing Process: Patient Care Plan for Cancer (Continued)

Nursing Assessment and Diagnoses	Outcomes and Evaluation Parameters	Planning and Interventions with *Rationales*
		• Provide clean liquids daily (e.g., denture cleaning solution, respiratory equipment fluid, drinking water).
		• Change solutions per protocol.
		• Avoid intramuscular injections.
		• Use strict aseptic technique when inserting medical devices (e.g., urinary catheters).
		Infection control practice.
		Instruct patient and family about infection prevention measures. *Reduces the risk of infection and encourages good infection control practices.*
Nursing Diagnoses:		***Interventions and Rationales:*** Evaluate baseline cardiac studies (e.g., echocardiogram, ECG, MUGAscan). *Provides baseline cardiac function to allow for future comparison.*
Ineffective Tissue Perfusion and Decreased Cardiac Output related to chemotherapy induced		Calculate and document cumulative dose of chemotherapeutic agents, if appropriate. *Provides ongoing information regarding maximum lifetime dosage.*

cardiac toxicity and capillary leak syndrome	**Outcome:** Normal tissue perfusion and cardiac output. **Evaluation Parameters:** Adequate peripheral perfusion as evidenced by: • Extremity pulses present by palpation and/or ultrasound • Capillary refill < 2 seconds on distal extremities • Color and temperature normal to extremities. Adequate urinary output evidenced by 30 mL/hr. Normal neurological function. No evidence of heart failure.	Assess for signs of congestive heart failure and report to health care provider: • Dyspnea • Tachycardia • Distended neck veins • Pedal edema • Crackles • Nonproductive cough • Extra heart tones (S_3) • Hepatomegaly. *Allows for prompt treatment.* Monitor vital signs for changes, and report to health care provider, such as: • Tachycardia • Tachypnea • Hypotension or hypertension.

(continued)

793

#36 Nursing Process: Patient Care Plan for Cancer (Continued)

Nursing Assessment and Diagnoses	Outcomes and Evaluation Parameters	Planning and Interventions with *Rationales*
		Allows for prompt treatment.
		Assess for syncope, dizziness, and weakness. *Indicates inadequate perfusion.*
		Monitor serum electrolytes. *Provides additional sources for alteration in cardiac function.*
		Administer medications to support cardiac function. (e.g., diuretics, inotropic agents, vasodilators, oxygen). *Maximizes cardiac function.*
		Position flat or with legs elevated. *Maximizes blood return to heart.* Encourage patient to adhere to dietary modifications (e.g., fluid restriction, sodium restriction, no alcohol, no tobacco). *Maximize cardiac function.*
		Instruct patient and family that cardiac effects may be irreversible. *Allows for time to consider lifestyle changes.*
		Collaborate with oncologist for reduced dosing of chemotherapy if ejection fraction is < 55%. *Minimizes exposure to toxic effect of antineoplastic agents.*
		Monitor peripheral perfusion by assessing:
		• Capillary refill (<3.0 seconds)
		• Pulses present and strong throughout
		• Skin dry, color pink, and temperature warm.
		Provides information about the quality of circulation.

Nursing Diagnoses: Risk for Impaired Gas Exchange and Ineffective Airway Clearance related to chemotherapy, biotherapy, and transplant-induced pulmonary toxicity

Outcome: Adequate gas exchange and airway clearance.

Evaluation Parameters: Normal ABGs. No dyspnea: unlabored respirations < 24/minute. Normal neurological status. Normal breath sounds. No signs of impaired tissue oxygenation. Oxygen saturation is within normal limits.

Monitor urinary output for normal (> 30 mL/hr). Report abnormal findings to health care provider. *Indicates adequate renal perfusion and allows for prompt treatment if necessary.* Monitor neurological status and report abnormalities to health care provider. *Indicates possible perfusion abnormalities and need for prompt intervention.*

Interventions and Rationales: Assess for adventitious or diminished breath sounds. *Indicates decreased gas exchange.*

Note depth, rate, rhythm, and effort of respiration. *Assesses for respiratory distress or increased work of breathing.*

Note presence of cough, amount, color, and consistency of sputum. *Assesses for development of respiratory infections or pulmonary edema.*

Monitor ABGs and oxygen saturation via pulse oximetry. *Determines adequacy of gas exchange.*

Monitor restlessness and confusion. *Indicators of inadequate gas exchange with resultant brain hypoxia.*

Assess skin and mucous membranes for color (dusky, ashen, or cyanotic). *Indicators of tissue hypoxia and need for prompt intervention.*

Instruct patient to cough and deep breathe. *Promotes gas exchange.*

Administer humidified oxygen therapy as prescribed. *Promotes airway clearance.*

(continued)

#36 Nursing Process: Patient Care Plan for Cancer (Continued)

Nursing Assessment and Diagnoses	Outcomes and Evaluation Parameters	Planning and Interventions with Rationales
		Monitor for complaints of chest pain and report to health care provider. *May indicate acute pulmonary event such as pulmonary embolism, pleural effusion, or pneumothorax.*
		Instruct patient and family about symptoms of pulmonary toxicity and to report findings to health care provider. *Allows for prompt intervention.*
		Instruct patient and family regarding possibility of irreversible pulmonary effects. *Allows patient to consider initiating lifestyle changes consistent with pulmonary function.*
Nursing Diagnosis: Potential for Deficient Fluid Volume related to bone marrow suppression, hepatotoxicity, hepatic veno occlusive disease (VOD), and hematologic laboratory abnormality induced by cancer treatments	**Outcome:** No evidence of bleeding. **Evaluation Parameters:** Platelet count will be within normal limits. Hemoglobin and hematocrit will be within normal limits. Hemodynamic status will be maintained.	*Interventions and Rationales:* Monitor platelet counts and report a count of < 50,000/mm³ to health care provider. *Identifies need for prompt treatment.* Monitor liver function tests and coagulation studies. *Identifies need for prompt treatment.* Assess for bleeding and report findings to the health care provider: • Decrease in hemoglobin and hematocrit • Prolonged bleeding or oozing from invasive procedures, venipunctures, cuts, or scratches • Presence of petechiae or ecchymosis • Presence of frank or occult blood in emesis, stool, or sputum

Patient will demonstrate appropriate self-care behaviors.	• Presence of blood from any body orifice
	• Change in mental status
	• Change in vital signs (e.g., ↑
	Early detection aids in early treatment.
	Perform venipunctures once daily for all laboratory tests. *Minimizes the risk of bleeding.*
	Avoid taking rectal temperatures; avoid use of suppositories or enemas. *Minimizes the risk of bleeding.*
	Apply direct pressure to injection and venipuncture sites for a minimum of 5 minutes. *Minimizes bleeding.*
	Instruct patient regarding ways to minimize the risk of bleeding:
	• Perform oral hygiene with soft toothbrush or toothettes.
	• Avoid use of commercial mouthwashes.
	• Avoid straight-edge razors.
	• File nails with emery board.
	• Avoid foods that are difficult to chew.
	Provides for appropriate self-care behaviors.

(continued)

#36 Nursing Process: Patient Care Plan for Cancer (Continued)

Nursing Assessment and Diagnoses	Outcomes and Evaluation Parameters	Planning and Interventions with Rationales
Nursing Diagnoses: Risk for Deficient Fluid Volume related to nausea, vomiting, diarrhea (due to pelvic radiation & cancer), hepatic VOD, and capillary leak syndrome *Risk for Excess Fluid Volume* related to hepatic VOD	*Outcomes:* Adequate hydration. Absence of skin breakdown. Normal electrolytes. *Evaluation Parameters:* Normal serum electrolytes. Skin surrounding anus remains intact. Cessation of diarrhea episodes. No evidence of dehydration or fluid overload. Absence of skin breakdown. Normal electrolytes.	*Interventions and Rationales:* Assess bowel pattern. *Determines baseline.* Record frequency of diarrhea and vomiting episodes. *Indicates degree of fluid loss.* Establish and maintain IV access. *Allows for fluid volume replacement if needed.* Administer IV fluids per protocol. *Determines need for fluid administration or restriction and prevents dehydration.* Record accurate intake and output. *Determines adequacy of fluid volume replacement.* Monitor daily weights using the same scale and with the same clothing. *Indicates fluid retention or loss.* Monitor serum electrolyte values, hemoglobin and hematocrit, liver function tests, and coagulation studies and notify health care provider of critical abnormalities. *To monitor hematologic changes associated with fluid changes.* Monitor for presence of edema. *Indicates fluid retention.* Measure abdominal girth daily and apply landmark indicators to abdomen. *Indicates presence of accumulating ascites and allows for accuracy and consistency in measurements.* Restrict sodium and water intake. *Prevents fluid retention in extracellular spaces.*

Monitor lung sounds. *Evaluates for fluid accumulation in lung, which may require prompt treatment.*

Place patient in semi-Fowler's position to avoid the patient lying flat. *Allows for optimal ventilation in the presence of ascites.*

Assess for excoriation of skin surrounding anus. *Identifies need for interventions.*

Instruct patient to cleanse area frequently. *Prevents skin breakdown.*

Instruct patient to notify health care provider if skin breakdown occurs. *Allows for prompt treatment.*

Administer antidiarrhea medication per protocol. *Reduces frequency of diarrhea episodes.*

Instruct patient to use low-residue diet and limit fat content. *Reduces amount of diarrhea.*

Interventions and Rationales: Inspect oral cavity daily. *Provides information needed to determine if treatment is necessary.*

Instruct patient regarding proper oral care:

- Brush and floss teeth as tolerated.
- Use moistening gauze or toothettes instead of toothbrush if needed, for instance, if platelet count is low (<40,000/mm³).
- Rinse with normal saline four times per day.
- Avoid commercial mouthwashes.
- Cleanse mouth before and after meals.

(continued)

Nursing Diagnosis:
Impaired *Skin Integrity* related to alopecia, stomatitis, xerostomia, skin reactions due to radiation therapy, invasive procedures and lines, biotherapy-induced dry desquamation, rashes, and pruritus, edema, cancer diagnosis and treatment

Outcomes: Maintain or restore skin integrity. Cope with hair loss. Mucous membranes are intact.
Evaluation Parameters: Minimal skin changes noted. Appropriate self-care behaviors are demonstrated. Skin infections are absent.

#36 Nursing Process: Patient Care Plan for Cancer (Continued)

Nursing Assessment and Diagnoses	Outcomes and Evaluation Parameters	Planning and Interventions with *Rationales*
	Social interaction is maintained.	*Prevents trauma and maintains oral hygiene.*
	Intact oral mucous membranes are maintained.	Administer cytoprotectives as ordered (e.g., Ethyol). *Promotes comfort and reduces incidence of mucous membrane breakdown.*
	Nutritional status is maintained.	Provide bland and soft diet. *Allows for ease of chewing and swallowing and reduces discomfort.*
	Patient is not suffering.	
	Skin integrity is maintained or restored.	Administer saliva substitutes and moisten food as needed. *Allows for ease of swallowing.*
		Instruct patient to report signs of stomatitis:
		• Burning
		• Pain
		• Areas of redness
		• Open lesions on the lips
		• Pain with swallowing
		• Intolerance to temperature extremes
		Identifies beginning stages of mucous membrane breakdown and facilitates prompt treatment.

Assist in oral hygiene during mild stomatitis:

- Normal saline rinses every 2 hours, every 6 hours during sleep.
- Use soft toothbrush or toothette.
- Avoid use of dentures except for meals.
- Maintain proper fit of dentures.
- Moisten lips with lubricating ointment.
- Avoid eating foods that are spicy, those with temperature extremes, and those that are difficult to chew.

Promotes hygiene, minimizes trauma, and provides for comfort.

Assist in oral hygiene during severe stomatitis:

- Discontinue use of dentures.
- Rinse with prescribed agent or irrigate oral cavity with mixture of saline, *anti-Candida* agent (Mycostatin), and topical anesthetic agent.
- Position patient properly for irrigations.
- Provide oral suction device.
- Use gauze or toothette with irrigation solution for cleansing.
- Lubricate lips.

Promotes hygiene and comfort.

Assess patient's ability to chew, swallow, and presence of gag reflex. *Identifies risk for aspiration.*

(continued)

#36 Nursing Process: Patient Care Plan for Cancer (Continued)

Nursing Assessment and Diagnoses	Outcomes and Evaluation Parameters	Planning and Interventions with *Rationales*
		Encourage use of pureed diet or liquid diet. *Promotes comfort and maintains nutrition.*
		Monitor for signs of infection and notify health care provider immediately. *Facilitates prompt treatment.*
		Obtain tissue cultures as needed. *Provides evidence of infection.* Administer analgesics, topical and systemic, as prescribed. *Promotes comfort.*
		Discuss patterns of hair loss and regrowth with patient and family. *Provides information so preparations for loss can begin and provides an understanding of the temporary nature of alopecia.*
		Encourage expression of concerns related to hair loss. *Facilitates coping.*
		Reduce or prevent hair loss:
		• Cut long hair prior to treatment.
		• Use mild shampoo, conditioner in small amounts.
		• Gently pat hair dry.
		• Avoid electric curlers, curling irons, dryers, clips, barrettes, hair sprays, hair dyes, or other hair chemicals.
		• Avoid excessive brushing or combing; use wide-tooth comb.
		• Use scalp tourniquets or hypothermia as appropriate.

Prevents hair loss as long as possible by decreasing the uptake of chemotherapy. Also maintains presence of hair as long as possible by reducing weight and manipulation.

Encourage patient to avoid actions that traumatize the scalp:

- Keep scalp lubricated to reduce itching (use vitamins A and D).
- Use sunscreen or hat when exposed to ultraviolet rays.

Prevents breakdown of the skin.

Offer ways to cope with hair loss:

- Obtain wigs or hairpieces prior to hair loss.
- Take photograph of hair loss to wig shop to improve matching of hair color.
- Contact American Cancer Society for available resources.
- Wear scarf, hat, or other device as needed.

Reduces changes in appearance.

Assess skin integrity. *Provides baseline information.*

Instruct patient regarding skin care of area within treatment field:

- Cleanse with lukewarm water.
- Avoid use of soap, powders, deodorants, and fragrances.
- Avoid shaving.
- Keep skinfolds dry and clean.
- Use devices to protect skin from sun, heat, and cold.

(continued)

#36 Nursing Process: Patient Care Plan for Cancer (Continued)

Nursing Assessment and Diagnoses	Outcomes and Evaluation Parameters	Planning and Interventions with *Rationales*
		• Avoid use of restrictive or tight-fitting clothing.
		• Avoid use of tape.
		• Avoid massaging, vigorous rubbing, or scratching.
		Minimizes skin trauma and provides protection.
		Instruct patient regarding skin care if dry desquamation occurs:
		• Cleanse with lukewarm water.
		• Avoid use of soap, powders, deodorants, cosmetics, ointments, and fragrances.
		• Avoid shaving.
		• Avoid rubbing or scratching.
		• Avoid hyperthermia or hypothermia treatments.
		• Avoid use of adhesive tapes.
		• Avoid exposure to sunlight or cold weather conditions.
		• Avoid use of restrictive clothing; use of cotton materials is preferred.
		• Apply hydrophilic moisturizing lotion or ointment two to three times per day (e.g., vitamins A and D ointment or Aquaphor).
		Prevents further skin damage and drying and aids in healing.

Instruct patient regarding skin care if moist desquamation occurs:

- Notify health care provider if blistering occurs.
- Keep blisters intact.
- Avoid frequent cleansing of the area.
- Apply saline irrigations or cold compresses three to four times per day.
- Apply dressings as prescribed (e.g., Vigilon).
- Apply zinc oxide or silver sulfadiazine with nonstick dressing if radiation treatments are being held.
- If area is draining, apply thin layer of gauze.

Provides for healing, decreases inflammation, and prevents infection.
Administer antihistamines per protocol. *Relieves itching associated with pruritus.*
Apply cold towels to affected area. *Relieves itching associated with pruritus.*
Instruct patient to maintain room humidity between 30% and 40%. *Relieves itching associated with pruritus.*

Nursing Diagnosis: *Activity Intolerance* related to fatigue, bone marrow suppression, anorexia, and hepatotoxicity.

Outcome: Able to perform activities of daily living (ADLs).

Evaluation Parameters: Maintain ADLs and minimize fatigue. Serum laboratory studies within normal limits.

Interventions and Rationales: Encourage frequent rest periods. *Energy is conserved and replenished.*
Encourage more sleep hours at night. *Restores energy levels.* Encourage patient to reorganize daily schedule of activities and seek assistance with shopping, cooking, housework, etc. *To minimize energy expenditure.*

(continued)

#36 Nursing Process: Patient Care Plan for Cancer (Continued)

Nursing Assessment and Diagnoses	Outcomes and Evaluation Parameters	Planning and Interventions with Rationales
	Adequate energy levels are maintained. Patient shows no evidence of suffering or discomfort. Adequate diet with recommended calorie and protein intake is maintained.	Encourage a temporary decrease in work hours. *Decreases physical and psychological stress and provides for rest.* Assess nutritional intake for adequate protein and calorie intake.
		Provides source of energy. Administer blood products per protocol. *Provides adequate oxygen availability, which will decrease fatigue.* Monitor fluid and electrolyte balance. *Provides information regarding nerve transmission and muscle function.* Assess for sources of discomfort and suffering. *Minimizes energy expenditure.*
Nursing Diagnosis: *Imbalanced Nutrition: Less Than Body Requirements* related to chemotherapy and biotherapy-induced nausea, vomiting, hepatotoxicity,	**Outcome:** Adequate nutritional status and maintenance of body weight. **Evaluation Parameters:** Patient experiences fewer episodes of nausea and vomiting.	**Interventions and Rationales:** Monitor accurate intake and output and record. *Indicates trends in intake pattern.* Perform nutritional assessment: • Calorie count • Ability to swallow • Food preferences • Patterns and behaviors related to eating

anorexia, and effects of pre- and post-transplant treatment

- Ethnic and cultural preferences.

Adequate calorie intake maintained.

Serum laboratory studies within normal limits.

Adequate energy levels are maintained.

Prescribed diet is tolerated.

Indicates adequacy of nutrition.

Monitor serum albumin, prealbumin, glucose, magnesium, sodium, and iron.

Assesses adequacy of nutritional intake.

Assess for signs of malnutrition:

- Muscle wasting
- Edema
- Changes in hair condition
- Changes in skin.

Indicates adequacy of nutrition.

Consult nutritionist to determine appropriate needs for individual.

Assists in establishing or maintaining adequate nutrition.

Provide meticulous oral care. *Prevents infection and promotes appetite.*

Administer antiemetics and appetite stimulants per orders.

Assists in improving appetite by reducing nausea and vomiting.

(continued)

#36 Nursing Process: Patient Care Plan for Cancer (Continued)

Nursing Assessment and Diagnoses	Outcomes and Evaluation Parameters	Planning and Interventions with *Rationales*
		Encourage small frequent meals that are high in calories and protein. *Such meals are more suitable for digestion, better tolerated.*
		Encourage adequate fluid intake, limiting fluids during mealtime. *Prevents the development of satiety.*
		Increase activity level as tolerated. *Activity stimulates the appetite.* Provide environment suitable for eating:
		• Pain free
		• Relaxed environment
		• Presentation of food tray.
		To increase appetite.
		Monitor tube feedings or IV total parenteral nutrition per protocol. *Determines tolerance of nutritional delivery system.*
		Administer cytoprotectives as ordered (e.g., Ethyol). *Promotes comfort and improved nutrition by preventing dry mouth.*
		Provide discharge teaching to patient and family regarding nutritional needs. *Maintains nutritional status at home.*

Nursing Diagnosis	Outcome / Evaluation Parameters	Interventions and Rationales
Nursing Diagnosis: *Pain related to skin reactions, cough from chest radiation, chemotherapy-induced pancreatitis, chemotherapy- and biotherapy-induced peripheral neuropathy and bone pain, mucositis, invasive procedures, and disease process*	**Outcome:** Pain is controlled. **Evaluation Parameters:** Patient verbalizes pain level and previous interventions that were successful in alleviating pain. Pain is reduced or absent as evidenced by patient denying presence or by nonverbal behaviors: no facial grimacing, restlessness, etc. Patient reports complementary strategies of pain control are effective.	**Interventions and Rationales:** Assess pain using pain scale (0–10) to quantify pain level. *Provides consistency for evaluating pain.* Assess discomfort characteristics: • Location • Quality • Frequency • Duration • Alleviating therapies *Provides baseline for assessing change.* Assess other factors contributing to pain: • Fear • Fatigue • Anger • Anxiety *Provides data about factors that decrease the patient's tolerance to pain* Ensure adequate fluid intake. *Minimizes frequency and intensity of cough.* Instruct patient to avoid irritants such as smoke. *Minimizes cough.* Instruct patient regarding the use of humidification in the air. *Minimizes cough.* Administer analgesics according to protocol. *Provides pain relief.* Monitor for side effects of analgesics and treat accordingly.

(continued)

#36 Nursing Process: Patient Care Plan for Cancer (Continued)

Nursing Assessment and Diagnoses	Outcomes and Evaluation Parameters	Planning and Interventions with *Rationales*
		Ensures tolerance of analgesics.
		Encourage use of pureed diet or liquid diet. *Promotes comfort and maintains nutrition.*
		Monitor for signs of infection and notify health care provider immediately. *Facilitates prompt treatment.*
		Administer analgesics prior to a procedure or treatment that may cause discomfort. *Controls increased pain level related to procedures and treatments.*
		Instruct patient to notify nurse when pain is not relieved or when pain begins to occur again. *Indicates need for additional pain management therapies or the administration of analgesics earlier in the pain cycle.*
		Collaborate with the patient and the multidisciplinary team when changes in pain management are necessary. *Increases the patient's sense of control and allows for agreement and input from all team members.*
		Instruct patient and family about complementary strategies to relieve pain and discomfort:
		• Guided imagery
		• Relaxation techniques
		• Distraction
		• Cutaneous stimulation. *Helps reduce anxiety and promotes relaxation.*

Nursing Diagnosis:	**Outcomes:** Social	**Interventions and Rationales:** Assess patient's feelings about body image
Disturbed Body Image re-	integration	and level of self-esteem. Validate concerns. *Provides baseline for evaluating*
lated to skin reactions,	Normal social interactions	*changes and determining effectiveness of interventions.*
alopecia, long-term venous	and acceptance of body	Advocate for participation in activities and decision making. *Facilitates a*
access devices, decreased	image changes	*sense of control.* Encourage patient to verbalize concerns. *Begins coping*
sexual function, role	**Evaluation Parameters:**	*process.*
changes, and other cancer	Participates in self-care	Provide personalized care. *Prevents depersonalization.*
treatments	activities.	Discuss patterns of hair loss and regrowth with patient and family.
	Demonstrates interest in	*Provides information so preparations for loss can begin and provides an under-*
	appearance.	*standing of the temporary nature of alopecia.*
	Resumes or continues in-	Assist in self-care when fatigue, nausea, vomiting, or other distressing symp-
	teractions with others in	toms occur. *Improves self-esteem by ensuring physical well-being.*
	established social net-	Help patient in selecting cosmetic devices that increase sense of attractive-
	work.	ness. *Promotes positive body image.*
	Explores alternative ways	Offer ways to cope with hair loss:
	of expressing concern	• Obtain wigs or hairpieces prior to hair loss.
	and affection with	• Take photograph of hair to wig shop to improve matching of hair color.
	partner.	• Contact American Cancer Society for available resources.
		• Wear scarf, hat, or other device as needed.
		(continued)

#36 Nursing Process: Patient Care Plan for Cancer (Continued)

Nursing Assessment and Diagnoses	Outcomes and Evaluation Parameters	Planning and Interventions with Rationales
Nursing Diagnosis: Impaired Urinary Elimination related to radiation therapy	**Outcomes:** Minimize cystitis. Able to urinate normally. **Evaluation Parameters:** Laboratory studies within normal limits. No evidence of discomfort or suffering. Adequate fluid intake maintained. Normal urinary patterns.	*Reduces changes in appearance.* Encourage dialogue between patient and partner regarding sexual function and alternatives. *Allows for affection and acceptance.* ***Interventions and Rationales:*** Assess for hematuria. *Indicates possible infection or cystitis.* Monitor fluid intake and encourage adequate intake. *Decreases incidence of cystitis.* Monitor for signs of urinary tract infection. *Promotes prompt treatment.* Obtain urine analysis and culture. *Evaluates for infection.* Assess for pain with urination. *Determines presence of symptoms needing further treatment.* Administer antibiotics, bladder analgesics, and antispasmodics as ordered. *To treat infection and pain.* Evaluate patient's understanding of cause of cystitis and measures to relieve symptoms. *Provides evidence of need for education.*

Nursing Diagnosis	Outcome	Interventions and Rationales
Nursing Diagnosis: *Risk for Impaired Swallowing* related to esophagitis or pharyngitis	**Outcome:** No difficulties with swallowing. **Evaluation Parameters:** Adequate nutritional status is maintained. Adequate pain management is maintained. Full course of radiation therapy is completed.	**Interventions and Rationales:** Instruct patient to follow a soft, bland, or liquid diet that is high in protein and calories. *Facilitates swallowing and promotes adequate nutritional intake.* Administer anesthetic and coating mouth rinses prior to eating. *Relieves discomfort associated with swallowing.* Administer analgesics per protocol. *Relieves discomfort associated with swallowing and allows for patient to continue with therapy.*
Nursing Diagnoses: *Risk for Sexual Dysfunction* related to radiation therapy of the pelvis *Altered Sexuality Patterns* related to late effects of transplantation	**Outcome:** Maintains sexual functioning as desired. **Evaluation Parameters:** Patient and partner understand rationale for treatment. Patient and partner maintain effective communication.	**Interventions and Rationales:** Assess level of dysfunction via patient interview. *Determines baseline and need for interventions.* Encourage patient to discuss concerns with partner. *Facilitates effective communication.* Facilitate consultation with urologist as needed, including patient education regarding rationale. *Provides treatment and education.* Monitor for symptoms that affect libido. *Allows for treatment and understanding of changes.*

(continued)

813

#36 Nursing Process: Patient Care Plan for Cancer (Continued)

Nursing Assessment and Diagnoses	Outcomes and Evaluation Parameters	Planning and Interventions with *Rationales*
	Sexual functioning is improved.	Assess for fear, anxiety, diminished self-image, and depression. *Indicates need for resources for coping.* Facilitate communication about sexual issues. *Promotes open communication between patient and partner.* Instruct patient on hygiene and contraceptive measures. *Prevents infections and pregnancy.*
Nursing Diagnosis: *Delayed Growth* and *Development* related to late effects of transplantation in children	***Outcome:*** *Normalized growth and development.* ***Evaluation Parameters:*** Growth patterns are normal according to standardized charts. Educational needs are being met. Identifies need to access support systems. Actively participates in recovery.	***Interventions and Rationales:*** Monitor patient's growth according to standard charts. *Helps determine if growth patterns are impaired.* Evaluate normal growth and development behaviors consistent with the patient's age. *Indicates need for possible treatment.* Monitor for learning disabilities. *Indicates need for special educational resources.* Administer growth hormone per protocol. *Assists in normalizing growth and development patterns.* Provide educational and emotional resources to patient and family. *Improves coping and ability to function with deficits.*

Nursing Diagnosis:	Outcome: Patient will	Interventions and Rationales: Assess patient's and family's understanding of
Ineffective Coping related to alopecia, fatigue, biotherapy induced depression, anxiety, transplant process, role changes, lifestyle changes, diagnosis of cancer	demonstrate effective coping skills. **Evaluation Parameters:** Demonstrates effective coping strategies for living with cancer. Identifies need to access support systems. Actively participates in recovery.	diagnosis, recommended treatment, and prognosis. *Provides information about need for further teaching if not consistent with actual diagnosis, treatment, or prognosis.* Encourage patient to express feelings. *Effective coping strategy.* Monitor aggressive behaviors. *May indicate ineffective coping.* Assess patient's and family's support systems. *Indicates need for recommendations.* Consult psychiatrist, psychologist, or spiritual counselor. *Provides expertise that will evaluate for effective coping and make recommendations for assistance.* Encourage family to use memory prompts with patient for orientation in regard to time, date, and location. *Allows for reorientation and participation in care.*
Nursing Diagnosis: *Deficient Knowledge* related to radiation therapy, chemotherapy, biotherapy side effects, and self-care needs	**Outcome:** Understand the use of radiation therapy for cancer and the self-care behaviors necessary to manage side effects. **Evaluation Parameters:** Patient verbalizes an	**Interventions and Rationales:** Assess patient's expectations and concerns about therapy. *Determines baseline knowledge.* Instruct patient and family about: • The purpose of using radiation therapy to treat cancer • Routines such as consultation, simulation, treatment schedules, routine appointments, and follow-up • Expected length of each visit

(continued)

815

#36 Nursing Process: Patient Care Plan for Cancer (Continued)

Nursing Assessment and Diagnoses	Outcomes and Evaluation Parameters	Planning and Interventions with *Rationales*
	understanding of the purpose for therapy, side effects, and measures used to minimize side effects, and protective measures. Patient demonstrates appropriate self-care behaviors. Patient understands the use of biotherapy and chemotherapy for cancer and the self-care behaviors necessary to manage side effects.	• Appearance of equipment and environment. *Decreases anxiety associated with treatment.* Instruct patient and family about the effects and side effects associated with radiation therapy. *Decreases anxiety associated with treatment.* Instruct patient and family about measures used to minimize side effects. *Provides for less distress associated with treatment, which maximizes chance of patient continuing with therapy.* Instruct patient and family about visiting restrictions and isolation requirements associated with internal radiation therapy. *Provides for an understanding of the need to protect others.* Instruct patient and family about: • The purpose of using chemotherapy and biotherapy, and transplantation to treat cancer • Routines such as appointments and follow-up treatments

	• Expected length of each visit
	• Appearance of infusion equipment and vascular access devices.
Patient understands the use of transplantation for cancer and the self-care behaviors necessary to manage side effects.	*Decreases anxiety associated with treatment.*
	Assess patient's expectations and concerns about transplantation.
	Determines baseline knowledge.
	Instruct patient and family about the effect and side effects associated with transplantation and associated conditioning.
Patient demonstrates appropriate self-care behaviors.	*Decreases anxiety associated with treatment.*
	Instruct patient and family about measures used to minimize side effects.
	Provides for less distress associated with treatment, which maximizes chance of patient continuing with therapy.

Sources: Bender, C., & Rosenzweig, M. (2004). Cancer. In S. Lewis, M. Heltkemper, & S. Dirksen (Eds.), *Medical–surgical nursing assessment and management of clinical problems* (6th ed.). St. Louis: Mosby; Iwamoto, R. (2001) Radiation therapy. In S. Otto (Ed.), *Oncology nursing* (4th ed.). St. Louis: Mosby; Keller, C. (2001). Bone marrow and stem cell transplantation. In S. Otto (Ed.), *Oncology nursing* (4th ed.). St. Louis: Mosby; Oncology Nursing Society. (2001). *Chemotherapy and biotherapy guidelines and recommendations for practice.* Pittsburgh: Author; Rokita, S. (2004). Oncology: Nursing management in cancer care. In S. Smeltzer & B. Bare (Eds.), *Brunner & Suddarth's textbook of medical–surgical nursing* (10th ed.). Philadelphia: Lippincott Williams & Wilkins; Wikle-Shapiro, T. (1998). Nursing implications of bone marrow and stem cell transplantation. In J. K. Itano & K. N. Taoka (Eds.), *Core curriculum for oncology nursing* (3rd ed.). Philadelphia: W. B. Saunders.

#37 Nursing Process: Patient Care Plan for Patient Receiving Noninvasive Positive Pressure Ventilation

Assessment for Selection, Initiation, and Assessment of Patient on NPPV

Subjective Data:
Do you think you could attempt a trial of NPPV?
Which interface would you prefer?
Are you experiencing any episodes of nausea or vomiting?
Have you ever had problems with claustrophobia?

Objective Data:
Level of consciousness.
Hemodynamic stability.
Ventilation.
Work of breathing.
Oxygen saturation.
Abdominal and genitourinary assessment.
Vital signs ABGs.

Nursing Assessment and Diagnoses	Outcomes and Evaluation Parameters	Planning and Interventions with Rationales
Nursing Diagnosis: *Ineffective breathing pattern that can be treated with NPPV related to Impaired Gas Exchange, Ineffective Airway Clearance, and Ineffective Breathing Pattern*	**Outcomes:** Patient is candidate for NPPV. Improved gas exchange on NPPV. **Evaluation Parameters:** Arterial blood gases improved within 3 hours of NPPV. Decreased work of breathing as exhibited by the patient. Alert and oriented.	**Interventions and Rationales:** Assess level of consciousness and ability to follow commands and co-operate *to determine the presence of cerebral hypoxia.* Assess compliance with keeping the mask in place to determine if the *treatment is being tolerated.* Assess level of sedation *to determine if more or less is needed to keep the patient comfortable.*

818

Assessment for Level of Consciousness and Patient's Ability to Communicate and Procedural Tolerance

Subjective Data:
What is your name, where are you, what is the date, and why are you here?

Objective Data:
Glasgow Coma Scale.
Follows commands.

Nursing Assessment and Diagnoses	Outcomes and Evaluation Parameters	Planning and Interventions with *Rationales*
Nursing Diagnosis: Tissue perfusion ineffective: cerebral related to decreased oxygenation and increased CO_2 levels	*Outcome:* Tolerance of NPPV until it is not needed. *Evaluation Parameters:* Able to follow commands. Responds correctly to questions of time and place. *Glasgow Coma Scale (GCS) < 10 and/or inability to follow commands would disqualify patient from receiving NPPV.*	*Interventions and Rationales:* Assess neurological status frequently after initiating NPPV. Increasing confusion related to increased CO_2 levels would signify failure of NPPV.

(continued)

#37 Nursing Process: Patient Care Plan for Receiving Noninvasive Positive Pressure Ventilation (Continued)

Assessment of Level of Comfort

Subjective Data:

What is your pain level at, using the 1–10 scale? A 1 is very little pain and a 10 is the worst imaginable pain.

What is your experience with pain?

Do you routinely take pain medications at home; if so, what for and what kind?

Are you allergic to any pain medication?

Do you have any cultural or religious beliefs that impact your pain control?

Does the pain get worse with deep inspiration?

Describe the pain: burning, sharp, aching, or any other term that is descriptive of it.

Objective Data:

Grimacing on movement.

Restlessness and irritability.

Taut facial expression.

Nursing Assessment and Diagnoses	Outcomes and Evaluation Parameters	Planning and Interventions with Rationales
Nursing Diagnosis: *Pain related to ventilation or other preexisting conditions*	**Outcomes:** Pain controlled with analgesia. Level of sedation is adequate. **Evaluation Parameters:** Appears relaxed. Expresses relief of pain.	**Interventions and Rationales:** Assess pain and sedation level. *Increasing levels of pain would require increased analgesics that might decrease respiratory drive.* Provide adequate sedation. *Increasing anxiety would prevent patient from tolerating NPPV. Too much sedation could decrease respiratory rate and prevent ability to cooperate.*

Assessment of Hemodynamic Stability

Subjective Data:

Do you become light-headed or pass out?

Do palpitations or light-headedness occur at the same time?

Do your feet swell and, if so, under what circumstances.

Objective Data:

Vital signs: BP and HR Oxygen saturation.

Level of consciousness.

ECG.

Lab values: electrolytes and measures of acidosis.

Cardiac output.

Lung/cardiac.

Urine output.

Nursing Assessment and Diagnoses	Outcomes and Evaluation Parameters	Planning and Interventions with *Rationales*
Nursing Diagnosis: Decreased cardiac output related to heart failure and hypotension	*Outcome:* Hemodynamically stable. *Evaluation Parameters:* Adequate blood pressure. Heart rate less than 100 beats per minute. Respiratory rate less than 18 breaths per minute while resting.	*Interventions and Rationales:* Monitor blood pressure and heart rate. *Hemodynamic instability, severe tachycardia, and/or hypotension (shock) would exclude patient. Uncontrolled ischemia or arrhythmias would also disqualify patient.* Auscultate heart sounds. Palpate pulses. Assess cardiac rhythm if patient is on monitor. Obtain 12-lead ECG to *further evaluate rhythm.* Administer antiarrhythmic and or beta-blockers as prescribed. Assess extremities for edema.

(continued)

821

#37 Nursing Process: Patient Care Plan for Receiving Noninvasive Positive Pressure Ventilation (Continued)

Urine output minimum of 30 mL/hr. Lungs clear to auscultation. Intake and output within normal limits.	Assess fluid status and JVD. Weigh patient. Administer diuretics. Monitor intake and output. *Fluid overload can prevent adequate gas exchange.*

Assessment of Respiratory Effort

Subjective Data: Do you feel short of breath? Is it becoming worse or better? How long have you been experiencing shortness of breath? Do you have it at rest or just with activities?	**Objective Data:** Oxygen saturation. ABGs. Skin color and temperature. Respiratory rate. Lung sounds.

Nursing Assessment and Diagnoses	Outcomes and Evaluation Parameters	Planning and Interventions with *Rationales*
Nursing Diagnoses: Ineffective breathing pattern, related to lung constriction, lung collapse, low tidal volumes	*Outcome:* Improved ventilation after application of NPPV. *Evaluation Parameters:* Decrease in respiratory rate, decreased use of accessory muscles, and decreased dyspnea.	*Interventions and Rationales:* Assess respiratory status for appropriateness of application of NPPV. *The following respiratory parameters would prompt the practitioner to not attempt NPPV:* *Inability to clear secretion* *Excessive secretions* *No cough or gag*

Oxygen saturation and ABGs within normal limits.	*Impaired swallowing*
Patient denies increased work of breathing.	*Respiratory arrest or unreliable respiratory drive.*
	Assess facial trauma or anatomic abnormalities that would prevent adequate mask fit.
	Assess breathing pattern, rate, and depth.
	Monitor respiratory rate and quality *to assess improvement in ventilation with NPPV.*
	Assess chest expansion. Note paradoxical respirations.
	Assess cough and ability to clear secretions.
	Assess use of accessory muscles during inspiration or prolonged expiratory phase.
	Assess nasal flaring or pursed-lip breathing.

Assessment for Sufficient Oxygen Saturation Related to Altered Blood Gas

Subjective Data:

Do you have any preexisting health problems such as heart or lung disease?

Objective Data:

Lung sounds.
Oxygen saturation.
Work of breathing, e.g., gasping, increased rate, loudness.
Vital signs.
Skin and nail bed color.
ABGs.
Oxygen saturation.

(continued)

#37 Nursing Process: Patient Care Plan for Receiving Noninvasive Positive Pressure Ventilation (Continued)

Nursing Assessment and Diagnoses	Outcomes and Evaluation Parameters	Planning and Interventions with Rationales
Nursing Diagnosis: *Impaired Gas Exchange* related to pulmonary disease/infection	**Outcome:** Improved oxygen saturation after application of NPPV. **Evaluation Parameters:** SpO_2 > 92% on room air. No increased work of breathing. Lungs sounds clear.	**Interventions and Rationales:** Review ABGs and monitor SpO_2. *Ensure that initial ABG/SpO_2 value does not require immediate intervention such as endotracheal intubation.* Severe acidosis (pH < 7.2) and hypoxemia (PaO_2 < 60) would require invasive intubation. Auscultate breath sounds. Note any adventitious sounds such as wheezes or crackles in the bases. Assess pulse oximetry for absolute value as well as adequacy of waveform. *Waveform should always be monitored with SpO_2 to ensure that SpO_2 is accurate. Dampened waveform can reflect probe displacement.* Maintain SpO_2 > 92% to provide appropriate level of oxygen therapy via mask. Obtain chest x-ray as ordered. Compare film to previous studies to assess lungs. Administer bronchodilators if appropriate to increase ventilation.

Assessment of Patient's Coping Abilities

Subjective Data:

How are you feeling about your health and illness?

Tell me what you are feeling about your illness and being on NPPV.

Who are the people in your life that are your support system? How have you handled fearful situations in the past?

Nursing Diagnosis: *Anxiety related to discomfort, inability to communicate, lack of adequate sleep, and use of analgesics and sedatives*

Outcome: *Reduced anxiety and confusion.*

Evaluation Parameters: *Calm demeanor; acceptance of therapy. Patient can communicate and eat. Mask fits appropriately.*

Objective Data:

Facial expressions.

Mood.

Verbalization of fear regarding injury, impact on family, and future.

Interventions and Rationales: *Provide constant observation and coaching of patient once NPPV therapy is instituted.*

Explaining procedure to patient and coaching will decrease anxiety and promote acceptance of therapy.

Select appropriate mask for patient.

Examine patient and note face size.

Discuss interfaces and plan for initiation with patient and team (health care provider, respiratory therapist, and patient).

Use of an oronasal or full-face mask with gel mask improves compliance and is more efficient for gas exchange and allows mouth breathing.

Transition to nasal mask if appropriate as patient improves.

(continued)

825

#37 Nursing Process: Patient Care Plan for Receiving Noninvasive Positive Pressure Ventilation (Continued)

Assessment of Soft Tissue Injury of Skin, Nose, Mouth, and Nasopharynx

Subjective Data:

Are you experiencing any pain around, under, or near the mask?

Objective Data:

Skin breakdown near and under mask.

Nursing Assessment and Diagnoses	Outcomes and Evaluation Parameters	Planning and Interventions with *Rationales*
Nursing Diagnosis: Risk for impaired skin integrity of face and nose related to poor fitting mask	*Outcome:* Absence of soft tissue injury. *Evaluation Parameters:* No tissue breakdown noted. Skin and soft tissue clear and intact.	*Interventions and Rationales:* Apply protective device on bridge of nose *to prevent skin breakdown.* Provide frequent oral care *to prevent mouth dryness and to prevent increase in plaque.* Keep dentures in place *to assist with mask fit.*

Assessment for Abdominal Pain

Subjective Data:

Are you having any abdominal pain?
Do you feel like you are swallowing air?
Are you nauseated?

Objective Data:

Abdominal girth.
Oxygen saturation.
Vomiting.
Bowel sounds.

Nursing Assessment and Diagnoses	Outcomes and Evaluation Parameters	Planning and Interventions with Rationales
Nursing Diagnosis: *Risk for Injury and abdominal distention related to high pressures, long-term ventilation, and predisposing abnormality*	**Outcome:** No abnormal abdominal distention noted. **Evaluation Parameters:** Abdomen soft and nontender. Bowel sounds present. Patient free of nausea and vomiting.	**Interventions and Rationales:** Assess abdomen for distention, pain, or tenderness. *Persistent nausea and vomiting would be a contraindication to NPPV. Lack of bowel sounds and/or a distended abdomen might increase risk of aspiration with NPPV* If abdomen is distended, consider obtaining order for placement of nasogastric tube *to decompress stomach.* Stop all feeding and oral intake until patient is stable on NPPV. Position patient with head of bed > 30 degrees.

Assessment for Aspiration Related to Insecure Airway

Subjective Data: Are you feeling like you are getting enough air? Do you feel more short of breath?	**Objective Data:** Lung sounds. Oxygen saturation. Vital signs. Increased work of breathing. Bowel sounds. Abdominal distention.

(continued)

#37 Nursing Process: Patient Care Plan for Receiving Noninvasive Positive Pressure Ventilation (Continued)

Nursing Assessment and Diagnoses	Outcomes and Evaluation Parameters	Planning and Interventions with Rationales
Nursing Diagnosis: Risk for Aspiration	**Outcome:** Free of aspiration. *Evaluation Parameters:* Clear lungs. Oxygen saturation within normal limits.	**Interventions and Rationales:** Instruct patient how to remove mask if vomiting occurs. *Aspiration is a significant risk for patients with NPPV.*

Assessment of Knowledge Deficit

Subjective Data:

What are your concerns about the diagnosis of respiratory disease in terms of prognosis, changes in lifestyle, and progression of disease?

Do you understand how to take medications and their potential side effects?

Do you understand what symptoms you might have and how to monitor them at home and when to contact the health care provider?

Objective Data:

Patients may be anxious, confused, and need repeated information.

Nursing Assessment and Diagnoses	Outcomes and Evaluation Parameters	Planning and Interventions with *Rationales*
Nursing Diagnosis: *Deficient Knowledge* related to the diagnosis, treatments, and long-term management	**Outcomes:** Patient/family understand: The diagnosis of respiratory disease. Their prognosis and treatments. Lifestyle changes. Symptoms to monitor. **Evaluation Parameters:** Patient/family will: Ask appropriate questions. Follow appropriate medication regimen. Call when their symptoms worsen for urgent evaluation when needed.	*Interventions and Rationales:* Discuss with patient/family the cause and prevention of respiratory disease. *This will enhance their understanding of risk factors and prevention.* Discuss how the NPPV works and how to prevent complications. *This will provide the fundamental treatment strategies and should increase compliance.* Discuss the common symptoms of respiratory disease with the patient and family, describing shortness of breath, cough, fatigue, activity intolerance, weight gain/edema, palpitations, chest tightness, and poor concentration. *This will enable patients to recognize their symptoms and reinforce calling early when their symptoms worsen, so they can be seen and have adjustments made in their medications, preempting an urgent hospitalization.*

#38 Nursing Process: Patient Care Plan for the Orthopedic Surgical Patient

Nursing Assessment and Diagnoses	Outcomes and Evaluation Parameters	Planning and Interventions with *Rationales*
Nursing Diagnosis: *Gas Exchange, impaired* related to anesthetic or narcotic effect, fluid overload, pulmonary or fat emboli, pneumonia, or preexisting pulmonary or cardiovascular disease exacerbation	**Outcomes:** Airway open. Adequate gas exchange. **Evaluation Parameters:** Breath sounds clear, without evidence of snoring or stridor. Oxygen saturation > 94% or as ordered by health care provider. Arterial blood gas demonstrates PaO_2 > 80 mmHg and $PaCO_2$ 35–45 mmHg. Respiratory rate 12–20 per minute, unlabored with good chest expansion. Alert and oriented to person, place, time, and situation.	*Interventions and Rationales:* Initially a jaw thrust maneuver may be necessary to maintain an open airway if the patient has snoring breath sounds indicating airway obstruction from tongue. If this maneuver is necessary, the patient may require additional reversal agents such as naloxone or flumazenil. The anesthesiologist or surgeon may need to be contacted for orders for these medications. *To maintain open airway.* Assess patient for adequacy of respiratory rate and depth, auscultate breath sounds, and monitor oxygen saturation. Analyze arterial blood gas when results are available. *Indicates gas exchange is adequate.* Assess patient's level of consciousness and orientation to person, place, time, and situation. *Confusion, agitation, restlessness, or difficult arousal may indicate hypoxia.* Encourage patient to perform incentive spirometry (ICS) every 1–2 hours for 10 breaths while awake. Have patient cough and deep breathe after utilizing ICS. Assist patient out of bed (OOB) to chair and ambulating at least three times a day. *To promote adequate gas exchange, promote airway clearance, and prevent atelectasis.*

Nursing Diagnosis:
Neurovascular Dysfunction, Peripheral: Risk for related to edema, vascular insufficiency, nerve damage, or surgical complication

Outcomes: Absence of neurovascular deficits. Skeletal structures in alignment.
Evaluation Parameters: Full strength.
Sensation intact.
No numbness, tingling, or pain.
Pulses 2–3 + palpated.
Skin warm, pink, and dry.
Capillary refill time < 3 seconds.

Interventions and Rationales: Perform neurovascular assessment every 2–4 hours. Assess bilateral extremities *to give indication of normal findings for patient.*
Elevate limb above level of heart in position of function *to decrease edema formation and prevent contracture.*
Evaluate sensation using a dermatome chart for patients with epidural anesthesia/catheters and patients with spinal surgery. *Dermatome chart describes level of anesthesia or deficit.*
Evaluate strength and range of motion during planned postoperative activities. *Postoperative exercise improves circulation, improves healing, and prevents contractures and deconditioning.*

Nursing Diagnoses:
Fluid volume, Deficient related to blood loss and inadequate fluid intake *Fluid volume, Imbalanced: Risk for* due to

Outcome: Adequate and balanced intake and output.
Evaluation Parameters: Vital signs within normal limits.
Intake and output balance.
Lungs clear.

Interventions and Rationales: Strict intake and output (I&O) to include all po liquids, IV fluid intake and urine, gastric, and wound drainage output. Maintain shift and ongoing totals. Assess wound drainage. Frankly bloody drainage may be present on the first postoperative day, but should change to serosanguinous after that. Notify health care provider of excessive blood loss *to give an accurate reflection of fluid balance.*

(continued)

#38 Nursing Process: Patient Care Plan for the Orthopedic Surgical Patient (Continued)

Nursing Assessment and Diagnoses	Outcomes and Evaluation Parameters	Planning and Interventions with Rationales
impaired renal function and fluid intake in excess of output	Urine output adequate. BUN and creatinine normal. Hgb and HCT stable. Drainage from wound < 50 milliliters in 25 hours.	Obtain vital signs as ordered. *Tachycardia and low blood pressure may indicate hypovolemia. Increased respiratory rate or adventitious breath sounds may indicate volume overload.* Monitor laboratory studies for signs of hypo-/hypervolemia. *The hemoglobin and hematocrit, BUN, and creatinine levels provide information on volume status.*
Nursing Diagnosis: Pain, Acute related to surgical procedure, compartment syndrome, osteoarthritis, or cerebrospinal fluid (CSF) leak (in spinal surgery patient)	*Outcomes:* Patient will have pain controlled and will be able to participate in all aspects of rehabilitation program. *Evaluation Parameter:* Pain scale score at or below predetermined comfort level score.	*Interventions and Rationales:* Medicate patient for pain score greater than comfort level. Notify health care provider if symptoms unrelieved by ordered medication. *Patients have a right to pain control within their described comfort level. Pain that is not relieved may indicate development of complications such as compartment syndrome.* Place spinal patient in supine position if he complains of headache. *CSF leak headache increases with drainage, upright position.*

Nursing Diagnosis: *Infection, Risk for* and delayed wound healing related to age, open surgery, compound fracture, and comorbid condition

Outcomes: Wound/bone healing within expected time frame.
No evidence of infection.
Evaluation Parameters: Surgical incision is clean, dry, and approximated, without redness.
Urine clear, no odor.
Vital signs within normal limits (WNL).
WBC count < 11,000/mcL

Interventions and Rationales: Obtain vital signs as ordered or every 4 hours, including temperature *to provide early indication of changes indicating infection.* Assess surgical site and drainage each shift *to provide early indication of changes indicating infection.* Monitor lab values, especially WBC count. *Elevations in WBC indicate infection.*

Nursing Diagnosis: *Self-Care, Readiness for Enhanced* related to surgery, pain, immobility, or decreased mental status

Outcome: Patient able to care for self.
Evaluation Parameters: Able to perform postoperative exercises including transfers, ambulation, and pulmonary toilet at prescribed intervals.

Interventions and Rationale: Patient should be assisted out of bed as soon as feasible. Follow health care provider orders/clinical pathway instructions for mobility and activities. If health care provider does not order progressive mobilization of the patient, notify health care provider to obtain activity orders *to prevent deconditioning and maintain or improve functional status.*

(continued)

#38 Nursing Process: Patient Care Plan for the Orthopedic Surgical Patient (Continued)

Nursing Assessment and Diagnoses	Outcomes and Evaluation Parameters	Planning and Interventions with *Rationales*
	Able to ambulate with walker 50 feet with steady gait; able to ambulate unassisted for 50 feet with steady gait. Able to complete toilet and hygiene functions unassisted.	
Nursing Diagnoses: Skin Integrity, Risk for Impaired related to decreased sensorium and immobility.	*Outcome:* Patient will have no evidence of skin breakdown. *Evaluation Parameters:* Skin surface clean, dry, pink, and intact. Patient position change is performed or observed at least every 2 hours while in bed or every 15 minutes while seated.	*Interventions and Rationales:* Turn and position patient every 2 hours while in bed (logroll, maintaining spinal alignment if patient with spinal surgery). Float heels off of bed with pillows or heel lift device. Follow hospital protocol for use of pressure relief mattresses and overlays *to prevent pressure ulcer development*. Assess skin integrity and document each shift and with each change in position. Assess areas over bony prominences, where prostheses, casts, traction, or splints contact *to provide early detection of potential for skin breakdown.*

Nursing Diagnoses:
Knowledge, Deficient of self-care needs and treatment plan related to postoperative delirium

Therapeutic Regimen Management, Ineffective related to postoperative exercises, administration of deep venous thrombosis (DVT) prophylaxis, and self-care activities without assistance related to age, obesity, decreased functional capacity, and lack of home support

Outcome: Patient is able to discuss a realistic plan for self-care after hospital discharge.

Evaluation Parameters:
Patient verbalizes knowledge of plan of care and goals. Patient demonstrates ability to perform postoperative exercises correctly in the appropriate frequency. Patient verbalizes a plan for assistance with activities of daily living (ADL) and ongoing therapeutic requirements if needed. Demonstration of ability to ambulate at least 100 feet and perform self-care activities.

Interventions and Rationales: Assess patient's readiness to learn and provide patient education regarding patient procedures, activities, medications, and care needs. *Assessment of patient readiness enables the nurse to provide education at appropriate times.*

Begin discharge planning on admission. Encourage significant other/family participation in plan. Evaluate care needs compared with patient abilities. Patient/significant other should be able to verbalize/demonstrate essential activities prior to discharge. *To ensure that sufficient time is allotted to provide education and training so that patient/family are able to perform activities after discharge.*

Prior to discharge, ensure that patient understands plan of care and is able to verbalize important aspects in her own words and to verbalize a plan for obtaining medications, equipment, and assistance in the home environment to *help ensure compliance with treatment plan.*

#39 Nursing Process: Patient Care Plan for Spinal Cord Injury

Assessment of Neurological Status

Subjective Data:
Are you able to move your arms, hand, legs, feet? Do you have numbness or tingling anywhere?

Objective Data:
Motor strength.
Sensory level.
Deep tendon reflexes.
Sphincter tone.

Nursing Assessment and Diagnoses	Outcomes and Evaluation Parameters	Planning and Interventions with Rationales
Nursing Diagnoses: Risk for constipation related to spinal cord injury *Disturbed Sensory Perception* related to spinal cord injury *Risk for Injury* due to spinal instability	**Outcomes:** Stabilization or improvement of neurological function. Maintenance of spinal alignment. **Evaluation Parameters:** Existing neurological function is preserved. Spine is immobilized with the appropriate orthotic device and mobility restrictions.	**Interventions and Rationales:** Spinal precautions maintained as ordered by the treating health care provider. *Measures to limit additional mechanical injury to the spinal cord.* Administer methylprednisolone per hospital protocol. *May limit inflammatory response and secondary injury to the spinal cord.* Maintain adequate oxygenation and MAP above 85 mmHg and systolic BP above 90 mmHg to prevent secondary injury due to *hypoxia and hypotension.* Monitor motor and sensory function *to assess for change in neurological function allowing for prompt medical attention if needed.*

Assessment of Pulmonary Function

Subjective Data:
Do you feel short of breath?
Do you feel like you are unable to clear your secretions?

Objective Data:
Lung sounds.
Monitor respiratory rate.
Use of accessory muscles for breathing.
Amount and character of secretions.
Adequacy of cough. Monitor pulse oximetry. Monitor arterial blood gases.
Change in mental status (i.e., anxiety, confusion, increased lethargy).

Nursing Assessment and Diagnoses	Outcomes and Evaluation Parameters	Planning and Interventions with Rationales
Nursing Diagnoses: *Ineffective Breathing Pattern* related to pulmonary complications of spinal cord injury *Ineffective Airway Clearance* related to the loss of spinal innervation of the respiratory muscles	***Outcome:*** Adequate gas exchange. ***Evaluation Parameters:*** Adequate oxygenation is achieved as evidenced by normal blood gases and pulse oximetry. Patient is able to clear airway secretions. Patient is without complaint of dyspnea. Lung sounds remain clear. Patient remains alert and oriented without anxiety or restlessness.	***Interventions and Rationales:*** Monitor respiratory status. *Evaluate for change indicative of declining respiratory function including increased use of accessory muscles, inability to clear secretions, drop in oxygen saturation, change in mental status, change in respiratory parameters (tidal volume, vital capacity, negative inspiratory force).* Institute pulmonary hygiene, including cough and deep breathing exercises, chest physiotherapy, assisted cough techniques, suctioning *to promote gas exchange and airway clearance.* Administer humidified oxygen as ordered *to increase oxygenation.* Report decline in respiratory function to the medical team. *Medical management including mechanical ventilatory support may be necessary.* *(continued)*

#39 Nursing Process: Patient Care Plan for Spinal Cord Injury (Continued)

Assessment of Cardiovascular Status

Subjective Data:
Are you dizzy or light-headed?

Objective Data:
Heart rate and rhythm.
Blood pressure.
Urine output.

Nursing Assessment and Diagnoses	Outcomes and Evaluation Parameters	Planning and Interventions with Rationales
Nursing Diagnosis: *Risk for Ineffective Tissue Perfusion* related to cardiovascular effects of neurogenic shock	**Outcomes:** Patient maintains hemodynamic stability. Patient is able to tolerate being in an upright position. **Evaluation Parameters:** MAP > 85 mmHg SBP > 90 mmHg HR > 50–60 Patient does not complain of dizziness or light-headedness.	**Interventions and Rationales:** *Monitor hemodynamic status to assess for change to allow for prompt medical intervention. Administer vasoactive agents and atropine as ordered to ensure adequate blood pressure, heart rate, and cardiac output. Monitor intake and output and replace intravascular volume to ensure adequate fluid status. Hypovolemia can contribute to hemodynamic instability.* Utilize abdominal binder and thigh-high compression stockings to *increase venous return to the heart and limit blood pooling in abdomen and lower extremities due to vasodilation. Transition patient slowly into an upright position to avoid orthostatic hypotension.*

Assessment of Peripheral Tissue Perfusion

Subjective Data:

Do you have any pain or pressure in your extremities?

Have you noticed any abnormal swelling or redness in your extremities?

Have you noticed change in temperature in one or more extremity?

Objective Data:

Peripheral pulses.

Temperature and color of the extremities.

Unilateral swelling in the extremities.

Nursing Assessment and Diagnoses

Nursing Diagnosis: Risk of Ineffective Peripheral Tissue Perfusion related to DVT

Outcomes and Evaluation Parameters

Outcome: Patient does not develop DVT.

Evaluation Parameters: The patient does not exhibit signs of DVT: redness, edema, change in temperature of extremity.

Patient does not complain of pain or tenderness.

Peripheral pulses remain intact.

Planning and Interventions with *Rationales*

Interventions and Rationales: Utilize antiembolic hose and sequential compression boots *to limit blood pooling in the lower extremities*.

Administer prophylactic dose of anticoagulant as ordered once cleared by the surgical team *to prevent formation of peripheral DVT*.

Begin mobilization of patient including range-of-motion exercises as soon as cleared by the surgical team *to limit the effects of prolonged immobility*.

Assess color, temperature, and size of extremities and check peripheral pulses. Report abnormalities to the medical team *to enable early detection and prompt treatment*.

(continued)

839

#39 Nursing Process: Patient Care Plan for Spinal Cord Injury (Continued)

Assessment of Gastrointestinal Function

Subjective Data:

Are you nauseous?

Do you have any abdominal pain?

When was your last bowel movement?

Objective Data:

Abdominal pain.

Abdominal distention.

Bowel sounds.

Frequency of bowel movements.

Guaiac stools.

Hematocrit.

Dietary intake.

Nursing Assessment and Diagnoses	Outcomes and Evaluation Parameters	Planning and Interventions with Rationales
Nursing Diagnoses: *Risk for constipation* related to impaired gastric motility due to spinal cord injury *Potential for Gastric Ulceration* related to stress of critical injury	*Outcomes:* Gastrointestinal function will be maintained. Patient will be without evidence of gastric stress ulceration. A regular pattern of bowel movements will be established.	*Interventions and Rationales:* Assess abdomen for tenderness and distention. Auscultate bowel sounds. *Evaluation of gastrointestinal function.* Monitor hematocrit and check stool for occult blood if drop in hematocrit noted without other explanation (i.e., surgery) *to assess for GI bleed due to gastric stress ulceration.* Use nasogastric tube if ileus is present *to provide for decompression of the stomach.*

| | Patient will receive adequate nutrition to meet caloric requirements. *Evaluation Parameters:* Abdomen will remain soft, nontender, and nondistended. Patient will be without complaints of nausea, vomiting, constipation, or epigastric pain. Hematocrit will remain stable. Nutrition will be implemented. | Administer stress ulcer prophylactic regimen as ordered by the medical team. Institute bowel regimen of stool softener, chemical stimulation such as a suppository, and mechanical (digital) stimulation *to establish a regular bowel elimination pattern.* Institute parenteral nutrition until patient is able to tolerate enteral feedings. Call for dietary consult *to determine patient's caloric needs.* |

Readiness for Enhanced Nutrition related to increased metabolic need and inadequate caloric intake

Assessment of Urinary Elimination

Subjective Data:

Are you able to urinate?
Do you feel like your bladder is full?
Have you had any incontinence of urine?

Objective Data:

Urinary output.
Bladder scan to assess for urinary retention.

Nursing Assessment and Diagnoses	Outcomes and Evaluation Parameters	Planning and Interventions with *Rationales*
Impaired Urinary Elimination due to neurogenic bladder	*Outcomes:* The patient will establish a normal pattern of urinary elimination. The patient will be	*Interventions and Rationales:* Use indwelling catheter during the acute period to allow for complete bladder emptying and accurate measurement of urinary output.

(continued)

#39 Nursing Process: Patient Care Plan for Spinal Cord Injury (Continued)

Nursing Assessment and Diagnoses	Outcomes and Evaluation Parameters	Planning and Interventions with *Rationales*
Nursing Diagnoses: *Risk for Autonomic Dysreflexia* related to autonomic dysfunction as a result of spinal cord injury	able to recognize the signs of autonomic hyperreflexia, identify potential causes, and describe treatment of hyperreflexia. *Evaluation Parameters:* The patient and caregiver can perform CIC. The patient and caregiver can verbalize common causes of hyperreflexia, common symptoms of hyperreflexia, and actions to take should hyperreflexia occur.	Check postvoid residuals by either intermittent catheterization or bladder scan *to assess for urinary retention.* Teach CIC to patient and caregiver *to encourage a consistent manner of bladder emptying.* Instruct patient and caregiver on common causes and signs of autonomic hyperreflexia and interventions to institute when these signs occur.

Assessment of Pain

Subjective Data:
Are you having pain?
Where do you hurt?

Objective Data:
Facial grimacing.
Crying.
Increased spasticity.
Elevated blood pressure.
Elevated heart rate.

Nursing Assessment and Diagnoses	Outcomes and Evaluation Parameters	Planning and Interventions with Rationales
Nursing Diagnosis: Readiness for enhanced comfort due to injury and/or surgical procedure	*Outcome:* Effective control of pain. *Evaluation Parameters:* The patient will report improvement of pain. The patient is able to participate in therapies.	*Interventions and Rationales:* Assess pain utilizing a pain scale to *provide a method of measuring degree of pain and response to pain control measures.* Administer analgesics as ordered *to provide pharmacologic treatment of pain.* Utilize distraction and repositioning techniques *to augment pharmacologic treatment of pain.*

Assessment of Psychosocial State

Subjective Data:
Are you feeling sad, depressed?
How have you dealt with stress in the past?
Who is your support person?

Objective Data:
Refusal to communicate.
Refusal to participate in activities.
Avoidance of eye contact.
Anger.
Crying.
Expressing feelings of hopelessness.

(continued)

#39 Nursing Process: Patient Care Plan for Spinal Cord Injury (Continued)

Nursing Assessment and Diagnoses	Outcomes and Evaluation Parameters	Planning and Interventions with *Rationales*
Nursing Diagnoses: *Ineffective Coping* related to loss of control over environment and uncertainty of the future	**Outcomes:** Patient will exhibit appropriate coping strategies. Patient will exhibit less anxiety. **Evaluation Parameters:** Patient reports improved mood. Patient participates in care. Patient is able to express feelings.	**Interventions and Rationales:** Encourage the patient to express her feelings *to provide for self-expression and identification of feelings. Allow* patient to participate in decisions *so the patient regains some control over self and the environment.* Request psychiatric consultation. *Assist with crisis counseling and to help the patient to identify appropriate coping strategies.* Administer antianxiolytics and antidepressants as prescribed.

Assessment of Adaptation

Subjective Data:

What are you able to do for yourself?

What adaptive equipment do you have available and what will be needed?

Objective Data:

Functional assessment based on preserved motor function.

Patient/caregiver knowledge of use of equipment.

Patient/caregiver knowledge of available resources.

Nursing Assessment and Diagnoses	Outcomes and Evaluation Parameters	Planning and Interventions with *Rationales*
Nursing Diagnoses: *Self-Care Deficit* related to spinal cord injury *Deficient Knowledge* regarding adaptation strategies and resources	**Outcome:** Patient will implement self-care strategies utilizing the appropriate adaptive devices within the limitations of his injury. **Evaluation Parameters:** The patient participates in his own care. The patient will be able to identify available resources to help him to be independent within the limitations of his injury.	**Interventions and Rationales:** Schedule nursing care around PT/OT sessions *to ensure patient is able to participate in rehabilitative activities.* Have adaptive equipment readily available and encourage patient to use the equipment in self-care activities. *Encourages self-care strategies and reinforces education on the use of the equipment.* Assist the patient in identifying available community resources *to assist in independent living.*

#40 Patient Teaching & Discharge Priorities for Spinal Cord Injury

Need	Teaching
Understanding of bowel/bladder regimen	The patient and family are taught how to perform CIC and how to perform bowel care including insertion of a suppository, digital stimulation of the bowel, and disimpaction of stool.
Prevention of complications	The patient and family are taught strategies such as frequent position changes and skin care to avoid the formation of pressure ulcers. The patient and family will understand the importance of maintaining a regular bowel and bladder regimen to avoid complications of UTI and bowel impaction.
Safety	Proper instruction on the use of adaptive equipment and transfer strategies will be given to the patient and family. The patient and family will be instructed on the signs and symptoms of autonomic hyperreflexia, common causes of hyperreflexia, and strategies to implement if autonomic hyperreflexia occurs.
Emotional adjustment of patient and family to psychosocial impact of SCI	The patient and family are encouraged to discuss their feelings openly. The patient and family will be able to identify supportive resources to help them cope with both the physical and psychosocial changes due to SCI.
Adaptation of environment	The patient and family will be provided instruction on necessary adaptation to the home environment and resources to assist with completion of environmental changes necessary to accommodate the patient's deficits and adaptive equipment. If the patient is unable to be discharged to a home environment, arrangements for an assisted living environment will be made.

#41 Nursing Process: Patient Care Plan for Acute Brain Disorders

Assessment of Altered Levels of Consciousness

Subjective Data:
Does the patient have any history of health problems, such as hypertension, heart disease, bleeding disorders, renal disease, or cancer? What were the patient's presenting symptoms/complaints? How long ago did the first symptoms present?

Objective Data:
Neurological assessment, including mentation, cranial nerve examination, motor and sensory examination. Imaging studies, including MRI, CT, and/or lumbar puncture. Laboratory data, including CBC, CMP, and drug levels.

Nursing Assessment and Diagnoses	Outcomes and Evaluation Parameters	Planning and Interventions with *Rationales*
Nursing Diagnoses: *Actual and Potential Alteration in Level of Consciousness* related to TBI, intracranial tumor, or infectious process	**Outcome:** Improvement to optimum level of function. **Evaluation Parameters:** Stable neurological examination. Glasgow Coma Scale. Laboratory tests, including serum sodium and cultures of blood and CSF if suspicious for infection.	**Interventions and Rationales:** Monitor neurological examination hourly, or as directed. *Allows early recognition of pending neurological deterioration.* Monitor lab values, including serum sodium levels and cultures. *Early recognition and treatment of hyponatremia or infection.*

(continued)

#41 Nursing Process: Patient Care Plan for Acute Brain Disorders (Continued)

Nursing Assessment and Diagnoses	Outcomes and Evaluation Parameters	Planning and Interventions with Rationales
Impaired Physical Mobility related to altered level of consciousness	*Outcome:* Improvement to optimum level of motor function. *Evaluation Parameters:* Neurological motor and sensory examination. Level of participation in therapies and ADLs.	*Interventions and Rationales:* Monitor motor strengths and limitations. *Allows early recognition of neurological changes.* Initiate therapies, such as physical and occupational unless contraindicated. *Early initiation of therapies helps to identify deficits and needed areas for improvement.* Initiate activity as tolerated, unless contraindicated. *Physical activity will increase strength and endurance, as well as decrease complications, such as pneumonia or blood clots.*
Ineffective Tissue Perfusion related to immobility	*Outcome:* Adequate tissue perfusion. *Evaluation Parameter:* Absence of DVTs or pulmonary embolus.	*Interventions and Rationales:* Encourage activity as tolerated, unless contraindicated. *Physical activity will prevent immobility and the formation of blood clots.* Apply thigh-high elastic stockings and sequential compression stockings *to increase venous circulation.* Administer subcutaneous injections of low-molecular-weight heparin, if indicated *to discourage the formation of blood clots.* Monitor lower extremities frequently for signs/symptoms of DVT. *Early recognition and treatment of a DVT may prevent extension of the clot or pulmonary embolus.*

Impaired verbal communication related to anatomical defect.	**Outcome:** Maximum level of communication. **Evaluation Parameter:** Ability to adequately communicate with others.	**Interventions and Rationales:** Assess type and degree of communication deficit *to determine patient needs and establish a baseline.* Arrange a speech therapy consult. *Early intervention and therapy optimizes results.*
Actual or Potential Alteration in Visual Perception related to TBI or brain tumor	**Outcome:** Maximum level of vision/visual acuity. **Evaluation Parameter:** Formal and informal vision screening including visual fields.	**Interventions and Rationales:** Assess vision by informal testing (i.e., counting fingers, reading the clock) *to assess type and degree of visual deficit present.* Institute safety measures, such as placing call light within reach, orienting patient to surroundings, *to prevent accidents/falls.* Obtain occupational therapy evaluation if warranted. *Evaluation of visual deficits and education regarding coping mechanisms.*
Ineffective Cerebral Tissue Perfusion related to electrolyte imbalances in TBI, brain tumors, or infectious process	**Outcome:** Optimum neurological function. **Evaluation Parameters:** Stable neurological examination. Electrolyte levels, specifically sodium.	**Interventions and Rationales:** Monitor serum sodium as indicated, at least daily *to assess for hyponatremia.* Conduct neurological assessments frequently *to assess for decreased level of consciousness.* Administer fluids as directed *to maintain adequate fluid balance.* Notify health care provider immediately of abnormal lab values or change in neurological examination. *Such changes may indicate hyponatremia.*

(continued)

#41 Nursing Process: Patient Care Plan for Acute Brain Disorders (Continued)

Assessment of Airway and Gas Exchange

Subjective Data:
Does the patient have any preexisting medical problems such as emphysema or asthma, or any cardiac diseases?

Objective Data:
Respiratory rate.
Oxygen saturation.
Arterial blood gases.
Vital signs.
Lung sounds.
Skin/nail bed/lip color.

Nursing Assessment and Diagnoses	Outcomes and Evaluation Parameters	Planning and Interventions with Rationales
Nursing Diagnoses: *Ineffective Airway Clearance* related to altered level of consciousness	**Outcome:** Adequate respiration status. **Evaluation Parameters:** Adequate arterial blood gases. Respiratory rate within normal limits. Normal oxygen saturation levels. Clear lung sounds. Mental status, such as confusion or agitation.	**Interventions and Rationales:** Monitor respiratory status (i.e, rate, rhythm, and quality). *Changes in respiratory rates or patterns may indicate pending respiratory failure. It may also indicate neurological change.* Monitor mental status. *Restlessness, agitation, or confusion may indicate hypoxia.* Monitor oxygen saturation *to assess adequacy of gas exchange.* Encourage deep breathing or use of an incentive spirometer to *promote adequate gas exchange.*

Position with head in neutral position, head of bed elevated at 30 degrees, unless contraindicated *to promote adequate gas exchange.*

Suction as necessary. *Patients with decreased neurological status may be unable to protect their airways.*

Report changes in respiratory patterns to health care provider. *Such changes indicate possible risk for respiratory failure.*

If patient not intubated, have necessary intubation equipment available. *Protecting the airway is the priority. Intubation may be necessary to protect airway.*

Interventions and Rationales: Keep NPO until alert and/or swallow reflex is assessed and deemed safe. *Altered level of consciousness may depress the cough and/or swallow reflex.*

Risk for Aspiration related to altered level of consciousness

Outcome: No aspiration.

Evaluation Parameters: Adequate oxygen saturation. Safe swallowing techniques.

Assessment of Hemodynamic Status

Subjective Data:

Does the patient have any preexisting cardiac or respiratory problems?

Objective Data:

Vital signs, including heart rate, blood pressure, respiratory rate, and central venous pressure, if available.

Oxygen saturation.

Skin, lips, and nail bed color.

Lung sounds.

Cardiac rhythm strips or EKG.

(continued)

#41 Nursing Process: Patient Care Plan for Acute Brain Disorders (Continued)

Nursing Assessment and Diagnoses	Outcomes and Evaluation Parameters	Planning and Interventions with Rationales
Nursing Diagnoses: *Decreased intracranial adaptive capacity related to increased intracranial pressure*	**Outcome:** Hemodynamic stability. **Evaluation Parameters:** Adequate blood pressure to maintain CPP. Stable vital signs, including CVP, Pulmonary Arterial Pressure PAP, and ICP.	**Interventions and Rationales:** Monitor vital signs as directed to establish a baseline and note changes in vital signs. Administer fluids and medications as directed to assist in maintaining blood pressure as ordered to maintain adequate CPP. Monitor EKG rhythm to assess for alterations in rhythm or rate. Monitor intake and output to assess fluid balance to maintain hemodynamic parameters. Notify health care provider of hemodynamic changes. *Medical intervention may be necessary to prevent hemodynamic instability leading to neurological decline.* Monitor neurological assessments closely. *Hemodynamic stability is closely related to CPP and ICP changes in neurologically compromised patients.*

Assessment of Pain

Subjective Data:
Does the patient complain of pain? Facial expressions (i.e., grimacing).

Objective Data:
Increased heart rate, blood pressure, or respiratory rate?

852

Nursing Assessment and Diagnoses	Outcomes and Evaluation Parameters	Planning and Interventions with *Rationales*
Nursing Diagnosis: Readiness for enhanced comfort related to brain tumor, head injury, meningitis, or surgical procedure	*Outcome:* Adequate pain control. *Evaluation Parameters:* Vital signs within normal limits. Patient verbalizes pain control.	*Interventions and Rationales:* Assess presence of pain or efficacy of pain control frequently *to ensure patient comfort.* Administer pain medications as ordered *to ensure patient comfort.*

Assessment of Coping

Subjective Data:
What are patient's complaints?
What is the patient's understanding of present condition or disease?
What are patient's concerns for the future?

Objective Data:
What is the patient's level of education? What is the patient's occupation? What is the patient's family support system? Does the patient have a religious affiliation?

Nursing Assessment and Diagnoses	Outcomes and Evaluation Parameters	Planning and Interventions with *Rationales*
Nursing Diagnoses: *Ineffective Coping* related to knowledge deficit	**Outcome:** Patient and family will have information needed.	

(continued)

#41 Nursing Process: Patient Care Plan for Acute Brain Disorders (Continued)

Readiness for Enhanced Family Coping related to neurological deficits

Evaluation Parameter: Discussions with patient, with verbalization of condition and treatment.

Outcome:
Family will have improved coping with neurological disability.

Evaluation Parameters: Discussions with patient and family with verbalization of concerns. Observation of family/patient interactions.

Involve family as appropriate. *Family support is important for recovery.*

Interventions and *Rationales:*
Reassure patient and family with honesty and compassion to *provide encouragement and information needed for coping.*
Encourage family members to voice concerns to *help with assessment of family needs.*
Provide family with support as needed, such as spiritual, therapies, or psychological. *Neurological disability affects the whole family and community.*

#42 Patient Teaching & Discharge Priorities for Acute Brain Disorders

Need	Teaching
Wound infection:	Assess surgical wound for signs/symptoms of infection.
Patient	Signs and symptoms of infection include:
	Redness
	Tenderness
	Exudate and/or odor
	Swelling
	Poor healing
	The presence of fever or any of the above symptoms should be reported.
Family support system	Assess family support for needed assistance.
Setting	
	Assess motor strengths and ability for ambulation.
	Obtain consults for physical and occupational therapy.
Mobility assistance:	Assess need for assistive devices, such as wheelchair, walker, or splints.
Patient	
Family support system	Assess availability of family for support with mobility and ADLs.
	Conduct family teaching.
Setting	Assess environment for risk factors.
Pain control:	Assess need for pain control.
Patient	Is present medication regimen adequate? Is pain controlled sufficiently to allow patient to participate in ADLs?
Family support system	Assess need for family intervention in dispensing pain medication.
Setting	Assess patient/family understanding of medication instructions.
	Assess patient cognitive status:
Safety:	Is patient a fall risk?
Patient	Assess safety awareness.
Family support system	Assess patient understanding of medication schedule and needs.
Setting	Assess patient need for supervision.
	Obtain consults for speech/cognitive evaluation.

(continued)

#42 Patient Teaching & Discharge Priorities for Acute Brain Disorders (Continued)

Need	Teaching
	Obtain social service consult.
	Obtain home health consult.
	Assess family involvement in patient's recuperative period.
	Conduct family teaching regarding possible cognitive impairments.
	Conduct family teaching regarding need for supervision.
	Assess environment for safety. May require home health or social service involvement.
Follow-up needs: Patient Family support system Setting	Assess need for follow-up appointments for needed therapies or interventions:
	Radiation therapy
	Outpatient therapies: physical, occupational, speech
	Health care provider appointments
	Laboratory visits for evaluation of drug levels or electrolytes
	Follow-up x-rays.
	Assess family understanding and need for further explanation.
	Assess availability of resources for follow-up.

INDEX

Page numbers followed by *t* indicate tables.